Research **Success**

A Q&A Review Applying Critical Thinking to Test Taking

Research **Success**

A Q&A Review Applying Critical Thinking to Test Taking

Geraldine N. Valencia Go, BSN, MA, PhD, RN, CGNS, BC
Faculty Emeritus
Consultant in Nursing Education
Certified Clinical Specialist in Gerontological Nursing

F.A. Davis Company • Philadelphia

F.A. Davis Company
1915 Arch Street
Philadelphia, PA 19103
www.fadavis.com

Printed in the United States of America

Last digit indicates print number: 10 9 8 7 6 5 4 3 2 1

Publisher, Nursing: Terri W. Allen
Director of Content Development: Darlene D. Pedersen
Content Project Manager: Jacalyn C. Clay
Electronic Project Editor: Sandra A. Glennie
Design and Illustration Manger: Carolyn O'Brien

As new scientific information becomes available through basic and clinical research, recommended treatments and drug therapies undergo changes. The author(s) and publisher have done everything possible to make this book accurate, up to date, and in accord with accepted standards at the time of publication. The author(s), editors, and publisher are not responsible for errors or omissions or for consequences from application of the book, and make no warranty, expressed or implied, in regard to the contents of the book. Any practice described in this book should be applied by the reader in accordance with professional standards of care used in regard to the unique circumstances that may apply in each situation. The reader is advised always to check product information (package inserts) for changes and new information regarding dose and contraindications before administering any drug. Caution is especially urged when using new or infrequently ordered drugs.

ISBN: 978-0-8036-3939-3

To nursing students and professional nurses who will make research a part of their lives.
— GVG

Reviewers

Marilyn E. Asselin, PhD, RN-BC
Associate Professor
College of Nursing
University of Massachusetts Dartmouth
North Dartmouth, Massachusetts

Louis A. Aurilio, PhD, RN-BC, NE-BC, CNE
Professor
Nursing Department
Youngstown State University
Youngstown, Ohio

Suzanne M. Barsness, RN, MSN, CCRC
Associate Professor
Northwest University
Kirkland, Washington

Sara Berger, MSN, RN-BC
Associate Professor
Sanford College of Nursing
Bismarck, North Dakota

Vicki Black, PhD, RN
Assistant Professor
Northern Arizona University
Flagstaff, Arizona

Flor C. Bondal, PhD, RN, CNS-BC
Associate Professor
Georgia College and State University
Milledgeville, Georgia

Diane M. Breckenridge, PhD, MSN, RN, ANEF
Professor and Director, Nursing Workforce, Strategies for Success Program
School of Nursing and Health Sciences
La Salle University
Philadelphia, Pennsylvania

Stephanie Chalupka, EdD, RN, PHCNS-BC, FAAOHN
Associate Dean for Nursing
Worcester State University
Worcester, Massachusetts

Sara L. Clutter, PhD, RN
Associate Professor of Nursing
Waynesburg University
Waynesburg, Pennsylvania

Lynne M. Connelly, PhD, RN
Director of Nursing
Benedictine College
Atchison, Kansas

Heather L. Evans, PhD, RNC-MNN, CLC
Assistant Clinical Professor and Director of International Programs
School of Nursing
University of Connecticut
Storrs, Connecticut

Vivienne Friday
Associate Professor of Nursing
Iowa Western Community College
Council Bluffs, Iowa

Barbara J. Hoerst, PhD, RN
Assistant Professor, Nursing
School of Nursing and Health Sciences
La Salle University
Philadelphia, Pennsylvania

Katherine Howard, MS, RN-BC, CNE
Nursing Instructor
Middlesex County College
Edison, New Jersey

James P. Humphrey, PhD, MSN, BSN, RN, CNS, CNL
Associate Professor Emeritus of Nursing
College of Nursing and Health Sciences, School of Nursing
Valdosta State University
Valdosta, Georgia

Peg Kerr, PhD, RN
Department Head, Nursing and Associate Professor
University of Dubuque
Dubuque, Iowa

Dorothy "Dale" M. Mayer, PhD, RN
Assistant Professor
College of Nursing
Montana State University
Missoula, Montana

Juleann H. Miller, RN, PhD
Associate Professor and Assistant Chair of the Nursing Department
St. Ambrose University
Davenport, Iowa

Kerry A. Milner, DNSc, MSN, RN
Assistant Professor
Sacred Heart University
Fairfield, Connecticut

Mary Minton, PhD, RN, CNS
Associate Professor of Nursing
South Dakota State University
Rapid City, South Dakota

Abigail Mitchell, DHEd, MSN, RN, CNE
Director of Graduate Nursing
D'Youville College
Buffalo, New York

Jessica Naber, RN, PhD
Assistant Professor
Murray State University
Murray, Kentucky

Sherry Obert, RN, BSN, MSN
Nursing Faculty
Mount Aloysius College
Cresson, Pennsylvania

Kristi Pfeil, MSN, RN
ADN Faculty
Victoria College
Victoria, Texas

Renee Pilcher, MSN, RN
Instructor of Nursing and Health
Clarke University
Dubuque, Iowa

Cheryl Riley-Doucet, RN, PhD, FGSA
Associate Professor
Oakland University
Rochester, Minnesota

Linda M. Schultz, PhD, CRRN
Assistant Professor
Maryville University
St. Louis, Missouri

Kristen Sethares, PhD, RN, CNE
Associate Professor of Nursing
University of Massachusetts Dartmouth
North Dartmouth, Massachusetts

Shellie Simons, PhD, RN
Associate Professor
University of Massachusetts Lowell
Lowell, Massachusetts

Cynthia Steinwedel, PhD, RN, CNE
Assistant Professor
Bradley University
Peoria, Illinois

Julia Vicente, MSN, BSN, RN, CCRN
Nurse Faculty
Chamberlain College of Nursing
Miramar, Florida

Susan Warmuskerken, MSN
Professor of Nursing
West Shore Community College
Scottville, Michigan

Camille M. Wendekier, MS, CRRN, CSN
Assistant Professor
Saint Francis University
Loretto, Pennsylvania

Melissa T. Williams, RN, MSN, EdS
Assistant Professor of Nursing
Georgia Regents University
Augusta, Georgia

Gracie S. Wishnia, PhD, RN, BC
Associate Professor
Spalding University
Louisville, Kentucky

Kathleen A. Wolff, PhD, APRN, CNS
Assistant Professor
Southwestern Oklahoma State University
Weatherford, Oklahoma

Acknowledgments

A writing project is never a solo endeavor. Here is the team. I am grateful to Robert Craven, Jr. and Robert Martone of F. A. Davis for taking the time and effort to launch this project and to Jacalyn Clay, who managed the many logistics and kept things moving smoothly. I am deeply indebted to Maggie Kelly, a most patient and talented editor who made my work sound great and gave me wonderful suggestions and constructive critiques. I also want to thank all the copy editors, especially Lisa Thompson, and Robert Butler, production manager, for their patience and perseverance. I am appreciative of all the suggestions and insightful questions posed by the reviewers. To my spouse, Richard, and daughter, Kimberly, for their understanding and support. To my colleagues and students who cheered and told me, "You can do it!"

GVG

Table of Contents

Critical Thinking and Research: Your Paradigm for Living and Working

TO THE NURSING INSTRUCTOR

Research is a "systematic inquiry that uses orderly methods to answer questions and solve problems" (Polit & Beck, 2014, p. 390). That sounds simple enough, given that our students are familiar with the nursing process with steps designed to solve problems. However, as students of nursing begin their undergraduate research course, many are intimidated by the new, abstract terms and concepts that are common, everyday language for researchers and experienced research consumers. Those of us who teach research find that the real challenge of the course is not teaching the content but rather getting students interested in and excited about a little-understood process. Students view research as merely a course, one in which a grade is to be earned to fulfill degree requirements. They often are not aware that research is something that will be part of who they are as practicing professionals. Students may not even realize how many tools and processes they use or learn about are the results of research. Generate a discussion of this topic by showing students the following list and asking what all these items have in common:

- The wheel
- The automobile
- Airplanes
- Spacecraft
- Calculators
- Computers
- X-ray machines
- Magnetic resonance imagers
- Penicillin
- The Braden Scale, for predicting pressure ulcers
- Kübler-Ross stages of loss

All of these developments have been possible because someone thought about doing something in a "better, more effective manner." Although at times outcomes were not always those expected by pioneers of knowledge, those who embarked on these projects were willing to take risks. All knowledge builds on prior knowledge; therefore, others use what is already known and are guided by previous successes and, yes, even failures.

Throughout their careers, students will likely assume many research-related roles, starting with the indirect role as consumers of research. For nursing as a profession to grow and adapt to new challenges, today's nursing students will need to become tomorrow's producers of research as they acquire the necessary knowledge and skills. Our job, as teachers of research, is to instill interest, to motivate, and to inspire confidence in these future researchers as well as to impart the knowledge and critical thinking skills they will need in this course and throughout their nursing careers.

To the Nursing Student

Critical Thinking. You will need to think critically throughout nursing school, your nursing career, and your life. But how do you learn to think critically? Critical thinking occurs in every level in the cognitive domain. This domain tests for the ability to know, understand, apply, analyze, synthesize, and evaluate information. The first four levels are used in this book because these are the levels addressed in the NCLEX-RN. Resources with more information about developing critical thinking skills are listed at the end of the introduction. These resources are useful because they specifically address critical thinking processes and applications for nursing students.

Critical Thinking and Test Taking. A practical application of critical thinking can be seen in test taking. Applying critical thinking to determine what is asked by the question and which option is the best answer is the first component. The second component is being "test smart," which means knowing and applying effective strategies for test taking. Let's look at some examples.

The first level in the cognitive domain, **knowledge**, entails "learning new facts and being able to recall them" (Hall, 2013, p. 331). Which of following is a qualitative research tradition?

1. Clinical trials
2. Correlational study
3. Phenomenology
4. Prospective study

To choose option 3, you need to recall a memorized fact. Although knowledge is considered a low critical thinking skill, it is an essential foundation for all the higher levels.

Comprehension, the second level in the cognitive domain, is the "ability to understand the meaning of learned material" (Hall, 2013, p. 331). Which of the following is the reason why a researcher would do a descriptive study?

1. There are insufficient funds to conduct a more advanced study.
2. The researcher has no expertise on the topic.
3. There is a dearth, or scarcity, of information on the topic.
4. There is a need to use findings to predict an outcome.

To select the best option, option 3, the test taker needs to understand, or comprehend, the different levels of purpose in research. Learned or memorized knowledge would also have to be recalled in order to answer the question correctly.

The third level in the domain, **application**, requires "using abstract newly-learned ideas in a concrete situation" (Hall, 2013, p. 331).

A researcher wants to protect the identities of her research participants. What measures would ensure their protection? **Select all that apply.** The researcher would

1. report only group data and not individual data.
2. avoid specifying the location of the research study.
3. make sure that participants know the risks of the study.
4. limit exposure of participants to research assistants.
5. use a coding system to identify participants.

To identify the correct options, the test taker needs to recall (knowledge) the rights of research participants. Second, the test taker needs to understand what those rights are (comprehension). Finally, the test taker applies this knowledge and understanding of those rights in the research study to get the correct options 1, 2, and 5.

The fourth level in the domain is **analysis**. This is the ability to discern the parts that make a whole in order to determine what is going on. One's knowledge, comprehension, and ability to apply the concepts are required in order to choose the correct option.

Research Study Information: "Quantitative studies in this review revealed significant associations between discrimination and health outcomes in Asian Americans" (Nadimpali & Hutchinson, 2012, p. 127). What does this information represent?

1. Research problem
2. Study recommendations
3. Study's significance
4. Study's findings

Arriving at the correct option, option 4, requires knowing the different parts of a published study and understanding the purpose of each part. Knowledge and comprehension allow the test taker to have applied the information in another concrete situation. The ability to analyze the information given and then to relate it to each of the options helps the test taker determine the best option.

Helpful Study Habits and Test-Taking Strategies

Preparing for a test starts as soon as a course begins or, even better, before it begins. Effective organizational skills will help you manage a demanding curriculum such as nursing. One key to success in any course is to **read the material before the actual class.** Having read the material allows you to ponder and reflect on the content and make a mental list of questions that you will need to ask in class.

Divide the material to be read into manageable segments. Perhaps reading 10 to 12 pages per day would be more effective than attempting to read 50 pages in several hours. Keep in mind that about 2 hours is the maximum amount of time most people can concentrate intensely. During class, **remove distractions.** That means turning off your cell phone and avoiding the Internet while using your laptop computer for note taking. **Ask thought-provoking questions** that stimulate critical thinking and listen to the questions of others and the faculty's responses. You will not learn much if you simply ask your instructor to repeat a definition (knowledge level) of a concept rather than to give an example (application). Remember to read the chapter summary and the case studies that help pull the chapter concepts together. **Practice test questions** are extremely helpful. Be sure you know the rationale for the correct option as well as for the incorrect ones.

Meet with the course faculty as often as possible. Faculty members often complain that students do not use posted office hours. Do not wait until you are worried about your grade. **Study with classmates** who have the "right chemistry." Writing test questions and exchanging them with classmates take effort, but the results are worthwhile.

Review your notes and slides for the test several days before. Attempting to reread the chapters will only lead to frustration (so many pages and only a few hours to review). Reread parts of the chapter only when you encounter something in your notes or slides that you forgot or did not understand. **Do something relaxing** the day or evening before the test and try to get a full night's **sleep.** Most students who study all night come to the test exhausted and are not able to think critically. Avoid substances that spike your energy on a temporary basis.

Report to the test room several minutes before the start time so that you have time to focus and take deep breaths. Carefully **follow the test directions.** During the test, do not dwell too long on one question (you might get it wrong) because you will not have enough time for other questions (that you could get correct). **Skip a question** you are having difficulty answering within 1 minute. Come back to it, if possible. Otherwise, make a good guess and move on. When you have finished and there is still time, go to those questions that you had difficulty with. Questions that you did not have difficulty doing the first time should be left alone. Changing your answers is not good practice because during the course of the test, you might have read something, and now this something will influence your original answer. Most often, students who change their original answers realize their errors after the test data are finalized.

How to Be "Test Smart"

A. **Look for key words** in the question, also called the stem.

1. What is the most important safeguard to protect the identities of research subjects?
   1. Allow no one to look at the data.
   2. Publish only group data.
   3. Have participants enter a back door.
   4. Select a remote site for the study.

The key words in the question are "most important." Eliminate the incorrect options, also called distractors, based on your knowledge and understanding of research concepts. Option 2 is the best option because this measure will protect the identities of research participants from the largest group (i.e., all readers of the published report).

B. **Eliminate as many options as you can** to increase probability of getting the correct option. Remember that there are no partially correct or partially incorrect options. Identify something incorrect in an option in order to eliminate it immediately.

2. Which of the following are tests of validity?
   1. Test–retest
   2. Split half
   3. Content
   4. Odd–even

Eliminate options 1, 2, and 4. *Reliability* means "consistency." In options 1, 2, and 4, the test is given twice, and a comparison is made between the first administration of the test and a retest as seen in option 1. In option 2, the first half of the test is given, then the second half. In option 4, the odd numbered items are given, then the even items. The only option that does not imply retesting for consistency is option 3.

C. **Pick the best option** from among all correct options. The best option would be the one that incorporates all or some of the other options.

3. Which of the following documents would provide evidence that research participants' rights are protected?
   1. Patient's Bill of Rights
   2. HIPAA
   3. Informed consent
   4. Research abstract

The correct option is option 3. Informed consent takes into consideration the provisions of HIPAA, and if the study is done on patients in a health-care facility, the Patient Bill of Rights is considered as well.

D. Working with fill-in-the-blank questions requires a different way of processing the information provided in the question. **Look for a synonym** if it is a concept or process that is being asked about. Apply knowledge and comprehension abilities in analyzing the information. In addition, identify key words that could provide clues to the answer.

4. ____________________ is a descriptive statistic and is the number that occurs most frequently in a distribution.

The correct answer is *mode*. Note "descriptive statistic" as a key phrase. Then recall knowledge of descriptive statistics. There is also the phrase "occurs most frequently."

E. Questions that require a select-all-that-apply response makes use of the strategies you know from single multiple choice questions. First, eliminate the options with incorrect parts. Second, review those that you might select as correct options. Third, look at the options you selected and make sure they are all correct.

5. What steps does a researcher take during the conceptual phase of a research study. **Select all that apply.** The researcher
   1. selects a research design.
   2. formulates the research problem.
   3. reviews the related current literature.
   4. identifies a method to recruit participants.
   5. writes the proposed hypothesis.

The correct options are 2, 3, and 5. You would first need to identify the key words in the question. Recall the definitions of each phase in the research process (Knowledge). Think of your understanding of each phase and the steps in the process (Comprehension) and how each step might be completed (Application). Finally, eliminate the options that do not belong (Analysis).

How to Use This Book

Research Success provides you with practice questions to review the concepts covered in your nursing research course. But that is only one way this book can support your learning. Pay attention to the critical thinking facilitators given after the answer rationales. Use the research studies in your core textbook or have on hand several different types of studies to complete these critical thinking activities. If you have a study group, each member can contribute one or two studies, each with a different design, to the group's pool of studies. These studies will be worthwhile to have because they can be referred to many times for different parts of the research process.

Please note that the number of test items in each chapter varies as determined by the extent of the topic covered. This in no way affects the comprehensiveness of questions that address content in most core textbooks. The final examination addresses topics not covered in the individual chapters. In addition, there are actual research studies, case studies, and hypothetical studies that are the bases for questions in the four levels of the cognitive domain. In the final examination, questions are not organized according to content area, so you can either select items as they pertain to your current topic or use the final examination as a course review to test your ability to know, comprehend, apply, and analyze research concepts.

As you go through each of the chapter questions, rationales, test-taking tips, and critical thinking facilitators, bear in mind that these all enhance critical thinking. Although nursing research is not tested on the NCLEX-RN, the critical thinking skills that you develop will increase your probability of success in the future. Success in your research course, your basic program, and the NCLEX-RN will give you a "new set of glasses" to view and enjoy the world from a different perspective—that of the professional nurse.

GVG

Establishing a Framework for Awareness and Understanding of Research

1

KEY WORDS

The following words include English vocabulary, nursing/medical terminology, concepts, principles, or information relevant to content specifically addressed in the chapter or associated with topics presented in it. English dictionaries, your nursing textbooks, and medical dictionaries such as *Taber's Cyclopedic Medical Dictionary* are resources that can be used to expand your knowledge and understanding of these words and related information.

Applied research
Basic research
Critical appraisal
Construct
Evidence-based practice
Levels of purpose of research
  Identification
  Description
  Explanation
  Prediction
Morbidity
Mortality
Purposive sample
Qualitative research
Quantitative research

QUESTIONS

Historical Milestones in Nursing Research

1. Which of the following explains why Florence Nightingale's work is considered the earliest milestone in nursing research? She:
   1. established the first schools that provided formal training for nurses.
   2. advocated for the recognition of nursing as a healthcare discipline.
   3. analyzed mortality and morbidity rates in the Crimean War.
   4. recommended many changes to improve public health.

2. Which of the following factors is the strongest influence on the advancement of the nursing profession through research?
   1. Increased numbers of nurses with advanced degrees
   2. Recognition of nursing as a scientific discipline
   3. Expansion of hospitals as social institutions
   4. Fiscal support from government and private organizations

Research and Its Role in Nursing Practice

3. Research is essential to the nursing profession for a number of reasons. **Select all that apply.**
   1. To demonstrate the accountability of nursing as a profession
   2. To build the scientific knowledge base of nursing
   3. To facilitate the adoption of evidence-based practice
   4. To use the expertise of nurses with advanced degrees
   5. To document the cost-effectiveness of nursing care
   6. To showcase the achievements of nurse researchers

Types of Research

4. In his study, a nurse educator wants to determine the effectiveness of preparatory skill review on the level of skill competency among beginning nursing students. This type of research can be categorized as
   1. descriptive.
   2. applied.
   3. basic.
   4. qualitative.
5. The researcher wants to explore the role of interferon in the initiation of the immune response system. Subjects were laboratory animals. This type of research can be categorized as
   1. applied.
   2. descriptive.
   3. qualitative.
   4. basic.
6. The researcher looked at the effects of guided imagery on mild hypertension among middle-aged African American women. This statement suggests that the study is an example of what type of research?
   1. Qualitative research
   2. Applied research
   3. Basic research
   4. Descriptive research
7. A researcher looked at the construct of academic integrity in relation to plagiarism and cheating on written examinations. The researcher then concluded that academic integrity is a phenomenon similar to the development of moral reasoning. This type of research could be classified as
   1. descriptive.
   2. applied.
   3. basic.
   4. qualitative.

Purposes of Research in Nursing

8. Research has many different levels of purpose. What level of research purpose is communicated by the following question: What are the demographic characteristics of 4-year college graduates who enroll in a nursing program?
   1. Explanation
   2. Description
   3. Prediction
   4. Identification

9. A researcher sought to find out about the phenomenon experienced by widowed older women as "taking stock of yourself," a feeling state that occurs during the first year of widowhood. The researcher will use a qualitative approach, and the level of purpose for this study would be
   1. explanation.
   2. description.
   3. identification.
   4. prediction.

Roles of Nurses in Research

10. The American Nurses Association Council of Nurse Researchers has identified the role of baccalaureate-prepared nurses relative to research. Which of the following is consistent with the primary role of baccalaureate nurses? They can
    1. design the research investigation.
    2. determine applicability of research in clinical practice.
    3. serve as the principal investigators of the study.
    4. identify potential areas for research.

11. Registered professional nurses with master's degrees are able to fulfill which primary research-related role? They can
    1. serve as the study's principal investigators.
    2. critically appraise validity of study findings.
    3. serve as experts on clinical topics.
    4. evaluate appropriateness of a research design.

The National Institute of Nursing Research

12. The establishment of the National Institute of Nursing Research (NINR) was a critical milestone for nursing research for which reason(s)? **Select all that apply.**
    1. The respectability of nursing research was increased.
    2. There was increased funding for research projects.
    3. Its mission was to decrease health disparities.
    4. There was growth in clinical research.
    5. There was increased support for advanced education.

Quantitative and Qualitative Approaches

13. Calzone et al. (2012) conducted a study that surveyed the integration of genomics into nursing practice. A convenience sample of practicing nurses responded to a questionnaire online. Data were analyzed using descriptive statistics. What type of study approach was used by the researchers?
    1. Qualitative
    2. Quantitative
    3. Experimental
    4. Correlation

14. Foley, Myrick, and Yonge (2012) explored a phenomenological perspective on preceptorship within an intergenerational context. Using a purposive sample, the researchers conducted unstructured interviews to collect data. Themes that emerged from the data included being affirmed, being challenged, and being in a pedagogical journey. What research approach did the researchers use?
    1. Qualitative
    2. Quantitative
    3. Experimental
    4. Correlational

The correct answer number and rationale for why it is the correct answer are given in **boldface blue type.** Rationales for why the other possible answer options are incorrect also are given, but they are not in boldface type.

1. 1. It is true that some of Nightingale's work included plans for establishing schools of nursing. However, this work was not related to her research.
   2. This is true of all the works of Nightingale, but this is not research related.
   3. **This is the correct option. This work is research related and was evident in her book, *Notes on Nursing*. Works that look at mortality and morbidity are considered research studies.**
   4. Nightingale could be credited with her recommendations for testing of public water and improving sanitation. However, these were her later works after the Crimean War.

   TEST-TAKING TIP: All of the options are correct statements regarding the contributions of Florence Nightingale. The key word in the question stem is "research." *Mortality* and *morbidity* are research-related terms. For instance, the National Center for Health Statistics of the U.S. Department of Health and Human Services is constantly involved in studies addressing the mortality and morbidity rates of different health problems affecting Americans. An example is a report by Heron (2010) that reported leading causes of deaths for 2009. Only option 3 is considered research.

   Content Area: *Historical Perspectives in Research;* ***Cognitive Level:*** *Analysis;* ***Question Type:*** *Multiple Choice*
   CRITICAL THINKING FACILITATOR: Go to the website of the Centers for Disease Control and Prevention (http://www.cdc.gov/nchs) and look at studies on mortality and morbidity. Why are studies on mortality and morbidity considered research?

2. 1. **This is the correct option. Much of the conduct and design of research requires advanced degrees (i.e., master's or doctoral degrees). Master's-prepared nurses can serve as clinical experts in research studies. Doctorally prepared nurses have major roles in conducting research that contributes to the scientific base for nursing practice. Graduates of baccalaureate programs are prepared to be consumers of research, not doers.**
   2. This statement might be a result of research. Research aims to build the scientific base of nursing that guides practice.
   3. This is a historical event that led to many changes in healthcare but is not related to nursing research.
   4. It is true that nursing research has seen increased support from the government and other private organizations. However, potential research studies are proposed and designed by nurses with advanced degrees. Funding sources consider the credentials and experience of researchers who submit research proposals. Proposals are competitive, and often novice researchers are sponsored by expert researchers, thus ensuring the completion and success of the project.

   TEST-TAKING TIP: Think about who designs and conducts research. Nurses need advanced degrees to be able to do these. BSN programs prepare nurses to be consumers of research, not doers of research.

   Content Area: *Introduction to Nursing Research;* ***Cognitive Level:*** *Analysis;* ***Question Type:*** *Multiple Choice*
   CRITICAL THINKING FACILITATOR: Advanced degrees facilitate the advancement of the discipline through research. What skills and experiences are essential requirements for nurses to do research?

3. 1. **This is a correct reason why research is essential to the nursing profession.**
   2. **This is a correct reason why research is essential to the nursing profession.**
   3. **This is a correct reason why research is essential to the nursing profession.**
   4. This is not a correct reason why research is essential. The goal states what is required to conduct research.
   5. **This is a correct reason why research is essential to the nursing profession.**
   6. Although the dissemination of completed research does showcase the achievement of researchers, it is not the reason why research is essential. **Statements 1, 2, 3, and 5 all address why nursing research is essential to the profession. Statement 4 indicates a process necessary to design and conduct a research study, but it is not a goal of research. Statement 6 is not related to the goal but might be a benefit for the nurse who does the research study.**

   TEST-TAKING TIP: The overall goal of research is the improvement of patient outcomes and the advancement of the profession. Specific goals such as cost-effective care and evidence-based practice improve patient outcomes.

Accountability is an essential component of nursing practice, and any endeavor that contributes to the knowledge base for nursing are inherent in the goal of research.

Content Area: *Introduction to Nursing Research;* ***Cognitive Level:*** *Analysis;* ***Question Type:*** *Multiple Response*

CRITICAL THINKING FACILITATOR: Look at all nursing activities in a particular unit of practice. Are these practices based on clinical protocols? How and where do these come from? One answer is through research and the processes related to evidence-based practice. Are patient outcomes improved with these clinical protocols in place?

4. 1. This is a specific type of quantitative research. The goal of descriptive research is to "observe, count, delineate, elucidate, and classify phenomena" (Polit & Beck, 2010, p. 22).

2. **This is the correct option. This study can be categorized as applied research. Applied research is "scientific investigation conducted to generate knowledge that will directly influence or improve clinical practice. The purpose of applied research is to solve problems, make decisions, or predict or control outcomes in real-life practice situations" (Polit & Beck, 2010, p. 22).**

   "This type of research is usually performed in actual practice conditions, on subjects who represent the group to which the results will be applied" (Fain, 2009, p. 21).

3. "Basic research is undertaken to extend the base of knowledge in a discipline" (Polit & Beck, 2010, p. 22). The researcher might not have immediate applications in mind. "Basic research closely resembles the work done in laboratories and is associated with scientists" (Fain, 2009, p. 21).

4. "Qualitative research is a systematic, subjective approach used to describe life experiences and give them meaning" (Burns & Grove, 2011, p. 73). The research purpose in the question stem expresses a relationship between an independent and a dependent variable. The relationship between the two is explicit and measurable. A quantitative approach is inherent in the purpose.

TEST-TAKING TIP: The two major types of research are basic and applied. Look at the title or description of the study. Rule out basic research by asking this question: Can the findings of this study have immediate applicability, or could these findings help solve a current problem in practice? If the answer is YES, then the research is applied and not basic.

Content Area: *Introduction to Nursing Research;* ***Cognitive Level:*** *Application;* ***Question Type:*** *Multiple Choice*

CRITICAL THINKING FACILITATOR: Look at the sample studies and determine which are applied or basic. After you have identified an applied research study, think about the applicability of its findings to practice. Ask yourself whether the study findings might be a solution to a clinical problem.

5. 1. Applied research is "scientific investigation conducted to generate knowledge that will directly influence or improve clinical practice. The purpose of applied research is to solve problems, make decisions, or predict or control outcomes in real-life practice situations" (Polit & Beck, 2010, p. 22). The described study in the question stem does not have immediate applicability to practice.

2. This is a specific type of quantitative research. The goal of descriptive research is to "observe, count, delineate, elucidate, and classify phenomena" (Polit & Beck, 2010, p. 22).

3. Qualitative research is "a systematic, subjective approach used to describe life experiences and give them meaning" (Burns & Grove, 2011, p. 73). This is not evident in the question stem.

4. **This is the correct option. Basic research is undertaken to extend the knowledge base in a discipline. Basic research does not have immediate applicability. The researcher's findings are not used as immediate solutions to problems.**

TEST-TAKING TIP: The two major types of research are basic and applied. Look at the title or description of the study. Can the findings of this study have immediate applicability, or could these findings help solve a problem in practice? If the answer is NO, then the research is basic and not applied.

Content Area: *Introduction to Nursing Research;* ***Cognitive Level:*** *Analysis;* ***Question Type:*** *Multiple Choice*

CRITICAL THINKING FACILITATOR: After you have identified a basic research study, ask yourself whether the findings can be applied as a solution to a clinical problem. Also think about what future studies (applied research) could be done using the knowledge from this basic study.

6. 1. "Qualitative research is a systematic, subjective approach used to describe life experiences and give them meaning" (Burns & Grove, 2011, p. 73). The research purpose in the question stem expresses a relationship between an independent and a dependent variable. The relationship between the two is explicit and measurable. A quantitative approach is inherent in the purpose.

2. **This is the correct option. This is an example of applied research. There is evidence from the research statement that findings have immediate applicability. Immediate applicability can be seen in the clinical practice of a nurse who, after a critical appraisal of the study findings, decides to implement guided imagery as a nonpharmacological approach to lowering blood pressure in patients she sees in a clinic.**

3. "Basic research is undertaken to extend the base of knowledge in a discipline" (Polit & Beck, 2010, p. 22). The researcher might not have immediate applications in mind. "Basic research closely resembles the work done in laboratories and is associated with scientists" (Fain, 2009, p. 21).

4. This is a specific type of quantitative research. The goal of descriptive research is to "observe, count, delineate, elucidate, and classify phenomena" (Polit & Beck, 2010, p. 22).

TEST-TAKING TIP: A clue in the question stem is the word "effects." The word "effects" indicates that the researcher did something (an intervention) to study participants and then determined the outcomes on a phenomenon of interest, in this case, mild hypertension.

Content Area: *Introduction to Nursing Research;* ***Cognitive Level:*** *Application;* ***Question Type:*** *Multiple Choice*

CRITICAL THINKING FACILITATOR: Focus on a study with an intervention (a program, an approach, a treatment modality) and see how the researcher looks at the effects of this on an outcome. This is applied research.

7. 1. This is a specific type of quantitative research. The goal of descriptive research is to "observe, count, delineate, elucidate, and classify phenomena" (Polit & Beck, 2010, p. 22).

2. This study can be categorized as applied research. Applied research is "scientific investigation conducted to generate knowledge that will directly influence or improve clinical practice. The purpose of applied research is to solve problems, make decisions, or predict or control outcomes in real-life practice situations" (Polit & Beck, 2010, p. 22). "This type of research is usually performed in actual practice conditions, on subjects who represent the group to which the results will be applied" (Fain, 2009, p. 21).

3. **This is the correct option. Basic research is undertaken to extend the knowledge base of the discipline. The researcher might not have immediate applications.**

4. "Qualitative research is a systematic, subjective approach used to describe life experiences and give them meaning" (Burns & Grove, 2011, p. 73). This is not evident in the question stem.

TEST-TAKING TIP: The research statement does express the intent of the researcher, which is to predict or explain an outcome. Look for indications that the findings might be applied immediately in an educational setting.

Content Area: *Introduction to Nursing Research;* ***Cognitive Level:*** *Application;* ***Question Type:*** *Multiple Choice*

CRITICAL THINKING FACILITATOR: Think about abstract ideas (concepts) that have not been studied extensively and about which knowledge is lacking. The initial research that will be done is mostly basic. Because nursing is a practice discipline, most research is applied.

8. 1. The study with a purpose of explanation is done to "clarify the relationships among phenomena and identify the reasons why certain events occur" (Burns & Grove, 2011, p. 8). There is no relationship expressed in the question.

2. **This is the correct answer. The purpose of description is to "observe, count, delineate, elucidate, and classify phenomena" (Polit & Beck, 2010, p. 22). The study findings would include characteristics such as age, gender, socioeconomic status, religious affiliation, employment, and so on.**

3. The study with a purpose of prediction is designed to "estimate the probability of a specific outcome in a given situation" (Chinn & Kramer, 2008; as cited in Burns & Grove, 2011, p. 9). There is no inherent prediction that could be proposed from the research question presented.

4. The study with a purpose of identification is done to clearly define, identify, or name the phenomenon. The qualitative approach is the most appropriate to use in this instance, and the study questions would be: "What is the phenomenon? What is its name?" (LoBiondo-Wood & Haber, 2010, p. 21).

TEST-TAKING TIP: A descriptive study is an important preliminary type of study to determine the basic characteristics of a particular phenomenon. There are no variables and relationships to be explored. Descriptive statistics are used to process the data from a study with description as its purpose.

Content Area: *Introduction to Nursing Research;* ***Cognitive Level:*** *Analysis;* ***Question Type:*** *Multiple Choice*

CRITICAL THINKING FACILITATOR: Look at the sample research studies in the Appendix of your core textbook and try to determine the level of purpose of each study by just looking at the title. Verify your answer by looking at the abstract. You will see a statement such as, "The purpose of this descriptive study is to . . ." or "The purpose of this correlational study is to . . .," which indicates the study's purpose.

9. 1. In qualitative studies, the purpose of explanation is explicit when the following questions are asked:
How does the phenomenon occur?
Why does it occur?
What does the phenomenon mean?
How did the phenomenon occur?
(Polit & Beck, 2010, p. 21)
2. The purpose of description is to "observe, count, delineate, elucidate, and classify phenomena" (Polit & Beck, 2010, p. 22). The study findings would include characteristics such as age, gender, socioeconomic status, religious affiliation, employment, and so on.
3. This is the correct option. The purpose of identification in qualitative research is to name or identify the phenomenon.
4. The study with a purpose of prediction is designed to "estimate the probability of a specific outcome in a given situation" (Chinn & Kramer, 2008; as cited in Burns & Grove, 2011, p. 9). There is no inherent prediction that could be proposed from the research question presented.

TEST-TAKING TIP: The purpose of identification in research is the most basic level in qualitative studies. Try to think of the appropriate types of questions if a researcher wants to describe or explore the phenomenon. Description and exploration are preceded by identification. Similarly, think about the problem-solving process. Identify the problem and then describe and explore it in that sequence.

Content Area: *Introduction to Nursing Research;* ***Cognitive Level:*** *Analysis;* ***Question Type:*** *Multiple Choice*

CRITICAL THINKING FACILITATOR: Look at samples of qualitative studies and try to determine the level of purpose of each.

10. 1. Baccalaureate graduates are prepared to be consumers of nursing research. The role of designing a study is one assumed by nurses with advanced degrees.
2. This is the correct option. Nurses prepared at the baccalaureate level, through their basic knowledge of the research process, are able to determine applicability of research in clinical practice. They do this through a critical appraisal of the research study. Knowing how to critically appraise a research study is a course objective in most undergraduate research courses.
3. Nurses with advanced degrees serve as principal investigators and are directly involved in designing and conducting the study. This is not a role of baccalaureate-prepared nurses.
4. This is every nurse's role regardless of educational preparation. Practicing nurses have many opportunities to identify areas of practice that improve patient outcomes and advance the science of nursing.

TEST-TAKING TIP: Think about the direct roles of nurses in research. The doers of research design and conduct the study from beginning to completion. The consumers of research evaluate the finished product using a set of guidelines in a process called critical appraisal. They then determine applicability to clinical practice. This indirect role in research is a primary role of baccalaureate nurses.

Content Area: *Introduction to Nursing Research;* ***Cognitive Level:*** *Comprehension;* ***Question Type:*** *Multiple Choice*

CRITICAL THINKING FACILITATOR: What are the other roles of baccalaureate-prepared nurses relative to research? What types of healthcare settings do they practice in? What are some specific roles of nurses in these practice settings?

11. 1. Nurses with master's degrees can serve as principal investigators, but this is not their primary role.

2. Nurses prepared at the master's level, are able to determine applicability of research in clinical practice. However, this is not their primary role.
3. **Nurses with master's degrees are considered experts in certain areas of practice. Therefore, their expertise in clinical topics is sought and this is their primary role relative to research.**
4. This role is part of the indirect role of research consumers who are baccalaureate prepared and higher. The research consumer needs to have the ability to critically appraise the different parts of a research study.

TEST-TAKING TIP: Nurses prepared at the master's level are considered clinical experts in specific areas of nursing practice. Therefore, they can serve as valuable resource persons in any health-care setting. Give examples of research studies where the clinical expertise of a master's-prepared nurse would be essential.

Content Area: *Introduction to Nursing Research;* ***Cognitive Level:*** *Analysis;* ***Question Type:*** *Multiple Choice*

CRITICAL THINKING FACILITATOR: Nurses prepared at the master's level are considered clinical experts in specific areas of nursing practice. Therefore, they can serve as valuable resource persons in any healthcare setting. Give examples of research studies where the clinical expertise of a master's-prepared nurse would be essential.

12. 1. **The statement is a correct reason why the establishment of the NINR was a milestone.**
2. **The statement is a correct reason why the establishment of the NINR was a milestone.**
3. The statement is incorrect. This was a goal of Healthy People 2010.
4. **The statement is a correct reason why the establishment of the NINR was a milestone.**
5. The statement is incorrect. Increasing funding for education is not a goal of the NINR.

TEST-TAKING TIP: "The mission statement of the NINR indicates support for clinical and basic research to establish a scientific basis for the care of individuals across the life span" (Nieswiadomy, 2009, p. 20).

Content Area: *Introduction to Nursing Research;* ***Cognitive Level:*** *Comprehension;* ***Question Type:*** *Multiple Response*

CRITICAL THINKING FACILITATOR: See whether your textbook describes the research priorities of the NINR. Take one of these areas and think about why it is a chosen priority by the NINR.

13. 1. Qualitative research is "a systematic, subjective approach used to describe life experiences and give them meaning" (Burns & Grove, 2011, p. 73). "Qualitative materials are narrative and subjective" (Polit & Beck, 2010, p. 17).
2. **This is the correct option. "Quantitative research is a formal, objective, rigorous and systematic process for generating numerical information about the world" (Burns & Grove, 2011, p, 34).**
3. An experimental study is a type of quantitative research. Experimental research is the most rigorous of all quantitative designs. The study described is a survey. "A survey obtains information about the prevalence, distribution, and interrelations of variables within a population. Survey data are used primarily in non-experimental correlational studies" (Polit & Beck, 2010, p. 294).
4. A correlation study is another type of quantitative research. Using correlation statistics, the researcher determines the relationship between or among variables. The information about the study does not identify any variables.

TEST-TAKING TIP: One excellent way to distinguish between a quantitative and a qualitative approach is to look at the study's data. Quantitative research collects and analyzes numerical data. Qualitative studies collect and analyze narrative data that are the participants' descriptions of their experiences. There are no statistical analyses done on the data.

Content Area: *Introduction to Nursing Research;* ***Cognitive Level:*** *Application;* ***Question Type:*** *Multiple Choice*

CRITICAL THINKING FACILITATOR: Look at the sample research studies in the Appendix of your core textbook. What do the data from the studies look like? How are the data presented in the studies?

14. 1. **This is the correct option. This study used a qualitative approach because study participants shared their experiences on preceptorship. Analyses of the**

narrative data shared by the participants yielded themes. The specific qualitative approach used is phenomenology. This is a "process of learning and constructing the meaning of human experience through intensive dialogue with persons who are living the experience" (Barroso, 2010, p. 102).

2. "Quantitative research encompasses the study of research questions and/or hypotheses that describe phenomena, test relationships, assess differences, and seek to explain cause and effect between variables and test for intervention effectiveness" (LoBiondo-Wood & Haber, 2010, p. 8).
3. "A true experimental design is an experiment in which the researcher tries to assess whether an intervention or treatment (independent variable) makes a difference in a measured outcome (dependent variable)" (Fain, 2009, p. 183).
4. "Correlational research involves the systematic investigation of relationships between or among variables. To do this the researcher measures the selected variables in a sample and then uses correlational statistics to determine the relationships among the variables" (Burns & Grove, 2011, p. 35).

TEST-TAKING TIP: A key word in the question is "phenomenological." A phenomenological study is one type of qualitative study that looks at the lived experience of individuals. The most common types of qualitative studies include grounded theory, historical, and ethnography.

Content Area: *Introduction to Nursing Research;* ***Cognitive Level:*** *Analysis;* ***Question Type:*** *Multiple Choice*

CRITICAL THINKING FACILITATOR: Look at sample studies in the Appendix of your core textbook. You can distinguish the qualitative studies by their titles. Titles of qualitative studies do not include variables. There will be a single phenomenon of interest, and at times the word "experience" will be included in the title, for example, "The Lived Experience of Chronic Illness." What do qualitative data look like? How were the data organized?

2 Creating the Foundation for Evidence-Based Practice

KEY WORDS

The following words include English vocabulary, nursing/medical terminology, concepts, principles, or information relevant to content specifically addressed in the chapter or associated with topics presented in it. English dictionaries, your nursing textbooks, and medical dictionaries such as *Taber's Cyclopedic Medical Dictionary* are resources that can be used to expand your knowledge and understanding of these words and related information.

Integrative reviews
Intuition
Levels of research evidence
Logical reasoning: deductive and inductive approaches
Meta-analysis
Meta-synthesis
Systematic reviews
Tradition
Trial and error

QUESTIONS

Evidence-Based Practice

1. Which of the following statements defines evidence-based practice (EBP)?
   1. "It is the systematic, rigorous, logical investigation that aims to answer questions about nursing phenomena" (LoBiondo-Wood & Haber, 2010, p. 6).
   2. "It is the empirical knowledge generated by the synthesis of quality study findings to address a practice problem" (Burns & Grove, 2011, p. 4).
   3. "It is the process of communicating and using empirical or research-generated knowledge to affect or change the existing practices in the healthcare system" (Burns & Grove, 2011, p. 547).
   4. "It is the collection, interpretation, and integration of valid research evidence combined with clinical practice and understanding of the patient and family" (LoBiondo-Wood & Haber, 2010, p. 7).

Sources of Nursing Evidence

2. There are many sources of information that nurses use to guide their practice. Tradition is one such source. Which of the following statements reflects using tradition as a source of information?
   1. "Let us try something else and see if it works."
   2. "I feel that we are headed in the right direction in resolving the issue."
   3. "The nurse manager said we should try to do it this way."
   4. "Let us do it like we always have in the past."

3. There are many sources of information that nurses use to guide their practice. One such source is logical reasoning that includes deductive or inductive approaches. Which of the following situations reflects deductive reasoning? A nurse
   1. is aware that a specific person has a traditional cultural background with an orientation to the past. The nurse believes all her patients who are from this culture are past oriented.
   2. knows that denial is often the first reaction of most patients diagnosed with a terminal illness. The nurse expects that a patient diagnosed with a terminal illness would initially deny having this diagnosis.
   3. assumes that all patients from a particular culture are stoic to pain based on his work experience with an individual from that culture who was stoic to pain.
   4. encounters a very rude New York City taxi driver. The nurse now believes that all New York taxi drivers are rude.

4. A nursing student spent some time during her clinical experience working with homeless persons. She assessed homeless persons' self-esteem to be very low during the first few weeks of homelessness. If this student encounters a newly homeless person and assumes that this person's self-esteem is low, what logical reasoning approach is the student using?
   1. Inductive
   2. Deductive
   3. Intuition
   4. Tradition

5. A nurse cared for a terminally ill client for a period of 1 year until the client died. Later, the nurse used her experience with this one client in guiding her care for all her clients with the same illness. It can be said that the nurse is using which logical reasoning approach?
   1. Inductive
   2. Deductive
   3. Intuition
   4. Tradition

Processes to Synthesize Research Evidence

6. There are several processes used to synthesize research evidence. Which process provides the strongest research evidence?
   1. Meta-summaries of qualitative studies
   2. A single randomized clinical trial
   3. Meta-analysis of correlational studies
   4. Systematic review of randomized clinical trials

7. One of the processes used to synthesize research evidence is an integrative review. What is included in an integrative review? **Select all that apply.**
   1. Research findings from quantitative studies
   2. Research findings from qualitative studies
   3. All quantitative studies for an intervention's efficacy
   4. Opinions of all expert clinicians on the intervention
   5. Reports of expert committees

8. Of the following levels of research evidence, which one is the weakest?
   1. An integrative review of experimental, quasi-experimental, and outcome studies
   2. A meta-analysis of correlational studies
   3. A single qualitative or descriptive study
   4. A single experimental study

9. Which of the following resources provides the most comprehensive source of information and the highest level of evidence, such as systematic reviews for EBP?
   1. The National Guideline Clearinghouse
   2. Annual Review of Nursing Research
   3. Cochrane Collaboration and Library
   4. Cumulative Index of Nursing and Allied Health Literature (CINAHL)

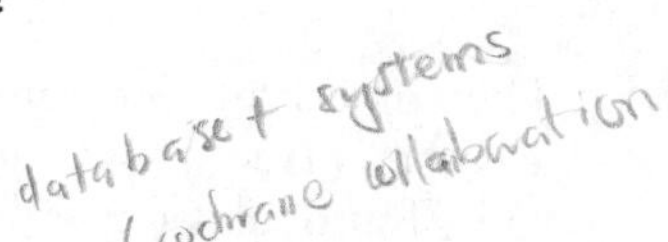

Barriers to Evidence-Based Practice

10. Melnyck and Fineout-Overholt (2010) identified barriers in adopting EBP. Some of these barriers are listed below. **Select all that apply.**
    1. Organizational constraints, such as lack of administrative support and incentives
    2. Lack of knowledge regarding EBP strategies
    3. Peer pressure to continue with practices steeped in tradition
    4. Pressure from the profession to adopt EBP
    5. Inadequate information in professional journals
    6. Overwhelming patient loads

Overcoming Barriers to Evidence-Based Practice

11. One of the major barriers to implementing EBP in the clinical setting is nurses' general lack of experience in reading and synthesizing research. Which of the following strategies could help overcome this barrier? **Select all that apply.**
    1. Collaborate with a nursing education program to access resources.
    2. Make a list of reasons why EBP should be valued.
    3. Use one familiar format for critical appraisals.
    4. Organize a journal club to discuss evidence.
    5. Listen to people's concerns about change.

ANSWERS AND RATIONALES

The correct answer number and rationale for why it is the correct answer are given in **boldface blue type**. Rationales for why the other possible answer options are incorrect also are given, but they are not in boldface type.

1. 1. This statement defines research.
   2. This statement describes best research evidence.
   3. This is a process known as research utilization.
   4. **This is the correct option because the statement includes the processes that are required for EBP. It is more than research utilization, and it is based on findings from valid research.**

   TEST-TAKING TIP: **EBP is a complex process that "promotes quality, cost-effective outcomes for patients, families, healthcare providers, and the health care system" (Burns & Grove, 2011., p. 4). Only option 4 is consistent with this statement.**

   Content Area: *Evidenced-Based Practice Basic Concepts;* ***Cognitive Level:*** *Comprehension;* ***Question Type:*** *Multiple Choice*

   CRITICAL THINKING FACILITATOR: Try to come up with examples of research, best research evidence, and research utilization based on your observations in clinical.

2. 1. This statement reflects trial and error. Alternate solutions to a problem are tried until a solution with positive outcomes is reached.
   2. Intuition is inherent in the statement. The "gut feeling" is used to select solutions to problems.
   3. The nurse manager is considered an authority figure and is therefore viewed as the best person to solve the problem. What the nurse manager says might be based on tradition, but it doesn't have to be.
   4. **This is the correct option. "What has worked in the past might work now" is the thinking reflected in the statement. Tradition, as it has in the past, will guide the solution to a problem.**

   TEST-TAKING TIP: **Nurses have a repertoire of traditions and practices that guide practice. Some are no longer current and appropriate. One example is bathing all patients in the morning without regard for the patient's preferences and care priorities. So when nurses say, "We have always done it this way," they are following tradition.**

   Content Area: *Sources of Evidence for Knowledge;* ***Cognitive Level:*** *Analysis;* ***Question Type:*** *Multiple Choice*

   CRITICAL THINKING FACILITATOR: Think of guidelines used by nurses in practice and decision making. Are their practices current? Are they able to provide a rationale for their actions and decisions?

3. 1. This is inductive reasoning. It is defined as "the process of developing generalizations from specific observations" (Polit & Beck, 2010, p. 13).
   2. **This is the correct option. Deductive reasoning is defined as" the process of developing specific predictions from general predictions" (Polit & Beck, 2010, p. 13).**
   3. This is inductive reasoning.
   4. This is inductive reasoning.

   TEST-TAKING TIP: **Deductive reasoning moves from a general premise to a specific situation. For example: All persons from this culture are stoic to pain. Patient A is from this culture. Therefore, he is stoic to pain.**

   Inductive reasoning moves from a number of specific examples to a general statement. Patient A is stoic to pain and is from Culture X. Patient B is stoic to pain and is from Culture X. Patient C is stoic to pain and is from Culture X. Therefore, based on these examples, one can generalize that persons from Culture X are stoic to pain.

   Content Area: *Nursing Sources of Evidence;* ***Cognitive Level:*** *Analysis;* ***Question Type:*** *Multiple Choice*

   CRITICAL THINKING FACILITATOR: Think about how you make certain decisions. What kind of reasoning do you use to arrive at your decision? If you think you arrive at your decision using a deductive approach, how did you process it?

4. 1. Inductive reasoning moves from the specific observations to general statements. The nursing student's initial assessment of homeless persons' sense of self-esteem was inductive: she made a generalization based on her assessment of numerous specific cases.
   2. **This is the correct option. Deductive reasoning moves from general premises to specific conclusions.**
   3. Intuition is not logical reasoning. This is a way of acquiring knowledge using a hunch or "gut feeling."
   4. Tradition is another way of acquiring knowledge. It is guided by beliefs based on

customs and usual way of doing things. It is not logical reasoning.

TEST-TAKING TIP: In the question stem , the student's experience with the general population of homeless persons guided her reasoning about a specific homeless person.

Content Area: *Nursing's Sources of Evidence;* ***Cognitive Level:*** *Analysis;* ***Question Type:*** *Multiple Choice*

CRITICAL THINKING FACILITATOR: Consider clinical situations in which you have had to make decisions and determine whether your logical reasoning in each situation was deductive or inductive. Think about how you use each approach.

5. 1. **This is the correct option. The nurse used the inductive approach, applying premises and conclusions from a specific situation to make general assumptions.**
2. Movement from general premises to a specific situation is deductive reasoning.
3. Intuition is a way to obtain evidence. This is also known as a hunch or a "gut feeling." It is not considered logical reasoning like inductive or deductive approaches.
4. Tradition is a way to obtain evidence. However, this is not logical reasoning like inductive or deductive approaches. The person using tradition relies on what has been done in the past to guide practice.

TEST-TAKING-TIP: The nurse's experience with a specific client was generalized to all clients with the same illness. Reasoning from specific premises to general ones is inductive reasoning.

Content Area: *Nursing's Sources of Evidence;* ***Cognitive Level:*** *Analysis;* ***Question Type:*** *Multiple Choice*

CRITICAL THINKING FACILITATOR: How many times have you used your experience with one individual and applied that to an experience with a group? What are the pitfalls of generalizing from a single experience?

6. 1. Meta-summaries of qualitative studies do not include quantitative studies. These are not the strongest levels of evidence.
2. A randomized clinical trial is a rigorous study that must follow specific criteria, but a single randomized clinical is still below the strongest levels of evidence that involve multiple studies and processes.
3. A meta-analysis of correlational studies is midpoint in the level of research evidence rigor.
4. **This is the correct option. The systematic review consists of many experimental studies. This is conducted by panels of expert researchers using rigorous criteria.**

TEST-TAKING TIP: A clue in the question is the word "systematic," which means that the processes were not haphazard but followed specific criteria. A systematic review is an inclusive process and involves all of the studies with the most rigorous designs.

Content Area: *Synthesis of Research Evidence;* ***Cognitive Level:*** *Comprehension;* ***Question Type:*** *Multiple Choice*

CRITICAL THINKING FACILITATOR: Visualize a diagram of the hierarchy of research evidence. The more advanced and complex the processes involved are, the higher the evidence is in the hierarchy. Similarly, the more types of research involved, the higher the level is. The more complex and rigorous the study, the higher is its level of evidence.

7. 1. **Research findings from quantitative studies are included in an integrative review.**
2. **Research findings from qualitative studies are included in an integrative review.**
3. Meta-analysis is the focus of all quantitative studies for intervention efficacy.
4. The opinions of expert clinicians provide the weakest form of evidence and are not included in integrative reviews.
5. Reports of expert committees provide the weakest form of evidence and are not included in integrative reviews.

TEST-TAKING TIP: A key word is "integrative." ***Integration*** **means "to bring together parts into a whole." The integrative review brings together qualitative and quantitative studies.**

Content Area: *Synthesis of Research Evidence;* ***Cognitive Level:*** *Analysis;* ***Question Type:*** *Multiple Response*

CRITICAL THINKING FACILITATOR: Know the basic definitions of the different processes for synthesizing research evidence. The weakest processes do not involve research studies but only the opinions of experts. Just like the levels of purpose of research (identification, description, exploration, prediction, and explanation), the more basic the purpose, the weaker in the level of evidence. For instance, a descriptive study is weaker than an experimental study with a purpose of prediction. Single studies are weaker than integrative, meta-analysis, and systematic reviews that involve many studies.

8. 1. An integrative review is one of the stronger processes to synthesize research evidence. It involves looking at many studies that have prediction and explanation as their purposes (experimental, quasi-experimental, and outcomes).
2. A meta-analysis of correlational studies is approximately at midpoint in the hierarchy of processes. This process would "determine the

type of relationship (negative or positive) and the strength of relationships among selected variables" (Burns & Grove, 2011, p. 24).

3. This is the correct option. This process is one of the weakest, only a step above opinions of experts (the lowest level). The level of purpose of a single qualitative or descriptive study is either identification or description. Both of these studies do not involve variables and are not looking at relationships between or among variables.

4. Although this is considered strong research evidence, it is still topped by integrative reviews, meta-analysis, and systematic reviews, processes that involve multiple studies that have very high levels of purposes (i.e., prediction and explanation).

TEST-TAKING TIP: A clue in the question is the phrase "weakest level." If the opinions of experts make up the weakest level, the next level has to be a beginning study that does not test a relationship between or among variables.

Content Area: *Synthesis of Research Evidence;* ***Cognitive Level:*** *Analysis;* ***Question Type:*** *Multiple Choice*

CRITICAL THINKING FACILITATOR: Recall the different levels of purpose of research. Studies with a purpose of identification or description are lower in the hierarchy of evidence compared with studies with a level of prediction or explanation.

9. 1. This is an agency that "provides varied audiences with easy-to-use mechanisms for objective, detailed information on clinical guidelines" (Burns & Grove, 2011, p. 495).

2. This is a publication that includes "experts' reviews of research organized into four areas: nursing practice, nursing care delivery, nursing education, and the nursing profession" (Burns & Grove, 2011, p. 13).

3. This is the correct option. The Cochrane Collaboration "seeks to provide timely up-to-date research evidence. The Cochrane Library is a database collection, providing access to systematic reviews, controlled trials, methodology registry, technology assessment and more" (Schmidt & Brown, 2009, p. 97).

4. The CINAHL database provides "authoritative coverage of the literature related to nursing and allied health" (Boswell & Cannon, 2014, p. 157).

TEST-TAKING TIP: Note the term "systematic reviews" in the question. This is the primary mission of the Cochrane Collaboration. Formed in the United Kingdom, the Cochrane Collaboration seeks "to conduct rigorous research summaries with the goal of making it easier for clinicians to learn what various studies found regarding the effectiveness of particular healthcare interventions" (Brown, 2009, p. 9).

Content Area: *Introduction to Evidence-Based Practice;* ***Cognitive Level:*** *Knowledge;* ***Question Type:*** *Multiple Choice*

CRITICAL THINKING FACILITATOR: Familiarize yourself with the different resources that facilitate research, such as agencies that provide research information or evidence. Also important are various print and nonprint resources that can be accessed for research information.

10. 1. Organizational constraints are barriers when practicing nurses are not supported or given incentives.

2. Lack of knowledge of EBP is a barrier because nurses need to know the processes involved in implementing EBP in the clinical settings.

3. Peer pressure to continue with practices based on tradition negates the value of EBP. Traditional ways lack the scientific and theoretical foundations of EBP.

4. The pressure from the profession is an incentive, not a barrier, to adopting EBP. EBP enables "clinicians to provide the highest quality of care as meeting the multifaceted needs of their patients and families" (Melnyck & Fineout-Overholt, 2010, p. 3).

5. Information and resources for EBP are increasing at a faster rate. Extramural and governmental resources and support facilitate the work of many scientists from health-care disciplines. These are not considered barriers to EBP.

6. Overwhelming patient loads are a barrier to adopting EBP because these workloads do not allow nurses time to read the latest professional literature or attend training in new practices unless they do so before or after their shift assignments.

TEST-TAKING TIP: Barriers to EBP are situations that prevent nurses from adopting new approaches (best practices) in improving patient care. Other barriers are those that inhibit or retard the implementation of EBP and make health-care providers rely on obsolete approaches to effective, high-quality patient care.

Content Area: *Evidence-Based Practice;* ***Cognitive Level:*** *Analysis;* ***Question Type:*** *Multiple Response*

CRITICAL THINKING FACILITATOR: Think about your time in clinical experience and identify possible barriers to high-quality nursing care that you have observed. These are very similar to barriers to EBP. New ways of thinking and doing things are always a threat to people's security, and this is a major barrier that brings with it a host of other barriers (e.g., not enough time, too much to do, lack of know-how).

11. 1. Collaboration is a strategy used to overcome the barrier of lack of resources.
2. Making a list of reasons why EBP should be valued would overcome the barrier of not valuing EBP.
3. Using a familiar format for critical appraisals of research studies is a strategy to overcome the barrier of the lack of experience in reading and synthesizing research.
4. Lack of experience in reading and synthesizing research can also be overcome by organizing a journal club, where more experienced nurses could assist and support those who lack the knowledge and skills to implement EBP.
5. Listening to people's concerns about EBP is a strategy to overcome the barrier of not valuing EBP.

TEST-TAKING TIP: Familiarize yourself with the different categories of barriers to research and EBP. There are clinician-related barriers, and there are organizational barriers.

Content Area: *Introduction to EBP;* ***Cognitive Level:*** *Comprehension;* ***Question Type:****Multiple Response*

CRITICAL THINKING FACILITATOR: Make a list of the barriers to EBP you have identified during your clinical experience and determine how each could be addressed.

3 Judging the Ethical and Legal Aspects of Research

KEY WORDS

The following words include English vocabulary, nursing/medical terminology, concepts, principles, or information relevant to content specifically addressed in the chapter or associated with topics presented in it. English dictionaries, your nursing textbooks, and medical dictionaries such as *Taber's Cyclopedic Medical Dictionary* are resources that can be used to expand your knowledge and understanding of these words and related information.

Assent
Autonomy
Beneficence
Code of ethics
Covert data collection
Implied consent
Informed consent
Institutional review board
Justice
Minimal risk
Right to anonymity and confidentiality
Right to fair treatment
Right to full dclosure
Right to protection from discomfort and harm
Right to self-determination
Risk–benefit assessment
Vulnerable populations

QUESTIONS

Historical Perspectives of Ethics in Research

1. From 1933 through 1945, the Nazi regime performed unethical medical activities and research on prisoners of war and Jews confined in concentration camps. Which of the following statements is true about these activities? These activities
   1. generated useful information on many common health problems.
   2. created a population of "racially pure" Germans.
   3. were brought to light in the Nuremberg trials of the experimenters.
   4. followed well-designed plans to achieve positive outcomes.

2. The Tuskegee Syphilis Study was conducted by the U.S. Public Health Service for 40 years. This study was considered highly unethical because of the following reason(s). **Select all that apply.**
   1. Only African American men with syphilis were selected to participate.
   2. Some who participated did not know the purpose of the study.
   3. Information on treatment for syphilis was withheld for some.
   4. The men received a stipend for participating in the study.
   5. Treatment was deliberately withheld for some.

Regulatory Aspects of Ethical Research

3. The Belmont Report was issued in 1978 by the U.S. Commission for the Protection of Human Subjects of Biomedical and Behavioral Research. Which of the following is true regarding the Belmont Report?
1. It differentiated therapeutic from nontherapeutic research.
2. Its basis was the Nuremberg Code.
3. It incorporates respect for persons, beneficence, and justice.
4. It stipulates full review of all studies involving humans.

4. Which of the following federal regulations address(es) directly the protection of human subjects in research? **Select all that apply.**
1. The Health Insurance Portability and Accountability Act (HIPAA) was enacted to protect health information in all areas, including research.
2. The Code of Federal Regulations (CFR) in 1973 provided for the protection of ill, mentally impaired, or dying individuals who have limited capacity to consent.
3. The Department of Health and Human Services (DHHS) Protection of Human Subject Regulations Title 45 CFR Part 46 protects the rights and welfare of subjects in DHHS funded studies.
4. The National Research Act established the National Commission for the Protection of Human Subjects for Biomedical and Behavioral Research.
5. The Declaration of Helsinki stipulated the access and provision of diagnostic and treatment procedures for research subjects.

5. One of the ethical principles addressed in the Belmont Report is beneficence. Which of the following actions by a researcher indicates adherence to the principle of beneficence?
1. Minimizing any harm or discomfort to the subjects
2. Respecting a participant's decision to withdraw
3. Distributing research benefits equally
4. Maintaining anonymity and confidentiality

6. One of the ethical principles addressed in the Belmont Report is respect for human dignity. Which of the following actions by a researcher indicates adherence to the principle of respect for human dignity?
1. Minimizing any harm or discomfort
2. Distributing research benefits equally
3. Making sure the participants know the risks involved
4. Maintaining anonymity and confidentiality

Rights of Research Participants

7. One of the rights of research participants is the right to anonymity. Which of the following behaviors of the researchers would protect this right of research participants? The researchers will
1. make sure that the informed consent was executed before the study.
2. hire trained data collectors for the study.
3. publish only group data and not individual data in the report.
4. explain the purpose of the study to the participants.

8. The right to confidentiality must be maintained by ethical researchers in their studies. This was evident in which of the following situations: The researchers
1. disclosed only the general location of the research site.
2. allowed only authorized personnel to have access to research data.
3. used a coding process to conceal the identity of each participant.
4. explained the nature and purpose of the study to the participants.

9. A researcher was doing a study on a new antihypertensive medication. A designated patient unit was the research site. A patient on the unit was hesitant to participate but finally consented because she thought that her care might be compromised if she refused. What right was compromised?
1. Right to confidentiality
2. Right to anonymity
3. Right to self-determination
4. Right to full disclosure

10. Some of the African American men who participated in the Tuskegee Syphilis Study were not informed of the purpose and procedures of the study. Which right of these study participants was violated?
1. Confidentiality
2. Anonymity
3. Full disclosure
4. Protection from harm

11. An implied consent is assumed to have been obtained when research participants
1. have adequate information about the study.
2. return a self-administered questionnaire.
3. are allowed to participate in making decisions.
4. know the risks involved in participating.

Protecting the Rights of Research Participants

12. Which initial major approach is used by researchers to protect research participants? Researchers
1. provide detailed information about the study procedures.
2. select the research participants carefully.
3. perform a risk–benefit assessment.
4. hire only qualified research assistants.

13. A researcher's intervention protocol entailed subjects climbing two flights of stairs to determine changes in their pulse rates. The researcher believes that the research participants were only subjected to minimal risk. Minimal risk is defined as
1. the benefits of the study outweighing the risks.
2. the risks outweighing the benefits of the study.
3. risks that are no greater than those encountered daily.
4. assessed risks and benefits are approximately equal.

14. Potential research participants exercise their right to self-determination before the start of a study. Which document provides evidence that this right was duly exercised?
1. HIPAA documents
2. Informed consent
3. Attendance records
4. Demographic information

15. Institutions with research programs and agencies that provide funding have institutional review boards (IRBs). Which of the following statements are true regarding the functions of IRBs?
Select all that apply.
1. IRBs decide whether research studies should get funded.
2. IRBs ensure that researchers do not engage in unethical behaviors.
3. IRBs examine the procedures for selecting research participants.
4. IRBs make sure that a process is in place for participants to give informed consent.
5. IRBs ensure that federal guidelines for research are followed.

16. Children who are potential research participants provide assent. Which of the following statements is consistent with assent? The researchers
    1. obtain the written consent of a legal guardian.
    2. get the child's affirmative agreement to participate.
    3. emphasize the voluntary nature of being a participant.
    4. use other methods to obtain consent such as videotaping.

17. Informed consent "is an ethical principle that requires researchers to obtain people's voluntary participation in a study after informing them of possible risks and benefits" (LoBiondo-Wood & Haber, 2010, p. 557). Which of the following are essential elements of informed consent? **Select all that apply.**
    1. Disclosure of essential study information to the participant or subject
    2. Comprehension of this information by the subject
    3. Competence of the subject to give consent
    4. Voluntary consent of the subject to participate in the study
    5. Contractual agreement by the subject to complete the study
    6. Willingness of the subject to disclose all personal information

18. A researcher, interested in cultural behaviors that occur during social gatherings, was a guest at a party and observed certain individuals interacting with other guests. Later this researcher wrote up the observations she obtained at the party and published her findings. In this instance, what right was violated by the researcher?
    1. Anonymity
    2. Self-determination
    3. Confidentiality
    4. Freedom from harm

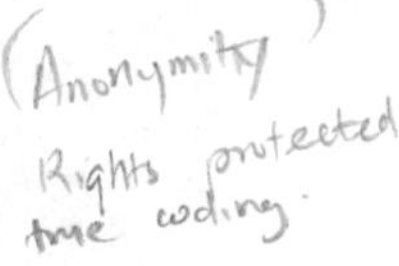

19. When research participant data are coded so that individual identities are protected, the researcher is safeguarding which right?
    1. Self-determination
    2. Anonymity
    3. Confidentiality
    4. Fair treatment

20. Mothers who had lost a young adult offspring were asked to share their experiences with the researcher. During the interviews, many of the mothers became extremely emotional in recounting their loss experience. If provisions were not in place, the researcher could be accused of violating which right of the participants?
    1. Self-determination
    2. Anonymity
    3. Freedom from harm or discomfort
    4. Fair treatment

21. A nurse educator asked her students to participate in a study on contraception. Students consented to participate because they thought that their nonparticipation might jeopardize their grades in the course. What right was violated?
    1. Freedom from harm
    2. Self-determination
    3. Fair treatment
    4. Informed consent

Research with Vulnerable Groups

22. Which of the following individuals are considered members of vulnerable groups relative to research? **Select all that apply.**
    1. A 70-year-old adult who is retired
    2. A 35-year-old self-employed woman
    3. A 40-year-old prison inmate
    4. An 18-year-old freshman college student
    5. A 50-year-old man in hospice facility

Ethics in Qualitative Research

23. Ethical issues in qualitative research differ from those in quantitative studies. Which of the following reasons would account for these differences? **Select all that apply.**
    1. Unanticipated issues might emerge because of the unpredictability of qualitative research.
    2. Anonymity is almost impossible to maintain in qualitative research because of the close interaction between the researcher and the participants.
    3. In qualitative research, the investigators maintain an objective, neutral position, removed from those being studied.
    4. The potential attrition of participants might influence the validity of the qualitative research study.
    5. The small sample size in a study conducted in a naturalistic setting might compromise the anonymity of participants.

24. The emergent and unpredictable nature of qualitative research demands that participants are constantly kept abreast of the study processes. To maintain the right to self-determination of participants, what must be executed as the study progresses?
    1. Informed consent
    2. Assent
    3. Full disclosure
    4. Process consent

ANSWERS AND RATIONALES

The correct answer number and rationale for why it is the correct answer are given in **boldface blue type.** Rationales for why the other possible answer options are incorrect also are given, but they are not in boldface type.

1. 1. The research studies were poorly designed. Consequently, there was little useful information generated from these studies.
2. This intent of the studies never came to fruition.
3. This is the correct option. The Nuremberg trials were about the atrocities committed against persons of Jewish affiliation and other prisoners of war. The trials also focused on unethical research and mistreatment of research subjects.
4. This is a false statement. The studies were poorly designed, and no ethical guidelines were followed.

TEST-TAKING TIP: A key word in the question stem is "unethical." This word indicates a violation of research participants' rights. In addition, the research subjects were prisoners of war and persons in concentration camps. These persons belonged to vulnerable groups, because they were confined and had little to no say on their own behalf.

Content Area: *Historical Perspectives of Ethics in Research;* ***Cognitive Level:*** *Comprehension;* ***Question Type:*** *Multiple Choice*

CRITICAL THINKING FACILITATOR: Review the historical events that served as the basis for regulations that protect the rights of research participants. Events in the early 1900s in other countries and in the United States have brought to light the important role of ethics in the conduct of research.

2. 1. This statement has to do with the sample of the study.
2. This is a reason why the study was considered unethical.
3. This is a reason why the study was considered unethical.
4. This is not a reason why the Tuskegee Syphilis Study was considered unethical.
5. This is a reason why the study was considered unethical.

TEST-TAKING TIP: The word "unethical" is a key word in the question stem. This term brings to mind physical and mental harm to persons, violating human rights, and exploiting people's vulnerability.

Content Area: *Historical Perspectives of Ethics in Research;* ***Cognitive Level:*** *Analysis;* ***Question Type:*** *Multiple Response*

CRITICAL THINKING FACILITATOR: Review the various rights of research participants. What rights were violated by the researchers in failing to inform participants about the study and risks involved? When known effective treatment was intentionally withheld from participants, what right was violated?

3. 1. This statement describes the Declaration of Helsinki.
2. This statement also describes the Declaration of Helsinki.
3. This is the correct option. The Belmont Report addresses the principles of beneficence, justice, and respect for persons.
4. This statement indicates a requirement of an IRB that determines whether research proposals are adhering to ethical standards for research.

TEST-TAKING TIP: The clue in the stem is the phrase "protection of human subjects of biomedical and behavioral research." Implicit in these words are rights of subjects that must be addressed. Note also that the Belmont Report is a document that guides the conduct of research.

Content Area: *Regulatory Aspects of Ethical Research;* ***Cognitive Level:*** *Knowledge;* ***Question Type:*** *Multiple Choice*

CRITICAL THINKING FACILITATOR: Think of other documents used in guiding ethical research. Professional organizations such as the American Nurses Association, American Medical Association, American Psychological Association, and others also have guidelines for researchers to consult in the design and conduct of research.

4. **1. This federal regulation directly addresses the protection of human subjects in research.**
2. This federal regulation directly addresses the protection of human subjects in research.
3. This federal regulation directly addresses the protection of human subjects in research.
4. This regulation is *indirectly* involved in the protection of human subjects. It created the National Commission for the Protection of Human Subjects for Biomedical and Behavioral Research.
5. This is not a federal regulation.

TEST-TAKING TIP: Key words in the question stem are "federal regulations." Explicitly, federal regulations are laws enacted by the government. Note also that the words "directly address" delineate

other regulatory aspects of human subject protection.

Content Area: *Regulatory Aspects of Ethical Research;* ***Cognitive Level:*** *Analysis;* ***Question Type:*** *Multiple Response*

CRITICAL THINKING FACILITATOR: Nursing is a scientific discipline. Therefore, research is an essential component of professional practice. Know the federal laws that govern nursing practice. Many of these address the design and conduct of research.

5. **1. This is the correct option. Beneficence is a principle of ethical research that "encourages the researcher to do good and above all do no harm" (Burns & Grove, 2011, p. 533).**
2. This action by researchers addresses protecting the right to self-determination.
3. This action by researchers addresses justice.
4. This action by researchers addresses respect for persons and their privacy.

TEST-TAKING TIP: Associate the uncommon word "beneficence" with the common, related word "beneficial," which can mean helpful. To demonstrate beneficence, one does something good and avoids hurting another.

Content Area: *Regulatory Aspects of Ethical Research;* ***Cognitive Level:*** *Application;* ***Question Type:*** *Multiple Choice*

CRITICAL THINKING FACILITATOR: Think of a research study that you are familiar with and identify its beneficial outcomes. What did the researcher do to adhere to the principle of beneficence?

6. 1. This is explicit in the principle of beneficence.
2. This is inherent in the principle of justice.
3. This is the correct option. Respect for human dignity includes the right to full disclosure. "Full disclosure means that the researcher has fully described the nature of the study, the person's right to refuse participation, the researcher's responsibilities, and the likely risks and benefits" (Polit & Beck, 2014, p. 84).
4. This is included as the right to privacy under the principle of justice.

TEST-TAKING TIP: The key word in the question stem is "respect." This term means that persons who are potential research subjects are entitled to be told what to expect. The principle puts the responsibility on the researchers, who must do everything to make sure research participants are kept fully informed and are able to maintain their autonomy and rights as human beings.

Content Area: *Regulatory Aspects of Ethical Research;* ***Cognitive Level:*** *Analysis;* ***Question Type:*** *Multiple Choice*

CRITICAL THINKING FACILITATOR: Think of a research study you are familiar with and determine whether the principle of respect for human dignity was considered in the conduct of the study. How did the researchers protect this right? Cite evidence from the study that this principle was upheld.

7. 1. This statement addresses the right to self-determination that is included under the principle of respect for human dignity.
2. This statement relates to the protocols of data collection.
3. This is the correct option. The identities of individual research participants are protected in several ways. One way is to report only group data and not individual data. Readers of the research report are not able to link data to any individual.
4. This statement reflects part of the responsibilities of researchers to protect the right to full disclosure.

TEST-TAKING TIP: Anonymity means that research data cannot be linked to any individual research participant. This protects the individual's right to privacy.

Content Area: *Rights of Research Participants;* ***Cognitive Level:*** *Analysis;* ***Question Type:*** *Multiple Choice*

CRITICAL THINKING FACILITATOR: What are other approaches to protect the anonymity of research participants? Look at any study and identify what strategies were used by the researchers to protect anonymity.

8. 1. This is a strategy to protect the anonymity of research participants. Disclosing the specific location of a research study jeopardizes privacy of research participants.
2. This is the correct option. "A promise of confidentiality is a pledge that any information participants provide will not be publicly reported in a manner that identifies them and will not be made accessible to others" (Polit & Beck, 2014, p. 89). Only authorized research personnel have access to the data.
3. This is another strategy to protect anonymity guaranteeing the right to privacy.
4. This pertains to the right to full disclosure.

TEST-TAKING TIP: Associate the word "confidentiality" with some common related words. Think about the statement "Someone confided in me." This means the information shared is not disclosed to anyone else. The dictionary lists "secret" as the meaning of "confidential."

Content Area: *Rights of Research Participants;* ***Cognitive Level:*** *Analysis;* ***Question Type:*** *Multiple Choice*

CRITICAL THINKING FACILITATOR: Look at any study. Is there any indication that confidentiality was not maintained? Who had access to the data?

9. 1. The right to confidentiality means that the researcher has a pledge to allow only duly authorized personnel access to study data.
2. The right to anonymity means that the researcher will protect individual identity and prevent linking of data with participants.
3. This is the correct option. The right to self-determination means that "prospective participants have the right to decide voluntarily whether to participate in a study, without risking penalty or prejudicial treatment" (Polit & Beck, 2010, p. 123).
4. The right to full disclosure means that participants have full knowledge of the study and its possible risks and benefits.

TEST-TAKING TIP: In the situation given, the patient is in a healthcare institution. This patient has a certain degree of vulnerability because she is dependent on others for her care. The patient worries that if she does not participate in the study, her care may suffer. The patient's vulnerability and her fear of retaliation are two reasons her right to self-determination might be compromised.

Content Area: *Rights of Research Participants;* ***Cognitive Level:*** *Analysis;* ***Question Type:*** *Multiple Choice*

CRITICAL THINKING FACILITATOR: Read over the methods section of any study. How were research participants recruited for participation? What procedures were instituted to protect their right to self-determination?

10. 1. This is not the right that was violated. The right to confidentiality means that participants' privacy will be protected by the researcher's pledge that only duly authorized research personnel will have access to the data.
2. This is not the right that was violated. The right to anonymity means that participants' privacy will be protected by not revealing participants' identities and preventing the linking of data to participants.
3. This is the correct option. The right to full disclosure was violated because some of the participants did not know the nature of the study nor the risks involved.
4. This right was violated during the Tuskegee Syphilis Study as well when some subjects did not receive the known treatment for syphilis. These subjects went untreated. However, this question is about informed consent and the right to full disclosure.

TEST-TAKING TIP: Key words in the question stem are "not informed." This means that research participants did not receive adequate information to make an informed decision to participate or not participate.

Content Area: *Rights of Research Participants;* ***Cognitive Level:*** *Application;* ***Question Type:*** *Multiple Choice*

CRITICAL THINKING FACILITATOR: Why might a researcher not obtain informed consent? What if the researcher expects to have difficulty in recruiting subjects if they are fully informed of the nature of the study? Does this provide a rationale for not gaining informed consent? Read over the methods section of any research study. How was the right to full disclosure ensured? What information was shared with potential participants before they signed the consent?

11. 1. This is a requirement to protect the right to self-determination.
2. This is the correct option. "The return of a completed questionnaire reflects the respondent's voluntary consent to participate" (Burns & Grove, 2010, p. 127).
3. This is called process consent.
4. This is part of the requirement to protect the right to full disclosure.

TEST-TAKING TIP: The key term in the question stem is "implied consent." The word "implied" means understood or indirectly stated. A questionnaire would have directions for completing and returning it. If someone did not wish to participate in a study, would he or she complete and mail in a questionnaire?

Content Area: *Rights of Research Participants;* ***Cognitive Level:*** *Comprehension;* ***Question Type:*** *Multiple Choice*

CRITICAL THINKING FACILITATOR: Think of situations when implied consent is applicable. For example, when you are feeling sick and you see your primary care physician, are you giving implied consent to treatment by virtue of your presence in her/his office?

12. 1. This approach protects the right to self-determination, and it is only one of the rights of research participants.
2. This approach is part of the methodology section on sample selection; it contains

more specific requirements that address the validity of a study.

3. **This is the correct option. This is a major strategy to protect research participants. Researchers need to conduct this process to determine "whether the benefits of participating in a study are in line with the costs be they financial, physical, emotional or social" (Burns & Grove, 2010, p. 125).**
4. This strategy addresses some ethical aspects of research but also issues in methodology, specifically in data collection or in the implementation of an intervention protocol.

TEST-TAKING TIP: Key words in the question stem are "initial" and "major." Assessment of the risk–benefit ratio will be a deciding factor in the design and conduct of a study.

Content Area: *Protecting the Rights of Research Participants;* ***Cognitive Level:*** *Comprehension;* ***Question Type:*** *Multiple Choice*

CRITICAL THINKING FACILITATOR: Read the background or introductory section(s) of a research article. Try to determine the benefits of participating in the study as well as the potential risks. In your opinion, what were the outcomes of the risk–benefit assessment done by the researchers? Also what safeguards were used to reduce risks of the participants?

13.
1. This is a positive outcome of the study and provides a rationale for conducting it (potential contribution to the knowledge base of the profession).
2. This is avoided in any research study because there are potential violations of human rights. No study should be conducted if the risks outweigh the benefits.
3. **This is the correct option. Minimal risk is defined as the "research subject's risk of harm anticipated in the proposed study that is not greater, considering probability and magnitude, than that ordinarily encountered in daily life or during performance of routine physical or psychological examination"(Burns & Grove, 2011, p. 542).**
4. This is not the definition of minimal risk.

TEST-TAKING TIP: The key word in the question stem is "minimal," which means the smallest. Climbing two flights of stairs is also an activity that most people do regularly.

Content Area: *Protecting the Rights of Research Participants;* ***Cognitive Level:*** *Knowledge;* ***Question Type:*** *Multiple Choice*

CRITICAL THINKING FACILITATOR: Think of other research activities that would entail minimal risk. Why do these entail only minimal risks? What safeguards are in place to ensure that there are only minimal risks for the research participants?

14.
1. HIPAA covers confidentiality and the anonymity of personal health information.
2. **This is the correct option. Informed consent "is an agreement by a prospective subject to participate voluntarily in a study after he or she has assimilated essential information about the study" (Burns & Grove, 2011, p. 540).**
3. This is not relevant to the question.
4. This is part of the research data that must be protected.

TEST-TAKING TIP: A key word is "self-determination." This relates to the person making decisions as an autonomous individual. Option 2 includes the word "consent," which means to agree.

Content Area: *Protecting the Rights of Research Participants;* ***Cognitive Level:*** *Knowledge;* ***Question Type:*** *Multiple Choice*

CRITICAL THINKING FACILITATOR: Think of other situations when a person has to make a decision. What processes are in place before a decision is made? After the decision is voluntarily made, what makes the decision official and legal? For example, people sign informed consents for surgery or major diagnostic tests just as they do to participate in a research study.

15.
1. This is not a function of an IRB but of the funding organization that requires studies to have IRB approval.
2. **This describes the functions of an IRB.**
3. **This describes the functions of an IRB.**
4. **This describes the functions of an IRB.**
5. **This describes the functions of an IRB.**

TEST-TAKING TIP: IRBs are primarily concerned with the ethical aspects of research. Therefore, all statements that have any relationship with ethics and protection of human rights are part of the functions of an IRB.

Content Area: *Protecting the Rights of Research Participants;* ***Cognitive Level:*** *Knowledge;* ***Question Type:*** *Multiple Response*

CRITICAL THINKING FACILITATOR: Inquire how research studies are reviewed in your clinical experience setting. How about your academic institution? Faculty, administration, and even students are involved in some type of research. Ask your nursing faculty if they are doing research. Find out about the review process necessary before a study involving human subjects can begin.

16. 1. This is the requirement for persons deemed to be incapable or incompetent to give consent.
2. This is the correct option. The statement describes assent.
3. This statement describes an element of recruiting participants according to ethical guidelines.
4. This statement might be considered a process used in providing necessary information to research participants.

TEST-TAKING TIP: The word "assent" means to agree. "By age 7, children can think in terms of concrete operations and can provide meaningful assent to participation as research subjects" (Burns & Grove, 2011, p. 112). Only option 2 is related to children as research subjects.

Content Area: *Protecting the Rights of Research Subjects;* ***Cognitive Level:*** *Knowledge* ***Question Type:*** *Multiple Choice*
CRITICAL THINKING FACILITATOR: Discuss with your classmates and instructors the ethical considerations of using children as research subjects. When do you think such use is appropriate? When is it inappropriate or unethical? Now investigate your institution's guidelines for the use of children as research subjects. How do these guidelines compare with the ideas generated in your discussion?

17. **1. This is an element of informed consent.**
2. This is an element of informed consent.
3. This is an element of informed consent.
4. This is an element of informed consent.
5. Potential research subjects have no obligation to complete the study. In fact, the right to self-determination guarantees that subjects may withdraw from the study without penalty.
6. Research subjects do not have to disclose all personal information. The information shared by research subjects is protected, and their right to privacy is safeguarded throughout the study and through the dissemination of study data.

TEST-TAKING TIP: An informed consent for research participation or for invasive procedures such as surgery and diagnostic tests brings with it the obligation to share essential information with the person involved. The information, after it is understood by the person, serves as a guide for making the decision.

Content Area: *Protecting the Rights of Research Participants;* ***Cognitive Level:*** *Comprehension;* ***Question Type:*** *Multiple Response*
CRITICAL THINKING FACILITATOR: Read a study's methods section and determine what processes were followed before informed consent was obtained. The description of the process of obtaining informed consent might be abbreviated in a published report. Look at a sample informed consent in any research textbook, and you will see the elements included in it.

18. 1. The researcher could easily maintain the subjects' anonymity. The right to anonymity means that research participants' identities will not be linked with their data.
2. This is the correct option. The right to self-determination means that potential research participants have the autonomy to consent to participate and to withdraw without penalty. The researcher did not seek the consent of the individuals she observed in her "study," and this is a clear violation of their rights. Hence, the behavior of the researcher is unethical.
3. The researcher could easily maintain confidentiality. The right to confidentiality means that participants' research data are protected, and only duly authorized personnel have access to them.
4. As long as anonymity and confidentiality apply, there is unlikely to be harm in this case. Right to freedom from harm means that participants must not be subjected to unnecessary risks and discomfort.

TEST-TAKING TIP: The situation described in the question is known as covert data collection, which means that data were collected without the subjects' awareness or knowledge. Informed consent was not obtained, and therefore subjects had no opportunity to make decisions about participation or nonparticipation.

Content Area: *Protecting the Rights of Research Participants;* ***Cognitive Level:*** *Analysis;* ***Question Type:*** *Multiple Choice*
CRITICAL THINKING FACILITATOR: Think of other situations when the right to self-determination might be violated. In some studies in which observation is the method of data collection, would the observed data be authentic if the subject knew of the observation? What would be an acceptable compromise for a study that follows ethical guidelines and at the same time generates authentic data?

19. 1. The right to self-determination means that persons are autonomous and can make their own decisions to participate or to refuse and withdraw at any time without penalty.
2. This is the correct option. When individual identities are protected and data cannot be linked to individual participants, the right to anonymity has been maintained.
3. Confidentiality means that data will not be publicly shared and that only duly authorized persons will have access.
4. This choice pertains to justice, which includes the right to fair treatment and the right to privacy.

TEST-TAKING TIP: The clause "individual identities are protected" pertains to anonymity—the status of being unknown.

Content Area: *Protecting the Rights of Research Participants;* ***Cognitive Level;*** *Comprehension:* ***Question Type:*** *Multiple Choice*

CRITICAL THINKING FACILITATOR: What are other strategies to protect the identity of research participants? How do published reports prevent disclosure of subjects' identities?

20. 1. Self-determination means that potential research subjects have the autonomy to decide whether or not to participate. This right can also be exercised when a research participant withdraws without penalty from a study.
2. Anonymity and confidentiality are relevant under the right to privacy.
3. This is the correct option. Freedom from harm and discomfort is covered under the principle of beneficence. "Harm and discomfort can take many forms; they can be physical (e.g., physical injury); emotional (stress); social (e.g., loss of social support); or financial (e.g., loss of wages)" (Polit & Beck, 2014, p. 83).
4. Fair treatment means that the researcher "must treat people who decline to participate in a study or who withdraw from it in a non-prejudicial manner" (Polit & Beck, 2010, p. 124).

TEST-TAKING TIP: Key words in the question stem include "extremely emotional." Reflect on a painful personal experience that you or someone else had. Does thinking about such an experience still hurt?

Content Area: *Protecting the Rights of Research Participants;* ***Cognitive Level:*** *Analysis;* ***Question Type:*** *Multiple Choice*

CRITICAL THINKING FACILITATOR: Look at the methods sections of several studies. If the study had an intervention, how was this implemented? Was there any possibility of harm to the participants? How was potential harm minimized or prevented?

21. 1. Freedom from harm means that the researcher takes measures to avoid, prevent, or minimize harm or discomfort. It is included under the principle of beneficence.
2. This is the correct option. A nurse educator is in a position to evaluate students. Therefore, students have some degree of vulnerability, and their ability to exercise autonomy is compromised. This pertains to the right to self-determination.
3. This question is not about fair treatment. Fair treatment means the researcher is nonprejudicial in the way someone is treated.
4. This question is not about informed consent. Getting informed consent is the ethical process before conducting a study. Informed consent is not a right but rather the evidence that the rights of participants have been protected and upheld.

TEST-TAKING TIP: A key phrase in the question stem is "jeopardize their grades." If the students believe that this is a compelling reason to participate in the study, then they are not fully exercising their right to self-determination. Fear of penalty or repercussions should not be reasons for participating in a study.

Content Area: *Protecting the Rights of Research Participants;* ***Cognitive Level:*** *Analysis;* ***Question Type:*** *Multiple Choice*

CRITICAL THINKING FACILITATOR: Obtaining informed consent means that researchers have considered how the rights of research participants could be protected and upheld. Consider why potential participants consent to participate. Are the potential benefits to a larger group a reason? Are potential participants thinking that their participation would make a significant contribution to the science of the profession?

22. 1. This individual is not considered vulnerable and can exercise full autonomy.
2. This individual is not considered vulnerable and can exercise full autonomy.
3. A prison inmate is in an institution and is not fully autonomous.
4. This individual is not considered vulnerable and can exercise full autonomy.
5. This man is also in an institution and is dependent on others for care.

TEST-TAKING TIP: The key word in the stem is "vulnerable." "Vulnerable subjects are special groups of people whose rights in studies need special protection because of their inability to provide meaningful informed consent or because their circumstances place them at higher-than-average-risk of adverse effects" (e.g., children, unconscious patients) (Polit & Beck, 2014, p. 394).

***Content Area:** Research with Vulnerable Groups; **Cognitive Level:** Analysis; **Question Type:** Multiple Response*

CRITICAL THINKING FACILITATOR: Relative to research, identify persons who belong to vulnerable groups. Provide a reason for their vulnerability.

23. **1. This is inevitable in qualitative research. Because the data in qualitative studies are descriptive and subjective, there is unpredictability. The researchers usually conduct personal interviews and become immersed in the data and their analysis. These are parts of the qualitative process. The sample is usually small because narrative, descriptive data are not statistically analyzed. Guidelines for a valid quantitative study, such as adequate or large samples, are not applicable in qualitative studies.**
    2. This is inevitable in qualitative research.
    3. This is true of quantitative studies.
    4. This is true of quantitative studies.
    5. This is inevitable in qualitative research.

TEST-TAKING TIP: Know that qualitative research is "the investigation of phenomena, typically in an in-depth and holistic fashion, through the collection of rich narrative materials using a flexible research design" (Polit & Beck, 2014, p. 389).

***Content Area:** Ethics in Qualitative Research; **Cognitive Level:** Comprehension; **Question Type:** Multiple Response*

CRITICAL THINKING FACILITATOR: Review the paradigms for quantitative and qualitative research. The paradigms are polar opposites in all the criteria.

24. 1. Informed consent is the evidence that potential participants have been given essential information to make their decision to participate in a study or not.
    2. Assent is given by children agreeing to participate in research.
    3. Full disclosure means the researchers have fully described the study, the potential risks and benefits, and the responsibilities of the participants.
    4. This is the correct option. Process consent is "an ongoing, transactional process of negotiating consent with participants, allowing them to collaborate in the decision-making about their continued participation" (Polit & Beck, 2014, p. 388).

TEST-TAKING TIP: The correct option contains the term "process," which suggests a continuous action. Also, the clause "as the study progresses" indicates that something can change. The unpredictability of qualitative studies necessitates a consent that is ongoing.

***Content Area:** Ethics in Qualitative Research; **Cognitive Level:** Comprehension; **Question Type:** Multiple Choice*

CRITICAL THINKING FACILITATOR: Take a look at a sample qualitative study in your core textbook. How was consent obtained? During the study, what did the researchers do to safeguard the participants' right to self-determination?

4 Exploring the Role of Quantitative Research in Evidence-Based Practice

KEY WORDS

The following words include English vocabulary, nursing/medical terminology, concepts, principles, or information relevant to content specifically addressed in the chapter or associated with topics presented in it. English dictionaries, your nursing textbooks, and medical dictionaries such as *Taber's Cyclopedic Medical Dictionary* are resources that can be used to expand your knowledge and understanding of these words and related information.

Assumption
Bias
Control
Critique
Disseminate
Extraneous variable
Generalizability
Inference
Paradigm
Random
Research design
Validity

QUESTIONS

The Positivist Paradigm

1. Which of the following assumptions is consistent with the positivist paradigm for research?
   1. Reality is something that is constructed by multiple individuals.
   2. Research focuses on the meaning of the participant's experiences.
   3. Research findings results from researcher–participant interactions.
   4. Values and biases are to be held in check; objectivity is desired.

2. Within the context of the positivist paradigm, a researcher doing a quantitative study must maintain a(n) ______________, ______________ position.

3. Data collected in quantitative studies are analyzed using ______________ methods.

4. In a quantitative study, ______________ reasoning guides the researcher.

5. Assumptions for doing research within the context of the positivist paradigm include which of the following? **Select all that apply.**
   1. There is a focus on the objective and quantifiable.
   2. The design is fixed from the beginning of the study.
   3. The researcher interacts with those being researched.
   4. The researcher seeks to understand the human experience.
   5. The study seeks to test a hypothesis.

Introduction to Quantitative Research

6. Which of the following hypothetical research questions can be answered by doing a quantitative study?
1. What are the effects of a structured tutoring program on the academic success of disadvantaged students in a BSN program?
2. What is the lived experience of young children orphaned by parents who have died from HIV/AIDS?
3. What are the experiences of young women who have undergone female genital mutilation?
4. How do young children integrate into a step family?

7. How does quantitative research influence evidence-based practice? **Select all that apply.**
1. Findings of quantitative research can be used to develop clinical protocols.
2. Quantitative research summaries can be part of systematic reviews.
3. Findings of a single quantitative study can provide the basis for evidence-based protocols.
4. Findings from a "single original study is the most basic form of research evidence" (Brown, 2014, p. 15).
5. No additional research is needed after a clinical protocol is in place.

8. What are the different levels of evidence that include quantitative studies in evidence-based practice? **Select all that apply.**
1. Review of the literature
2. Meta-analysis
3. Meta-synthesis
4. Critical appraisal
5. Systematic review

9. What are some examples of quantitative research designs? **Select all that apply.**
1. Quasi-experimental
2. Correlation
3. Ethnographic
4. Grounded theory
5. Experimental

Evaluation and Dissemination

10. What are the main ways of disseminating findings from quantitative studies to the professional community? **Select all that apply.**
1. Peer-reviewed journal articles
2. Research presentations in conferences or conventions
3. Faculty lectures in academic settings
4. Poster sessions in conferences or conventions
5. Journal clubs in practice settings

11. When quantitative studies are published in professional journals, ________________ format is used to organize and present the information.

12. How do nursing students as research consumers evaluate research studies? They
1. ask the opinions of authority figures.
2. do an appraisal called a critique.
3. use the problem-solving approach.
4. depend on the reputation of the publisher.

Concepts and Processes in Quantitative Research

13. A researcher wants to find out whether there is accessible and adequate parking in a small commuter college. Which of the following research activities would reduce bias in this study? The researcher will
1. survey the first 100 people who pass through the main gate of the college before 7:00 AM.
2. ask two persons from each department to answer the questionnaire.
3. select at random members of the college community to respond.
4. survey those who come to campus only 2 days a week.

14. ________________ is a "process of preventing those involved in a study (participants, intervention agents, or data collectors) from having information that could lead to a bias, e.g., knowledge of which treatment group a participant is in" (Polit & Beck, 2014, p. 375).

15. How are controls imposed in quantitative studies? **Select all that apply.**
1. The researchers design the intervention protocols very carefully.
2. Research assistants undergo training and are monitored by the researchers.
3. There is at least one group of participants who serve as a control group.
4. The researchers interact intensively with the research participants.
5. Research participants must all sign the informed consent.

16. A researcher wants to determine the relationship between teaching approach and skill competency among sophomore nursing students. If there is no control for students' previous experience with the skill, there will be a(n) ____________________ variable in this study.

17. ______________________ is "a quality criterion referring to the degree to which inferences made in a study are accurate and well-founded" (Polit & Beck 2014, p. 394).

18. "The degree to which the research methods justify the inference that the findings are true for a broader group than study participants" (Polit & Beck, 2014, p. 381) is called ________________.

ANSWERS AND RATIONALES

The correct answer number and rationale for why it is the correct answer are given in **boldface blue type.** Rationales for why the other possible answer options are incorrect also are given, but they are not in boldface type.

1. 1. The statement is not consistent with the positivist paradigm. One assumption of the paradigm is that reality already exists (Polit & Beck, 2014).
   2. The statement is not consistent with the positivist paradigm. The meaning of participants' experiences is consistent with the constructivist paradigm.
   3. Researcher–participant interactions are part of the findings in qualitative studies that support the beliefs of the constructivist paradigm.
   4. **This statement is consistent with the beliefs of the positivist paradigm. There is an emphasis on "controls over context" (Polit & Beck, 2014, p. 7). The researcher has to maintain a neutral position in relation to research subjects to maintain objectivity.**

   TEST-TAKING TIP: The key word in the question stem is "positivist," derived from "positivism," which emphasizes the rational and scientific. To the positivists, "phenomena are not haphazard, but rather have antecedent causes" (Polit & Beck, 2014, p. 7).

   Content Area: *The Positivist Paradigm;* ***Cognitive Level:*** *Analysis;* ***Question Type:*** *Multiple Choice*
   CRITICAL THINKING FACILITATOR: Think of beliefs of the positivist paradigm and how these beliefs are consistent with quantitative research. What are some of the processes that guide quantitative research?

2. **independent, objective**

   TEST-TAKING TIP: The key words in the stem are "positivist" and "quantitative." By staying independent, the researcher imposes control as a measure to reduce bias.

   Researcher–participant interactions might produce bias and influence the objectivity of the researcher. Because positivists value objectivity, they "use orderly, disciplined procedures with tight controls over the research situation to test hunches about the nature of phenomena being studied and the relationships among them" (Polit & Beck, 2014, p. 7).

   Content Area: *The Positivist Paradigm;* ***Cognitive Level:*** *Comprehension;* ***Question Type:*** *Fill-in-the-Blank*
   CRITICAL THINKING FACILITATOR: Where would measures to control extraneous variables be initially imposed? Would they start with the people involved such as the researchers and participants?

3. **statistical**

   TEST-TAKING TIP: A key word in the question stem is "quantitative," which means capable of being measured. Think of the word "quantity," which means number. In research, numbers are analyzed using statistical methods.

   Content Area: *The Positivist Paradigm;* ***Cognitive Level:*** *Knowledge;* ***Question Type:*** *Fill-in-the-Blank*
   CRITICAL THINKING FACILITATOR: Look at the results section of a sample quantitative study. How were data analyzed? Were descriptive or inferential statistics used?

4. **deductive**

   TEST-TAKING TIP: A key word in the stem is "quantitative." Because quantitative researchers value the beliefs of the positivist paradigm, they seek generalizations about phenomena. Therefore, they start with general premises and move to specific ones. This approach is consistent with deductive reasoning.

   Content Area: *The Positivist Paradigm;* ***Cognitive Level:*** *Knowledge;* ***Question Type:*** *Fill-in-the-Blank*
   CRITICAL THINKING FACILITATOR: Review the concepts of deductive and inductive reasoning in your textbook. Think of an everyday situation in which you might use a deductive approach.

5. 1. **The statement is consistent with obtaining best evidence within the context of the positivist paradigm.**
   2. **The statement is consistent with obtaining best evidence within the context of the positivist paradigm.**
   3. The statement is not consistent with the assumptions of the positivist paradigm. The researcher maintains an independent, objective position in relation to the research participants.
   4. The statement is not consistent with the assumptions of the positivist paradigm. Understanding of the human experience is possible only with intense dialogue with participants who share descriptions of their experiences (qualitative data) with the researcher. On the other hand, the quantitative researcher collects numeric data that are then subjected to statistical analysis.

5. The statement is consistent with obtaining best evidence within the context of the positivist paradigm. Quantitative researchers test relationships between and/or among variables (hypothesis).

TEST-TAKING TIP: A key word in the question stem is "assumptions." An assumption is a "principle that is accepted as being true based on logic or reason, without proof" (Polit & Beck, 2014, p. 374).

Content Area: *The Positivist Paradigm;* ***Cognitive Level:*** *Analysis;* ***Question Type:*** *Multiple Response*

CRITICAL THINKING FACILITATOR: Positivists believe in objective reality. Therefore, the conduct of quantitative research is influenced by their assumptions about what would be the "best methods for obtaining evidence" (Polit & Beck, 2014, p. 7).

6. 1. This statement is a research question for quantitative research. There are two variables, namely, a structured tutoring program (the independent variable) and academic success (the dependent variable). There are no variables in qualitative research.
2. This question can be best addressed using a qualitative approach because it is asking for the lived experiences of the participants. The data shared by participants will be narrative descriptions, not numeric data.
3. This question can be best addressed using a qualitative approach because the researcher is interested in the experiences of the participants. Participants will share their experiences through narrative descriptions.
4. This question can be best addressed using a qualitative approach. Children will share their experiences with the researcher, who will then analyze the descriptive data to answer the research question.

TEST-TAKING TIP: "Quantitative study" is the key term in the question stem. A quantitative study has variables, and the researcher determines the relationship between or among these variables. In contrast, a qualitative study looks at the participants' experiences and seeks to give these meaning (Burns & Grove, 2011). The experiences and their meaning are realities constructed by the researchers along with the participants. This statement is consistent within the context of the constructivist paradigm for research.

Content Area: *Introduction to Quantitative Research;* ***Cognitive Level:*** *Analysis;* ***Question Type:*** *Multiple Choice*

CRITICAL THINKING FACILITATOR: Look at a sample study and see how each research question is presented. Contrast the questions asked in quantitative studies with those asked in qualitative studies.

7. 1. Research findings, after several transformations, "become the basis for clinical protocols that guide clinicians' decisions and actions" (Brown, 2014, p. 5). "Clinical protocols are standards of care in that they define care that should be given to patients who are part of a defined population" (p. 6).
2. Systematic reviews include summaries of quantitative studies. A systematic review is a "research summary that produces conclusions by bringing together and integrating the findings from all available original studies" (Brown, 2014, p. 20).
3. Systematic reviews are not based on one sole quantitative study. All available findings from quantitative studies on a specific healthcare topic are included to "determine the best research evidence available for expert clinicians to use to promote evidence-based practice" (Burns & Grove, 2011, p. 550).
4. Basic building blocks for evidence-based practice are findings from a single study. Findings must be examined separately because each finding might have different levels of support by the study (Brown, 2014).
5. The statement is erroneous. "Agencies develop protocols to promote effective clinical management and to reduce variability in the care of their high-volume and high-risk patient groups" (Brown, 2014, p. 7). Not every protocol works best for every patient. Nurses should evaluate whether there are good outcomes for protocols. Change is imperative when a protocol is not effective.

TEST-TAKING TIP: The key term in the question stem is "evidence-based practice," which means "practice that involves making clinical decisions on the best evidence available, with an emphasis on evidence from disciplined research" (Polit & Beck, 2014, p. 380). Those options that indicate use of findings to form the basis for making decisions in the development of clinical protocols and systematic reviews are all influenced by quantitative research.

Content Area: *Introduction to Quantitative Research;* ***Cognitive Level:*** *Analysis;* ***Question Type:*** *Multiple Response*

CRITICAL THINKING FACILITATOR: Review the hierarchy of research evidence. You will find that quantitative research can be found at almost every level. Look at some examples of research studies you have encountered and determine where they would fit in the hierarchy.

8. 1. A review of the literature is a step in a study. It is not considered a part of the level of evidence.
   2. A meta-analysis is a level in the hierarchy of evidence. It is a "technique for quantitatively integrating the results of multiple studies addressing the same or highly similar research question" (Polit & Beck, 2014, p. 384).
   3. Metasynthesis consists of "grand narratives or interpretive translations produced from the integration or comparison of findings from qualitative studies" (p. 384).
   4. A critical appraisal or critique is an objective assessment of a study's strengths and limitations. This is not considered a level in the hierarchy of evidence.
   5. A systematic review is "a rigorous synthesis of research findings on a particular research question, using systematic sampling and data collection procedures and a formal protocol" (p. 393).

TEST-TAKING TIP: The key words in the question stem are "level of evidence." The word "evidence" means proof. Because quantitative research tests hypotheses, the findings from these studies serve as "proof" for the existence of a relationship between and/or among variables.

Content Area: *Introduction to Quantitative Research;* ***Cognitive Level:*** *Comprehension;* ***Question Type:*** *Multiple Response*

CRITICAL THINKING FACILITATOR:
Search the literature for research studies that are meta-analyses and systematic reviews. Why do you think these studies are essential in establishing evidence?

9. **1. A quasi-experimental study is a "type of quantitative research conducted to explain relationships, clarify why certain events happen, and examine causality between selected independent and dependent variables" (Burns & Grove, 2011, p. 545).**
   2. A correlational study "is a systematic investigation of relationships between two or more variables to explain the nature of relationships in the world; does not examine causality" (p. 535).
   3. An ethnographic study is a type of qualitative research that investigates cultures. "The research involves collection, description, and analysis of data to develop a theory of cultural behavior" (p. 537).
   4. The researcher who does a grounded theory study seeks to "understand the interaction between self and the group from the perspectives of those involved" (p. 78).
   5. An experimental study is "an objective, systematic, controlled investigation to examine probability and causality among selected variables for the purpose of predicting and controlling phenomena" (p. 537).

TEST-TAKING TIP: A key word in the question stem is "quantitative," which means relating to numerical data. Identify those answer choices where numerical data are gathered. Eliminate answer choices in which researchers were interested in people's descriptions of their experiences (i.e., that yield narrative data).

Content Area: *Introduction to Quantitative Research;* ***Cognitive Level:*** *Comprehension;* ***Question Type:*** *Multiple Choice.*

CRITICAL THINKING FACILITATOR:
Look at a sample study and try to determine the researcher's purpose for the study. If the researcher is seeking to find a relationship between and among variables and is testing hypotheses, then the design is quantitative.

10. **1. Quantitative studies and other types of studies are published in journals, specifically research journals, that have a high probability of reaching professionals interested in research.**
    2. Research presentations are also major ways of disseminating research to the professional community. Professionals interested in research attend these conferences and conventions.
    3. Faculty lectures in academic settings are not main ways of disseminating research to the professional community. Information might be shared by faculty as part of the regular course content. Of course, faculty teaching research courses are more likely to give out more research information compared to others.
    4. Poster sessions are another major way of disseminating findings from quantitative studies and other types of studies. Poster sessions in conferences and conventions provide a more extensive way to disseminate information because of open and easy access to presenters/researchers. Attendees have opportunities to dialogue with researchers and obtain specific information about the studies. There is also the opportunity for continuing contact

with researchers who are extremely receptive to conference participants.

5. Journal clubs in practice settings are not major ways of disseminating findings. Journal clubs might focus on a wide range of topics, not just research. Also, not all staff members are able to attend these on a regular basis.

TEST-TAKING TIP: A key word in the question stem is "main," meaning chief or leading. In the dissemination of research findings, main ways are those that would reach the largest number of professionals.

Content Area: *Evaluation and Dissemination;* ***Cognitive Level:*** *Comprehension;* ***Question Type:*** *Multiple Response*

CRITICAL THINKING FACILITATOR: Think of ways information is disseminated. Large gatherings such as conferences and conventions ensure that many people gain access to research findings. Publications, print or online, are also major ways of sharing information. In your institution, how is information disseminated to larger numbers of persons?

11. **IMRAD (Introduction, Method, Results, Analysis, and Discussion)**

TEST-TAKING TIP: Look at the abstract of a published study, and you can see that the main headings are formatted as IMRAD.

Content Area: *Evaluation and Dissemination;* ***Cognitive Level:*** *Knowledge;* ***Question Type:*** *Fill-in-the-Blank*

CRITICAL THINKING FACILITATOR: Think of how information is organized to facilitate understanding. You are familiar with a nursing care plan. How does a nurse present the information so that it is easily understood?

12. 1. The opinions of experts do not allow the research consumer to evaluate a research study.
    2. **"A research critique is an objective assessment of a study's strengths and limitations. Critiques usually conclude with the reviewer's summary of the study's merits, recommendations regarding the value of the evidence, and suggestions about improving the study or the report" (Polit & Beck, 2014, p. 67). By doing a critique, nursing students strengthen their ability to think critically and apply learned research skills (Polit & Beck, 2014).**
    3. Some of the steps in the problem-solving approach might be used in doing the critique. However, a critique goes through the steps of "comprehension, comparison, analysis, and evaluation" (Burns & Grove, 2011, p. 535).
    4. Reliance on the reputation of the publisher of the report does not constitute a critical appraisal of a research study.

TEST-TAKING TIP: A key word in the question stem is "evaluation." To evaluate means to find the worth or value of something, to conduct an appraisal. The term "appraisal" appears in option 2.

Content Area: *Evaluation and Dissemination;* ***Cognitive Level:*** *Analysis;* ***Question Type:*** *Multiple Choice*

CRITICAL THINKING FACILITATOR: Look at the guidelines for doing a critique in your textbook. The guidelines consist of criteria for evaluating the worth of the study. Writing a research critique could be compared to the process of writing a movie review. A critique of a study looks at strengths and weaknesses of a study, rather than a movie, and makes an evaluation of its research value, rather than its entertainment value.

13. 1. Surveying the first 100 people will produce, not reduce, bias. Those 100 people might have "something" that the other people do not have, "something" that might influence the overall results of the study. Selecting people through a nonrandom process produces bias.
    2. Selecting two persons from each department will not reduce bias because the two who are selected might have "something" that the others do not have. Selecting persons by preference rather than using a random process produces bias.
    3. **The random selection process would eliminate bias. Randomness is "an important concept in quantitative research involving having certain features of the study established by chance rather than by design or personal preference" (Polit & Beck, 2014, p. 390).**
    4. Personal preference was used in selecting the study participants. This nonrandom process produces bias.

TEST-TAKING TIP: The key word in the question stem is "bias." A bias is "an influence or action in a study that distorts the findings or slants them away from the true or expected" (Burns & Grove, 2011, p. 533).

Content Area: *Issues in Quantitative Research;* ***Cognitive Level:*** *Analysis;* ***Question Type:*** *Multiple Choice*

CRITICAL THINKING FACILITATOR: Think of situations in which bias might be a problem. For instance, would you treat all your patients equally and fairly if you were biased? If you were biased, would you evaluate your team members objectively?

14. Blinding or masking

TEST-TAKING TIP: The key word in the question is "preventing," which means to keep from happening. In this case, the blinding process prevents bias when certain information is withheld. Would research assistants treat research subjects differently if they knew information about them?

Content Area: *Issues in Quantitative Research;* ***Cognitive Level:*** *Comprehension;* ***Question Type:*** *Fill-in-the-Blank*

CRITICAL THINKING FACILITATOR: What would be the effects of subjects knowing which group (control or experimental) they were in? Would treatment of subjects in the two groups differ if the research assistant knew who belonged to which group?

15. 1. Intervention protocols are designed carefully to provide consistency and avoid bias.
2. Training and monitoring of research assistants provide consistency and fidelity of research procedures, thus avoiding bias and error.
3. Having a control, or comparison, group is one form of control. The control group does not receive the experimental intervention. If the subjects were selected by a random process (by chance), bias is eliminated. The researcher would attribute the outcome, or the dependent variable, to the intervention, or the independent variable.
4. A researcher's interaction with subjects or participants is not a form of control. In quantitative studies, a researcher's interactions with the participants might produce bias that could then lead to error.
5. Signing an informed consent is a requirement of ethical research and not a form of control.

TEST-TAKING TIP: The key word in the question stem is "control." In research, this means "the imposing of rules by the researcher to decrease the possibility of error and increase the probability that the study's findings are an accurate reflection of reality" (Burns & Grove, 2011, p. 515).

Content Area: *Issues in Quantitative Research;* ***Cognitive Level:*** *Analysis;* ***Question Type:*** *Multiple Response*

CRITICAL THINKING FACILITATOR: Review the assumptions of the positivist paradigm for research. "Positivists prize objectivity. Their approach involves the use of orderly, disciplined procedures with tight controls over the research situation to test hunches about the nature of phenomena being studied and relationships among them" (Polit & Beck, 2014, p. 7). Think of other controls that a researcher might impose on a study to control bias and avoid errors.

16. extraneous

TEST-TAKING TIP: The key words in the question are "no control." No control for students' previous experience could lead to errors and affect the reliability and validity of the study's findings. The prefix *extra-* means outside. So an *extraneous* variable is one that is not part of the study but that "can affect the measurement of the study variables and the relationships among these variables" (Burns & Grove, 2011, p. 538).

Content Area: *Issues in Quantitative Research;* ***Cognitive Level:*** *Comprehension;* ***Question Type:*** *Fill-in-the-Blank*

CRITICAL THINKING FACILITATOR: Your project in a community health course is to come up with a program to increase adherence to their therapeutic regimen by people with diabetes. How would you go about considering all the factors that might influence adherence and nonadherence to the regimen? What measures would you take to address these factors in your planning to ensure some degree of success?

17. Validity

TEST-TAKING TIP: The key word in the statement is "accurate," which means without error, or precise.

Content Area: *Issues in Quantitative Research;* ***Cognitive Level:*** *Comprehension;* ***Question Type:*** *Fill-in-the-Blank*

CRITICAL THINKING FACILITATOR: How would you differentiate validity from reliability? Think of situations where something might be reliable but not valid.

18. generalizability

TEST-TAKING TIP: The key phrase in the statement is "broader group than study participants." This means that study findings have wide application to a larger group, that they can be generalized to a larger population.

Content Area: *Issues in Quantitative Research;* ***Cognitive Level:*** *Comprehension;* ***Question Type:*** *Fill-in-the-Blank*

CRITICAL THINKING FACILITATOR: When are clinicians able to generalize research findings? Why do researchers caution research consumers about generalizing the findings to other populations or situations? In the lay world, when someone indicates you are generalizing (in the negative sense), what does he or she mean?

Getting Familiar with Quantitative Research Studies

5

KEY WORDS

The following words include English vocabulary, nursing/medical terminology, concepts, principles, or information relevant to content specifically addressed in the chapter or associated with topics presented in it. English dictionaries, your nursing textbooks, and medical dictionaries such as *Taber's Cyclopedic Medical Dictionary* are resources that can be used to expand your knowledge and understanding of these words and related information.

Abstract
Concept
Conceptual framework
Data
Dissemination
Generalizability
Hypothesis
Instruments
Operational definition
Population
Primary source
Principal investigator
Research question
Sample
Secondary source
Theoretical definitions
Theoretical framework
Variables
  Dependent variable
  Independent variable

QUESTIONS

Quantitative Research Terminology

1. Which of the following is (are) true about concepts? **Select all that apply.**
Concepts are
1. "the building blocks of a theory" (Fain, 2009, p. 71).
2. "the pieces of information gathered in a study" (Polit & Beck, 2014, p. 45).
3. "an image or symbolic representation of an abstract idea" (LoBiondo-Wood & Haber, 2010, p. 58).
4. "predicted relationships between variables" (Polit & Beck, 2014, p. 382).
5. "a systematic explanation about relationships among phenomena" (p. 393).

2. Hypothetical research information: Majority of the research participants had at least 2 years of college education. What does the information communicate?
1. Interpretation
2. Data
3. Statistics
4. Recommendations

3. Which of the following reflects data in a research report? The researchers
   1. submitted the research proposal to an institutional review board (IRB) of the university.
   2. presented in a table the outcomes from the intervention.
   3. discussed several limitations of the study.
   4. described the recruitment procedures to obtain a sample.

4. Which of the following statements is true regarding a conceptual model or framework? A conceptual model or framework
   1. "is a set of interrelated concepts, definitions, and propositions that presents a systematic view of phenomena for the purpose of explaining and making predictions about those phenomena" (LoBiondo-Wood & Haber, 2010, p. 587).
   2. "has valid and reliable methods of measuring each concept, and its relational statements or propositions have been tested through research and found to be valid" (Burns & Grove, 2011, p. 242).
   3. "is a set of interrelated concepts or abstractions assembled together in a rational scheme by virtue of their relevance to a common theme" (Polit & Beck, 2014, p. 376).
   4. "is a scientific process that validates and refines existing knowledge and generates knowledge that directly and indirectly influences clinical nursing practice (Burns & Grove, 2011, p. 543).

5. Which of the following is an example of an operational definition?
   1. Fetzer (2013) defined a relapsing fever as one characterized by "periods of febrile episodes and periods with acceptable temperature values" (p. 446).
   2. The characteristics of a workplace were measured using the Practice Environment Scale of the Nursing Work Index (Lansiquot et al., 2012).
   3. Aggressive workplace behaviors are those considered to inhibit the creativity and productivity of workers, lower their self-esteem, and negate worker contributions to the overall goal of the enterprise.
   4. Beck (2004) defined traumatic childbirth as "an event occurring during the labor and delivery process that involves actual or threatened serious injury or death to the mother or her infant" (p. 28).

6. Which of the following is a theoretical definition?
   1. "Normal uncomplicated grief is a common, universal reaction characterized by complex emotional, cognitive, social, physical, behavioral, and spiritual responses to loss and death" (Yancey, 2013, p. 709).
   2. Kwok et al. (2012) defined acculturation factors (English proficiency and length of stay in Australia) and cultural beliefs and having a mammogram using the Chinese Breast Screening Beliefs Questionnaire.
   3. Infertile women's psychosocial health problems and their infertility-related beliefs were measured by the Fertility Belief Questionnaire (Naab et al., 2013).
   4. The Practice Environment Scale of the Nursing Work Index measured quality of care delivery in ambulatory oncology settings (Friese & Manojlovich, 2012).

7. Which of the following is a research question?
   1. The researcher wants to determine the incidence of HIV infection among persons age 65 years and older who emigrated from Asia.
   2. What would be the design of a study that wants to look at the relationship between exercise and cardiovascular efficiency?
   3. What is the relationship between the use of storygrams on the skill competency of sophomore-level nursing students in a baccalaureate program?
   4. There is a positive correlation among level of nursing education of practicing nurses and mortality rates in a tertiary care facility.

8. Which of the following is a hypothesis?
1. Commitment will be the independent variable, and weight loss will be the dependent variable in the study that will test the relationship between the two.
2. There is a relationship between a structured exercise program and cardiovascular efficiency of adults age 45 years and older.
3. The purpose of the study is to explore the lived experience of adults with diabetes who have undergone an above-knee amputation.
4. The potential participants were recruited from inner city outpatient clinics located in ethnic enclaves.

9. What is the study population?
1. "It is the entire set of individuals or objects having some common characteristics" (Polit & Beck, 2014, p. 387).
2. "They are the individuals who participate and provide data in a study" (p. 393).
3. "An individual who provides information to researchers about a phenomenon under study" (p. 382).
4. They are the persons who assist the researcher in research-related activities such as the recruitment of subjects and collection of data.

10. Which of the following is (are) true about an independent variable? **Select all that apply.**
1. It is also known as the treatment or experimental variable.
2. It is the variable the researcher is interested in describing, explaining, or predicting.
3. It is the variable that is manipulated by the researcher.
4. It is also known as the response or outcome variable.

11. Read this title of a report: Su, C. P., et al. (2013). A randomized clinical trial of listening to noncommercial music on quality of nocturnal sleep and relaxation indices in patients in medical intensive care unit. What is the independent variable as expressed in the title?
1. Nocturnal sleep and relaxation indices
2. Patients in medical intensive care unit
3. Listening to noncommercial music
4. A randomized clinical trial

12. Read this title of a report: Kaplan, B. (2012). The effects of participation vs. observation of a simulation experience on testing outcomes: Implications for logistical planning for a school of nursing. What is the dependent variable as expressed in the title?
1. Implications for logistical planning
2. Testing outcomes
3. Participation
4. Observation of a simulation experience

13. What part of the study report presents all the main points of the study?
1. Title
2. Background information
3. Abstract
4. Discussion

14. How does the research consumer identify the principal investigator (PI) of the study? The PI is the person who
1. has the most credentials listed.
2. has the highest credential listed.
3. is listed first in the authors' byline.
4. has the clinical expertise on the topic.

Parts of a Published Research Report

15. Which of the following is (are) included in the introduction section of a published study? **Select all that apply.**
1. Procedures for measuring the variables
2. Nature and scope of the problem
3. Review of the literature
4. Significance of the study
5. Implications of the findings for nursing

16. Procedures for recruitment of subjects can be found in which section of the research report?
1. Introduction
2. Discussion
3. Results
4. Methods

17. Limitations of the study such as a small sample size will be included in which section of the research report?
1. Introduction
2. Discussion
3. Methods
4. Results

18. Descriptions of the instruments and their properties will be found in which section of the report?
1. Methods
2. Discussion
3. Results
4. Introduction

Phases of a Quantitative Research Study

19. In the conceptual phase of a research study, the researcher might undertake the necessary fieldwork. This means that the researcher will
1. identify a researchable problem that is significant to the discipline.
2. search for what is already known about the problem.
3. determine reliable and valid measurements.
4. seek clinical insights into the problem.

20. Selecting a research design means that the researcher
1. develops the intervention protocols that will be used.
2. specifies the sampling procedures to be followed.
3. selects a plan to answer the research question.
4. identifies a plan for analyzing the data.

21. What is (are) the purpose(s) of a review of the literature? **Select all that apply.**
1. Determine what is known or not known about a topic
2. Facilitate in formulating the research question
3. Identify potential research instruments
4. Present the impressions of researchers on the topic
5. Establish the significance of the topic to nursing

22. Which of the following titles suggests theoretical literature?
1. Bandura, A. (1985). Social foundation of thought and action: A social cognitive theory.
2. Craig, P., et al. (2013). Predictors of successful transition to registered nurse.
3. Arieti, D. (2013). Emotional work and diversity in clinical placements of nursing students.
4. Cohen, R. A., et al. (2013). Strategies used by adults to reduce their prescription drug costs.

23. Which of the following titles suggests data-based literature?
1. Plow, M., et al. (2011). Correlates of stages of change for physical activity in adults with multiple sclerosis.
2. Rogers, M. E. (1994). The science of unitary human beings: Current perspectives.
3. Newman, M. (1997). Evolution of the theory of health as expanding consciousness.
4. Johnson, J. E. (1999). Self-Regulation Theory and coping with physical illness.

24. Which of the following titles suggests a primary source?
1. Pender, N., et al. (2011). Health promotion in nursing practice.
2. Wang, P. (2013). The effectiveness of cranberry products to reduce urinary tract infections in females: A literature review.
3. Hellstrom, A. (2011). Promoting sleep by nursing interventions in healthcare settings: A systematic review.
4. Sakraida, T. J. (2002). Theories and middle range theories: Nola J. Pender: The health promotion model.

25. Which of the following titles suggests a secondary source?
1. Orem, D. E. (2001). The self-care deficit theory of nursing: A general theory.
2. Cahill, J., et al. (2012). Brain tumor symptoms as antecedents to uncertainty: An integrative review.
3. Harris, A., et al. (2013). Parental influences of sexual risk among urban African American adolescent males.
4. Lam, S. C., et al. (2012). Pedometer-determined physical activity and body composition in Chinese working adults.

26. The analytic phase of a research study includes
1. preparing the data for analysis.
2. collecting the data.
3. interpreting the results.
4. communicating the findings.

27. The discussion section of a research report includes which element(s)? **Select all that apply.**
1. Description of the statistical procedures
2. Recommendations for future studies
3. Clinical and research implications
4. Limitations
5. Procedures for sample recruitment

ANSWERS AND RATIONALES

The correct answer number and rationale for why it is the correct answer are given in **boldface blue type**. Rationales for why the other possible answer options are incorrect also are given, but they are not in boldface type.

1. **1. A theory is built from concepts. A theory "consists of an integrated set of concepts and relational statements that present a view of a phenomenon and can be used to describe, explain, predict, or control the phenomenon" (Burns & Grove, 2011, p. 45).**

2. Data are pieces of information in a study. Whereas in a quantitative study, the data are in numeric forms, in a qualitative study, the data are descriptive statements provided by the participants.

3. Abstract ideas are represented by concepts. "Concepts are formulated in words that enable people to communicate their meanings about realities in the world" (Kim, 2000, as cited in Fain, 2009, p. 71).

4. A hypothesis is a statement of relationship between two or more variables.

5. "Theories pull together the results of observations, allowing researchers to make general statements about variables and the relationships among variables" (Fain, 2009, p. 64).

TEST-TAKING TIP: When you think of a concept, you might come up with an idea. An idea is the beginning of something. Then you might want to give that idea a name. A concept is just that. It is a beginning, a building block, and it represents something abstract to which you give a name.

Content Area: *Basic Terminology;* ***Cognitive Level:*** *Comprehension;* ***Question Type:*** *Multiple Response*

CRITICAL THINKING FACILITATOR: Think of the concepts you learn in class such as communication, nursing process, decision making, patient satisfaction, nursing outcomes. These are all abstract ideas that have names. They form the building blocks of models or theories. For instance, these concepts could all be parts (building blocks) of a model of healthcare delivery.

2. 1. Interpretation means "making sense of the study results and examining their implications" (Polit & Beck, 2014, p. 52).

2. Data are pieces of information in a study.

3. Statistics are procedures used to analyze the data.

4. Recommendations are statements made for the application of research findings to clinical practice, education, or research.

TEST-TAKING TIP: The key word in the question stem is *information* which means "something learned or acquired." In a research study, what are learned or acquired by some method or process are called data.

Content Area: *Basic Terminology;* ***Cognitive Level:*** *Knowledge;* ***Question Type:*** *Multiple Choice*

CRITICAL THINKING FACILITATOR: Think of a process that you use in nursing practice such as history taking. What does this process yield? When you take a patient's history, you acquire information, also called data. Think of other processes you use to obtain data.

3. 1. Submission of the research proposal to an IRB does not constitute data. This is a requirement for the conduct of ethical research.

2. The outcomes of the intervention in a study would be measured and reported in numeric values that are subjected to appropriate statistical methods. These are the data of the study, and tables are one way to present the data.

3. Limitations of the study are presented by the researcher under the discussion section. Limitations are not considered data of the study.

4. Recruitment of the sample is information included under the methods section of the published report.

TEST-TAKING TIP: A key word in the correct option is *table*. A table implies information presented in a compact manner. Also, the term *outcomes* means "results." These are the data from the study.

Content Area: *Basic Terminology;* ***Cognitive Level:*** *Analysis;* ***Question Type:*** *Multiple Choice*

CRITICAL THINKING FACILITATOR: Familiarize yourself with the ways data are presented in the literature. Figures, graphs, and boxes are common ways you would see data presented in journal articles and textbooks.

4. 1. This statement is the definition of theory.

2. This statement describes a scientific theory.

3. This statement describes conceptual models or frameworks. Conceptual

models or frameworks provide a structure for "communicating a particular perception of the world. They represent ideas or notions that have been put together in a unique way to describe a particular area of concern" (Fain, 2009, p. 72).

4. This statement describes nursing research.

TEST-TAKING TIP: *Assembled together* is a key phrase, and it means the researcher has selected the concepts in order to study a phenomenon by "looking through someone else's glasses or walking in someone else's shoes" (Fain, 2009, p. 72).

Content Area: *Basic Terminology;* ***Cognitive Level:*** *Comprehension;* ***Question Type:*** *Multiple Choice*

CRITICAL THINKING FACILITATOR: Some published research reports might include a section on the conceptual framework or theoretical framework of the study. As you read this section, identify the key concepts as expressed in the title, the research question, or both.

5. 1. This definition is theoretical because it describes an "abstract or theoretical meaning of a concept under study" (Polit & Beck, 2014, p. 376).

2. This definition is an operational one because it includes the tool to measure the concept. An operational definition is the "definition of the concept or the variable in terms of the procedures by which it is to be measured" (p. 386). The tool to be used is the Practice Environment Scale of Nursing Work Index

3. This definition is theoretical.

4. This definition is theoretical.

TEST-TAKING TIP: In each of the options, identify a specific measurement for the variable. Research measurements will include terms such as *tool, scale, inventory, questionnaire,* or *checklist*.

Content Area: *Basic Terminology;* ***Cognitive Level:*** *Analysis;* ***Question Type:*** *Multiple Choice*

CRITICAL THINKING FACILITATOR: Look at a sample study in the appendix of your core textbook and identify operational definitions of concepts in them.

6. **1. This definition is theoretical because it is an "abstract or theoretical meaning of a concept under study" (Polit & Beck, 2014, p. 376).**

2. This definition is operational. The measurement is the Chinese Breast Screening Beliefs Questionnaire.

3. This definition is operational. The measurement is the Fertility Belief Questionnaire.

4. This definition is operational. The tool is the Practice Environment Scale of the Nursing Work Index.

TEST-TAKING TIP: Eliminate the options that specify a measurement for the concept or variable. Look for terms that indicate a research instrument such as *tool, inventory, scale, checklist,* or *questionnaire*. The definition that does not have a specific measurement of the concept or variable is a theoretical one.

Content Area: *Basic Terminology;* ***Cognitive Level:*** *Analysis;* ***Question Type:*** *Multiple Choice*

CRITICAL THINKING FACILITATOR: Consult a sample study and look for theoretical definitions. You could find these under the background information, the review of the literature, or the conceptual or theoretical framework sections.

7. 1. This statement is a purpose of the study.

2. Although this is an interrogative statement, it does not fulfill the criteria for a research question.

3. The research question is the interrogative statement that needs to be answered in the study. The research question expresses the variables, both independent and dependent, as well as the population to be addressed.

4. This statement is not a research question. This is an example of a hypothesis, a statement that expresses a relationship between or among two or more variables.

TEST-TAKING TIP: Determine what is being asked. Is the question an inquiry about a phenomenon or variables? Other research questions could ask about the effects or the influence of something (independent variable) over something (dependent variable).

Content Area: *Basic Terminology;* ***Cognitive Level:*** *Analysis;* ***Question Type:*** *Multiple Choice*

CRITICAL THINKING FACILITATOR: Differentiate a research problem from a research question. A research problem is "a disturbing or perplexing condition that can be investigated through disciplined inquiry" (Polit & Beck, 2014, p. 390). An example of a research problem is the high attrition rate among freshman nursing students in a baccalaureate nursing program. During the conceptual phase of the study and upon completion of the different steps involved, the researcher might come up with a research question such as: "What is the relationship of a mentoring program on the retention of freshman nursing students in a baccalaureate nursing program?"

8. 1. This statement identifies the plan of the researcher for the variables in a study.
2. This statement is a hypothesis because it is proposing a relationship between two variables, namely a structured exercise program and cardiovascular efficiency.
3. This statement is a purpose for a qualitative study.
4. This statement is information regarding sample recruitment.

TEST-TAKING TIP: Recall that a hypothesis is a statement about a relationship and it involves at least two variables. Also a hypothesis is often commonly known as "an educated guess." This means that it is a statement of a prediction.

Content Area: *Basic Terminology;* ***Cognitive Level:*** *Comprehension;* ***Question Type:*** *Multiple Choice*
CRITICAL THINKING FACILITATOR: Think of a situation that has happened and formulate a statement that might explain what happened. Although you do not have research data to support it, you nevertheless used some other processes such as previous experiences to support your statement (your hypothesis).

9. **1. This statement is a definition of a population.**
2. This statement describes the sample for a study.
3. This statement describes a subject or a participant in a research study.
4. This statement describes research assistants.

TEST-TAKING TIP: The everyday meaning of *population* can be applied in answering the question. A population is *all* of something—people, records, incidents, and so on. Members of a population share common characteristics. For instance, the population of a country is *all* the people who live there. Another example is the population of patient records at a clinic is *all* the records of a given period of time such as 2005 to 2010.

Content Area: *Basic Terminology;* ***Cognitive Level:*** *Knowledge;* ***Question Type:*** *Multiple Choice*
CRITICAL THINKING FACILITATOR: Look at the sample of a study and determine what the population would be. Remember that a sample should be representative of the population.

10. **1. This statement refers to the independent variable.**
2. This statement refers to the dependent variable.
3. This statement is about the independent variable.
4. This statement refers to the dependent variable.

TEST-TAKING TIP: Think of the independent variable as the "cause." If one varies the "cause," would the "effect" be different? Varying the cause is one way of "manipulating" it. For instance, if an educator changed her approach in teaching a concept (cause), will the degree of learning be different (effect)?

Content Area: *Basic Terminology;* ***Cognitive Level:*** *Knowledge;* ***Question Type:*** *Multiple Response*
CRITICAL THINKING FACILITATOR: Think of situations when you could identify a cause and a resulting effect. For instance, if you change your sleeping patterns (cause), will you see a change in your energy level (effect) during the day? Changing your sleeping patterns is your intervention, and your outcome is energy level.

11. 1. The two dependent variables of the study are nocturnal sleep and relaxation indices because these are the variables the researchers are interested in describing, explaining, or predicting.
2. The patients in medical intensive care are the subjects.
3. Listening to noncommercial music is the independent variable. It is the intervention or the variable that was manipulated to "cause an effect" on the dependent variables.
4. The randomized clinical trial represents the design of the study.

TEST-TAKING TIP: Remember that the independent variable is the variable that is manipulated by the researcher. It is the "cause" that is expected to produce an "effect." In experimental research, the independent variable is also known as the intervention.

Content Area: *Basic Terminology;* ***Cognitive Level:*** *Analysis;* ***Question Type:*** *Multiple Choice*
CRITICAL THINKING FACILITATOR: Look at a study that has an experimental or quasi-experimental design. Identify the variables expressed in the research question. The dependent variable would be the variable of interest. Ask yourself: "If I do something to one variable (vary it), what would happen to the other variable?" The variable that changes is the dependent variable. Try writing some sample problem statements related to a clinical problem. What would your intervention be (independent variable), and what would you expect as an outcome (dependent variable)?

12. 1. Implications include recommendations of the researcher for education, practice, or research.
   2. Testing outcomes represent the dependent variables. The dependent variable is the variable the researcher is interested in describing, explaining, or predicting.
   3. A variation of the independent variable is participation.
   4. Another variation of the independent variable is simulation experience. The researcher manipulated or "varied" simulation experience by having subjects either participate in the simulation or just observe the simulation experience.

TEST-TAKING TIP: A clue in the question stem is *testing* outcomes. Outcomes are dependent variables. They are seen as the "effects" of the manipulation of the independent variable or the "cause."

Content Area: *Basic Terminology;* ***Cognitive Level:*** *Analysis;* ***Question Type:*** *Multiple Choice*
CRITICAL THINKING FACILITATOR: Identify dependent variables in experimental or quasi-experimental studies in the appendix of your core textbook. What are the outcomes observed with an intervention?

13. 1. The study title could give one a general idea about the research study, but information would be limited. The title informs the reader of the variables and the sample and, possibly, the design.
   2. The background information of a study would include statistics on the phenomenon of interest, the significance of the study, and a review of the literature.
   3. The abstract includes essential information on the research question, methodology, results, discussion, and implications of the study. The abstract is usually set off from the rest of the article by a different font, and it always precedes the introduction or background of the study. The abstract is always included in any database because it informs the reader whether the study would be useful for the searcher's purposes.
   4. The discussion is the last section in a published report of a study, and it includes information on the meaning of the data in relation to the hypothesis(es); the limitations of the study; and the implications or recommendations for education, practice, and future research.

TEST-TAKING TIP: A clue in the question stem is *main points*. Study reports include the introduction, methods, results, analysis, and discussion (IMRAD). All of these are summarized in the abstract of a report.

Content Area: *Basic Terminology;* ***Cognitive Level:*** *Knowledge;* ***Question Type:*** *Multiple Choice*
CRITICAL THINKING FACILITATOR: Look at a sample research study. Can you locate the abstract and identify IMRAD?

14. 1. The person with the most credentials is not always the principal investigator. At times this person could be a mentor of the first author. The mentor is not listed first.
   2. The person with the highest credential is not always the principal investigator. This person could be a consultant and could serve as a member of the research team.
   3. The first author listed is the principal investigator. The principal investigator is the primary person responsible for the design and conduct of the study.
   4. The person with the clinical expertise might not be listed first. However, the person with the clinical expertise is listed first if he or she is the principal investigator.

TEST-TAKING TIP: There is a hierarchy in every project, and a research study is no exception. The first author listed is the leader of the project.

Content Area: *Basic Terminology;* ***Cognitive Level:*** *Knowledge;* ***Question Type:*** *Multiple Choice*
CRITICAL THINKING FACILITATOR: Look at the authors' credentials in a sample research study. In most instances, the lead author, as the principal investigator, has the most experience in studying the topic. An exception would be when the most experienced person might be listed last. This could indicate that this person is a mentor of the principal investigator and lead author.

15. 1. Procedures for measuring the variables are described under the methods section.
   2. The introduction section of a published research study includes the nature and scope of the problem.
   3. The introduction section includes the review of the literature, although there could be a separate subheading for these in some journals.
   4. The introduction section also includes the significance of the study.
   5. Implications of the findings for nursing are found under the discussion section.

TEST-TAKING TIP: The word *introduction* implies a start of something such as a topic or an idea. It is therefore logical

that the introduction section of a published report would orient the reader to the background of the study.

Content Area: *Parts of a Quantitative Study Report;* ***Cognitive Level:*** *Knowledge;* ***Question Type:*** *Multiple Response*

CRITICAL THINKING FACILITATOR: Use the IMRAD format of research reports in journals to familiarize yourself with the areas included in each section. Look at a sample research study and identify the included areas in each major section.

16. 1. The introduction section of a published report does not include a description of the recruitment of subjects.
2. The discussion section does not include a description of the recruitment of subjects. It can, however, include recommendations relative to the sampling for future studies.
3. The results section describes the data collected, and the researcher usually presents the data in tables or graphs.
4. The methods section includes information on how subjects were recruited for the study and what criteria were used in selecting them.

TEST-TAKING TIP: A key word in the question stem is *procedures*. Procedures mean methods or courses of action.

Content Area: *Parts of a Quantitative Study Report;* ***Cognitive Level:*** *Knowledge;* ***Question Type:*** *Multiple Choice*

CRITICAL THINKING FACILITATOR: Identify the methods section of a sample study and determine what is included.

17. 1. The introduction does not include a discussion of the limitations of the study.
2. Limitations of the study, such as issues in the collection of data or in the sample, are described in the discussion.
3. "The methods section includes a description of the research design, the sampling plan, methods of measuring variables and collecting data, study procedures, including procedures to protect human rights, and data analysis methods" (Polit & Beck, 2014, p. 63).
4. The results section "presents the findings that were obtained by analyzing the study data" (p. 63).

TEST-TAKING TIP: The key word in the question stem is *limitations*. Limitations are "theoretical and methodological restrictions in a study that may decrease the generalizability of the findings" (Burns & Grove, 2011, p. 541).

Content Area: *Parts of a Quantitative Study Report;* ***Cognitive Level:*** *Knowledge;* ***Question Type:*** *Multiple Choice*

CRITICAL THINKING FACILITATOR: Read the discussion section of any study and identify the content of the discussion section.

18. **1. The methods section includes descriptions of the instruments used to measure the variables. Included is a brief discussion of their properties, reliability, and validity and a mention of studies that have used these instruments.**
2. The discussion section of a published research report would include "an interpretation of the results, clinical and research implications, study limitations and ramifications for the believability of the results" (Polit & Beck, 2014, p. 65).
3. The results section would include a description of findings.
4. The introduction would include the nature and scope of the problem, significance of the study, and a review of related literature.

TEST-TAKING TIP: A key word in the question stem is *instruments*. Variables are measured by instruments, or research tools. The use of instruments implies that a process, or method, is in place; in fact, research instruments are described in the methods section of a research report.

Content Area: *Parts of a Quantitative Study Report;* ***Cognitive Level:*** *Knowledge;* ***Question Type:*** *Multiple Choice*

CRITICAL THINKING FACILITATOR: Locate the methods section of a research study. The research instruments and descriptions should be included in that section, and in some published reports, there might be a separate subheading on the tool(s) used. Identify the tool used in the study and determine the variable it will measure.

19. 1. Identifying a researchable problem means that the researcher has focused on a specific phenomenon of interest that is significant to the discipline.
2. The review of related literature would indicate what is already known about the phenomenon of interest.
3. Determining the availability of reliable and valid instruments is done during the literature review.

4. **Clinical insights into the problem or phenomenon are gained by spending time in the field.**

TEST-TAKING TIP: A key word in the question stem is *field*. The field in nursing practice is a clinical setting.

Content Area: *Phases in a Quantitative Research Study;* ***Cognitive Level:*** *Analysis;* ***Question Type:*** *Multiple Choice*

CRITICAL THINKING FACILITATOR: There are several steps in the conceptual phase of a quantitative research study, and these are logically sequenced. Determine how a researcher would progress through each step to get to the next phase.

20. 1. An intervention or treatment (the independent variable) may be "physiologic, psychosocial, educational, or a combination of these. The specific steps or components of the intervention need to be carefully planned and a rationale is given for providing the intervention in a particular way" (Burns & Grove, 2011, p. 282). Although an intervention is a requirement of some designs, it is not the design of the study.
2. The sampling plan is the "process of selecting a group of people, events, behaviors, or other elements that are representative of the population being studied" (p. 548). Although the type of sampling plan is determined by the type of research design, sampling is not the design.
3. **The plan to answer the research question is the design. "The purpose of a design is to maximize control over factors that can interfere with the validity of the study findings" (p. 253).**
4. Plans for analyzing the data are not the research design but are determined by the type of design selected by the researcher to answer the research question.

TEST-TAKING TIP: A key word in the question stem is *design*, and a key word in option 3 is *plan*. A plan or design is a scheme. Researchers need the plan to guide them in making decisions about the different aspects of the study such as how to select the sample, what kinds of controls to use, how to analyze and interpret the data, and so on.

Content Area: *Phases in a Quantitative Research Study;* ***Cognitive Level:*** *Comprehension;* ***Question Type:*** *Multiple Choice*

CRITICAL THINKING FACILITATOR: Look at the abstracts of several research studies you have and identify the design of each study. After you have done this, identify some of the key features of the design. You will see that the studies will have considered these features. That is what a design does. It serves as a plan or blueprint for the study.

21. 1. **Through a review of the literature, the researcher is able to determine what is known and unknown about the phenomenon of interest.**
2. **Through the literature review, the researcher is able to formulate the research question after knowing what is known about the phenomenon.**
3. **The researcher is also able to identify potential instruments to measure the variables through a review of the literature.**
4. Impressions of researchers about the phenomenon are subjective perspectives and do not belong in a review of the literature.
5. The review of the literature might be included in the introduction section of the published study. The introduction might also include the significance of the topic to nursing and healthcare. In some journals, the review of the literature might have its own subheading.

TEST-TAKING TIP: A key word in the question stem is *review*, which means "to look again." The researcher would "look again" at what has been done to help focus on the specific research problem, to determine what is already known, and to identify available resources.

Content Area: *Phases in a Quantitative Research Study;* ***Cognitive Level:*** *Knowledge;* ***Question Type:*** *Multiple Response*

CRITICAL THINKING FACILITATOR: Think of a class assignment that required you to search the literature. What is the purpose of this process? Although a search for research instruments was not one of your purposes, you were still able to find out what research instruments were available on your chosen topic and to determine if a topic lacked suitable research instruments.

22. 1. **Bandura's work is considered theoretical literature. "Theoretical literature includes concept analyses, models, theories, and conceptual frameworks that support a selected problem and purpose" (Polit & Beck, 2014, p. 190).**
2. The title suggests data-based literature. "Data-based literature consists of reports of research and includes published studies,

usually in journals or books and unpublished studies such as master's theses and doctoral dissertations" (p. 190). A key word in the title is *predictors*. Independent variables are also called predictor variables (Burns & Grove, 2011).
3. The title suggests data-based literature because this is a report of a study done on nursing students who were the research participants.
4. The title suggests data-based literature. This is a study with strategies as independent variables and prescription drug use as the dependent variable. The term *impact* in the title suggests a "cause and effect" relationship between the variables.

TEST-TAKING TIP: A key word in the question stem is *theoretical*. The term suggests no research data were collected from subjects or participants.

Content Area: *Phases in a Quantitative Research Study;* ***Cognitive Level:*** *Analysis;* ***Question Type:*** *Multiple Choice*

CRITICAL THINKING FACILITATOR:
Look at the references of a research study. Identify theoretical literature. Eliminate titles that have words suggesting a research study such as *influence*, *relationship*, *effects*, and *factors*. Also ask yourself: "Were data collected from subjects or participants? What does the study's title suggest?"

23. **1. The title suggests data-based literature. A key word in the title is *correlate*, which implies a relationship between variables.**
2. The title suggests theoretical literature. Science suggests laws or theories for verification.
3. The title suggests theoretical literature. The key word in the title is *theory*.
4. The title suggests theoretical literature. The key word in the title is *theory*.

TEST-TAKING TIP: A key word in the question stem is *data based*. The title suggests data would have been collected from a sample (persons, records, situations, and so on). Also, the correct option uses the word *correlates*. *Correlates* is a term for variables in correlational research. Correlational research is a "systematic investigation of relationships between two or more variables to explain the nature of relationships in the world" (Burns & Grove, 2011, p. 535).

Content Area: *Phases in a Quantitative Research Study;* ***Cognitive Level:*** *Analysis;* ***Question Type:*** *Multiple Choice*

CRITICAL THINKING FACILITATOR:
Look at the references of a research study, and try to identify data-based literature. The titles will have some key words such as *study*, *effects*, *influence*, *factors*, or *relationship*. In addition, you should be able to identify at least two variables in the title.

24. **1. The title suggests this is the author's original work on her model. The work is considered primary because a primary source is "written by the person who originated or is responsible for generating the ideas published" (Burns & Grove, 2011, p. 191).**
2. The title suggests a secondary source. A key term in the title is *literature review*. The author did a "summary of theoretical and empirical sources to generate a picture of what is known and not known about a particular problem" (p. 541). Primary sources were used by the author. Because the reader does not have direct access to these sources, he or she is relying on the current author's material for information.
3. The title suggests a secondary source. A systematic review is a "rigorous synthesis of research findings on a particular research question, using systematic sampling and data collection procedures and a formal protocol" (Polit & Beck, 2014, p. 393). The researcher doing the systematic review uses primary sources to do the review. The research consumer using such a review does not have direct access to the original works but relies on the review of the researcher for information about the studies.
4. This is a not a primary source. It is someone else's description of a theorist's work.

TEST-TAKING TIP: *Literature review* and *systematic review* are key terms in the options. The authors used the works of others to write the article. Option 4 is a synopsis of an author's original work written by someone else.

Content Area: *Phases in a Quantitative Research Study;* ***Cognitive Level:*** *Analysis;* ***Question Type:*** *Multiple Choice*

CRITICAL THINKING FACILITATOR:
Examine the references of a research article. Are you able to identify primary sources? These are original works by the authors or reports by the researchers who conducted the study.

25. 1. The title suggests the work was originated by the author.

2. The title suggests a secondary source. A key term in the title is *integrative review*. An integrative review of the literature is "a rigorous analysis and synthesis of results from independent quantitative and qualitative studies and theoretical and methodological literature to determine the current knowledge (what is known and not known) for a particular concept, measurement methods, or practice topic" (Burns & Grove, 2011, p. 540).

3. The title suggests an original work by the authors. This is a published research study by the researcher and is considered a primary source.

4. The title suggests an original work by the author. This is a published research study by the researcher and is considered a primary source.

TEST-TAKING TIP: The correct option has the key words *integrative review*. The other two works listed are research reports by the researchers, and the third is theoretical literature by the original author.

Content Area: *Phases in a Quantitative Research Study;* ***Cognitive Level:*** *Analysis;* ***Question Type:*** *Multiple Choice*

CRITICAL THINKING FACILITATOR:
Look at the references of a research report. Look at words such as *integrative review, review of the literature, systematic review, critiques, meta-analysis,* or *secondary analysis*. These terms indicate secondary sources.

26. 1. Preparing the data for analysis is in the empirical phase.

2. Collection of data is also in the empirical phase.

3. Interpretation of the findings is in the analytic phase. Interpretation involves "making sense of study results and examining their implications" (Polit & Beck, 2014, p. 52).

4. Communicating the findings of a study is in the dissemination phase. The term *disseminate* means "to scatter or promulgate."

TEST-TAKING TIP: A key word in the question stem is *analytic*, derived from *analysis*, which means "the organization and synthesis of data so as to answer the research question and test the hypothesis" (Polit & Beck, 2014, p. 374).

Content Area: *Phases in a Quantitative Research Study;* ***Cognitive Level:*** *Comprehension;* ***Question Type:*** *Multiple Choice*

CRITICAL THINKING FACILITATOR:
What are the activities in the different phases of a quantitative study? How does each activity contribute to the overall research process?

27. 1. Statistical procedures of a study are described in the methods section.

2. Recommendations for future studies are described in the discussion section.

3. Implications for clinical practice and research are included in the discussion section.

4. Limitations in the sample or aspects of the methodology are some of the topics included in the discussion section.

5. Procedures for sample recruitment belong under the methods section.

TEST-TAKING TIP: The discussion section of a research report is the last section. Therefore, one would expect recommendations and implications for practice. Limitations of the study guide consumers in generalizing the findings. They facilitate the work of future researchers.

Content Area: *Phases in a Quantitative Research Study;* ***Cognitive Level:*** *Knowledge;* ***Question Type:*** *Multiple Response*

CRITICAL THINKING FACILITATOR:
The discussion section of a research report is an important section because it summarizes the findings in light of the hypotheses and within the context of current research. Recommendations and implications might be found under subheadings, but limitations are always within the discussion section. Look for these in a discussion section of a report.

Examining Research Problems, Purposes, and Hypotheses

6

KEY WORDS

The following words include English vocabulary, nursing/medical terminology, concepts, principles, or information relevant to content specifically addressed in the chapter or associated with topics presented in it. English dictionaries, your nursing textbooks, and medical dictionaries such as *Taber's Cyclopedic Medical Dictionary* are resources that can be used to expand your knowledge and understanding of these words and related information.

Associative
Causal
Complex
Dependent variable
Directional
Feasibility
Hypothesis
Independent variable
Nondirectional
Null (statistical)
Problem statement (research purpose, research question)
Significance
Simple

QUESTIONS

Problem Statement

1. Which of the following statements best describes a problem statement? A problem statement is
   1. "a clear, concise statement of the specific goals of focus of a study" (Burns & Grove, 2011, p. 146).
   2. "a formal statement of the expressed relationship between two or more variables in a specified population" (p. 539).
   3. "a concept or broad issue that is important to nursing" (p. 145).
   4. a statement that "explains the need for the study" (Polit & Beck, 2014, p. 100).

2. Which of the following is an example of a problem statement?
   1. "Substance abuse problems by nurses are of critical public health importance because these professionals pose a direct threat to themselves and those in their care. Understanding the scope of the problem is paramount, but it is difficult to estimate the actual number, beyond purely anecdotal evidence" (Monroe et al., 2008, as cited in Monroe et al., 2013, p. 10).
   2. "The primary objectives of this study were to estimate the 1-year prevalence of employed nurses requiring an intervention for substance abuse problems in the United States and to estimate the 1-year prevalence of nurses enrolled in substance abuse monitoring programs" (Monroe et al., 2013, p. 11).
   3. "Of the 59 member boards sampled, an average of 128 nurses per board each year was identified as having a substance abuse problem. Moreover, an average of 41 nurses per board each year enrolled in disciplinary monitoring programs" (p. 12).
   4. "The current findings also suggest that regulatory boards and agencies of nursing throughout the world can better protect the public and help more nurses by using the ATD [alternative to discipline] paradigm to address substance abuse problems in nursing professionals and students" (p. 14).

Research Purpose and Question

3. A(n) __________ is the researcher's summary of the overall goal of the study.

4. The study seeks to "describe the characteristics of hospital-based registered nurses in the subregion, and to determine the relationships among practice environment characteristics and turnover intention" (Lansiquot, Tullai-McGuinness, & Madigan, 2012, p. 187). This statement is a
1. problem statement.
2. purpose.
3. hypothesis.
4. research problem.

5. A research question can be identified as the statement that addresses
1. "the specific query the researcher wants to answer to address a research problem" (Polit & Beck, 2014, p. 390).
2. "the area of concern in which there is a gap in the knowledge base needed for nursing practice" (Burns & Grove, 2011, p. 146).
3. "the potential to generate knowledge or refine relevant knowledge for practice" (Brown, 2009; as cited in Burns & Grove, 2011, p. 155).
4. "the expressed relationship between two or more variables in a specified population (Burns & Grove, 2011, p. 539).

6. **Research Study Title:** "Parenting Enhancement, Interpersonal Psychotherapy to Reduce Depression in Low-Income Mothers of Infants and Toddlers" (Beeber et al., 2013, p. 82). Which of the following would be an appropriate research question for the study?
1. Why do "depressive symptoms limit low-income mothers' ability to manage stressors effectively and interfere with their use of education and work training programs" (p. 82)?
2. What are the critical issues in collecting data in low-income mothers with depressive symptoms particularly during the immediate postpartum period?
3. What is the relationship of parenting enhancement and interpersonal psychotherapy on depression among low-income mothers of infants and toddlers?
4. How will parenting enhancement and psychotherapy be implemented in a controlled environment to measure depressive symptoms of low-income mothers of infants and toddlers?

7. What makes a study significant? **Select all that apply.**
1. The study addresses an area of concern to nursing education and practice.
2. The study could be completed with minimal time and effort.
3. The study contributes to nursing knowledge for evidence-based practice.
4. The study uses the experience and expertise of nurse researchers.
5. The study builds on past research studies.

Research Hypothesis

8. A hypothesis is a "formal statement of a(n) ________________ between two or more variables in a specified population" (Burns & Grove, 2011, p. 167).

9. Which of the following is an appropriately worded hypothesis?
1. Research participants would "exhibit greater activation of noncompliance and health risk stereotypes after subliminal exposure to Hispanic faces compared with non-Hispanic White faces" (Bean et al., 2013, p. 5).
2. Research participants would exhibit an appropriate level of "noncompliance and health risk stereotype after subliminal exposure to Hispanic faces compared with White faces" (p. 5).
3. "Yoga may improve mood status and quality of life for women undergoing detoxification for heroin addiction. Yoga can be used as an auxiliary treatment with traditional hospital routine care for these women" (Zhuang, An, & Zhao, 2013, p. 260).
4. "Patients in the control group received routine hospital care without exercise or guidance or practice" (p. 262).

10. Which of the following is a simple hypothesis?

1. Research participants would "exhibit greater activation of noncompliance and health risk stereotypes after subliminal exposure to Hispanic faces compared with non-Hispanic White faces" (Bean et al., 2013, p. 5).
2. Study participants will show a significant decrease in pain intensity levels and improved body posture after participation in Back School consisting of active therapy, ergonomics, and education (Jaromi, Nemeth, Kranicz, Lacczko, & Betlehem, 2012).
3. The student registered nurse anesthetists exposed to patient safety vignettes will exhibit superior clinical performance during simulated crisis compared to a matched group exposed to written case studies plus standard lecture (McLain, Biddle, & Cotter, 2012).
4. "Yoga may improve mood status and quality of life for women undergoing detoxification for heroin addiction. Yoga can be used as an auxiliary treatment with traditional hospital routine care for these women" (Zhuang, An, & Zhao, 2013, p. 260).

11. **Hypothesis:** The student registered nurse anesthetists exposed to patient safety vignettes will exhibit superior clinical performance during simulated crises compared with a matched group exposed to written case studies plus standard lecture (McLain, Biddle, & Cotter, 2012). In the hypothesis, what is the dependent variable?

1. Patient safety vignettes
2. Clinical performance
3. Simulated crisis
4. Written case studies plus standard lecture

12. **Hypothesis:** Lin (2013) hypothesized that increasing fluid intake would significantly decrease the incidence of bacteriuria in nursing home residents in southern Taiwan. In the hypothesis, what is the independent variable?

1. Bacteriuria
2. Significantly decrease
3. Nursing home residents
4. Fluid intake

13. A complex hypothesis states a relationship among ____________ independent or dependent variables.

14. Which of the following is a complex hypothesis?

1. The student registered nurse anesthetists exposed to patient safety vignettes will exhibit superior clinical performance during simulated crises compared with a matched group exposed to written case studies plus standard lectures (McLain, Biddle, & Cotter, 2012).
2. Research participants with care coordination will have significantly better health outcomes (cognitive functioning, depressive symptoms, functional status, and quality of life) over time compared with those in the control group (Marek et al., 2013, p. 269).
3. "Playing an avatar-based reality technology game can strengthen peer resistance skills" (Norris et al., 2013, p. 25).
4. Increasing fluid intake will significantly decrease the incidence of bacteriuria in nursing home residents in southern Taiwan (Lin, 2013).

15. **Hypothesis:** "Women with coeliac disease who participate in a patient education with an active method would experience increased psychological well-being compared with women with coeliac disease acting as controls" (Jacobson, Friedrichsen, Goranson, & Hallert, 2011, p. 768). In the hypothesis, what is the independent variable?

1. Women with coeliac disease
2. Psychological well-being
3. Patient education with an active method
4. Women acting as controls

16. Which of the following describes a nondirectional hypothesis? It is a hypothesis that
1. states no relationship exists between the variables in the study.
2. makes a specific prediction about the direction of the relationship between two variables.
3. does not state the direction of the expected relationship between the study variables.
4. states the anticipated relationship between variables in the study.

17. A directional hypothesis is evident when the hypothesis statement uses which of the following terms? **Select all that apply.**
1. Related to
2. Less than
3. Greater than
4. Not related to
5. Difference

18. Which of the following is a nondirectional hypothesis?
1. There is a relationship between critical thinking and performance on the NCLEX examination.
2. Graduates who take a formal review class on NCLEX preparation have a higher probability of passing the examination than graduates who review on their own.
3. There is no relationship between critical thinking and performance on the NCLEX examination.
4. BSN graduates who do not take a formal review course will have a lower probability of passing the NCLEX than those who took a formal review course.

19. Which of the following is a directional hypothesis?
1. "Playing an avatar-based reality technology game can strengthen peer resistance skills" (Norris et al., 2013, p. 25).
2. There is a "relationship between quality of work life (QWL) and nurses' intention to leave their organization (ITLorg)" (Lee, Dai, Park, & McCreary, 2013, p. 160).
3. The examination performance level of students who participate in regular tutoring sessions is different from the performance level of students who study by themselves.
4. Rheumatoid arthritis–related fatigue is related to depressive symptoms, perceived health improvement, and satisfaction with abilities (Franklin & Harrell, 2013).

20. Which statement is a null hypothesis?
1. There is a "relationship between quality of work life (QWL) and nurses' intention to leave their organization (ITLorg)" (Lee, Dai, Park, & McCreary, 2013, p. 160).
2. There is no relationship between regular exercise and cardiovascular efficiency in older adults without hypertension.
3. Older adults who have a regular program of daily exercise will score higher on a tool measuring cardiovascular efficiency than older adults who exercise only sporadically.
4. There is a difference in the examination performance level of students who participate in regular tutoring sessions compared with students who study by themselves.

21. Which of the following statements describes an associative hypothesis? An associative hypothesis
1. "proposes relationships among variables that occur or exist together in the real world, so that when one changes, the other changes" (Reynolds, 2007; as cited in Burns & Grove, 2011, p. 167).
2. "states the nature (positive or negative) of the interactions between two or more variables" (p. 174).
3. "clearly predicts the relationships among variables and contains variables that are measurable or able to be manipulated in a study" (p. 175).
4. "states that a relationship exists but does not predict the nature of the relationship" (p. 173) between the variables in the study.

22. Which of the following is an associative hypothesis?
    1. There is a relationship among age, gender, and ethnicity on the attitudes toward older adults among practicing registered nurses in a community health setting.
    2. A cardiac exercise program will significantly improve the self-efficacy of middle-aged men who have survived a myocardial infarction.
    3. Graduates of advanced practice programs who take a formal structured review course will show a higher level of performance on the certification examination than graduates who reviewed on their own.
    4. Nursing students who practice the nonproctored foundations of nursing examinations will earn significantly higher course grades than students who do not do the practice tests.

23. A causal hypothesis is one that "proposes a(n) ____________ interaction between two or more variables that are referred to as independent and dependent variables" (Burns & Grove, 2011, p. 170).

24. Which of the following is a causal hypothesis?
    1. There is no found difference between the rate of substance abuse among nurses and the general population.
    2. There is a difference in the patient falls classification relative to units, hospitals, and individuals (Simon, Klaus, Gajewski, & Dunton, 2013).
    3. There is a "relationship between the quality of work life (QWL) and nurses' intention to leave their organization [ITLorg]" (Lee et al., 2013).
    4. Research participants with care coordination will have significantly improved health outcomes (cognitive functioning, depressive symptoms, functional status, and quality of life) over time compared with those in the control group (Marek et al., 2013, p. 269).

Feasibility of a Study

25. Which of the following factors would be considered in determining the feasibility of a study? **Select all that apply.**
    1. Ethical considerations
    2. Researcher experience
    3. Extensive literature
    4. Availability of resources
    5. Potential influence on practice
26. A novice researcher gets a mentor to work with him on his research project. What feasibility factor was addressed in this situation?
    1. Availability of resources
    2. Researcher experience
    3. Funding
    4. Potential influence on practice

27. A researcher wants to determine whether there is a difference in pain perception among male research participants. She considers a design that ensures no harm to research subjects. In doing so, this researcher is considering what aspect of feasibility?
    1. Researcher expertise
    2. Availability of subjects
    3. Access to equipment
    4. Ethical considerations

Significance of a Study

28. Which of the following would make a study significant? **Select all that apply.**
1. The study builds on previous research on the topic.
2. Findings would improve delivery of healthcare.
3. The expertise of the researcher would be enhanced.
4. Priorities of the nursing profession are addressed.
5. The study assures the protection of subjects' rights.

Critiquing Research Problems and Hypotheses

29. Which of the following questions is appropriate to ask in critically appraising a study's research problem?
1. Was the problem statement approved by an institutional review board?
2. Did the problem statement express a relationship between two variables?
3. Did the problem statement indicate the significance of the topic to nursing?
4. Did the problem statement indicate the appropriate design to be used?

30. Which question is appropriate in critically appraising a study's hypothesis?
1. Was the hypothesis derived directly from the purpose of the study?
2. Did the hypothesis express how subjects were recruited for the study?
3. Did the hypothesis clearly express a relationship between two variables?
4. Did the hypothesis address the significance of the study to nursing?

ANSWERS AND RATIONALES

The correct answer number and rationale for why it is the correct answer are given in **boldface blue type.** Rationales for why the other possible answer options are incorrect also are given, but they are not in boldface type.

1. 1. This statement defines a purpose for the research study. A clue in the option is the word "goals."
   2. This statement is the definition of a research hypothesis. A clue in the option is the phrase "relationship between two or more variables."
   3. An issue or concept might be the research topic. This is not the problem statement.
   4. **The statement is the definition of a problem statement.**

   TEST-TAKING TIP: The correct option has the word *need*, which indicates a lack of something. This lack of something presents a problem.

   Content Area: *Problem Statement;* ***Cognitive Level:*** *Knowledge;* ***Question Type:*** *Multiple Choice*
   CRITICAL THINKING FACILITATOR: To familiarize yourself with the terminology, look at the definitions of *research topic, research problem,* and *problem statement.* Most textbooks provide tables of these with specific examples. Also, be sure to look at a sample research study and see whether you can locate these elements in a study.

2. 1. **This statement from a study indicates the problem and also the need to investigate it. The statement is appropriate as a problem statement.**
   2. This statement is an expressed objective, or purpose, of the study. Note the word "objective" in the statement.
   3. This statement describes some of the data from the study and is not a problem statement.
   4. This statement is a recommendation by the researchers. A clue in the statement is the word "suggest." which is synonymous with "recommend."

   TEST-TAKING TIP: Knowing the definition of a problem statement would definitely help in selecting the correct option. Only option 1 articulates the problem and why there is a need for the investigation.

   Content Area: *Problem Statement;* ***Cognitive Level:*** *Application;* ***Question Type:*** *Multiple Choice*
   CRITICAL THINKING FACILITATOR: A problem statement expresses an identified issue that needs to be investigated. A rationale is provided for the need. Physically locating the problem statement is easy. It is usually found at the end of a brief presentation of statistics about the problem. Locate a problem statement in a sample research study.

3. **research purpose**

   TEST-TAKING TIP: A key word in the statement is "goal," which is synonymous with "purpose."

   Content Area: *Research Purpose;* ***Cognitive Level:*** *Knowledge;* ***Question Type:*** *Fill-in-the-Blank*
   CRITICAL THINKING FACILITATOR: Understanding the definition of a research purpose facilitates understanding other key concepts in research. Identify the research purpose in a sample study. Differentiate the study's research purpose from its problem statement.

4. 1. This statement is not a problem statement because it does not express a problem and the need for the investigation.
   2. **This statement expresses the goals, or objectives, of the study. This is the research purpose.**
   3. This statement is not a hypothesis because a hypothesis expresses a proposed relationship between or among variables in a study.
   4. This statement is not a research problem because it does not identify an issue or concern about a particular topic significant to the profession.

   TEST-TAKING TIP: The key words in the statement are "describe" and "determine," which are terms used to identify the purpose of a study.

   Content Area: *Research Purpose;* ***Cognitive Level:*** *Comprehension;* ***Question Type:*** *Multiple Choice*
   CRITICAL THINKING FACILITATOR: Review the levels of research purposes such as to identify, to describe, to explore, to test, and to predict. Recall that the purpose of a study is one factor in deciding what approach will be used to answer the research question.

5. 1. **This statement describes a research question. A clue in the option is the word "query," which means *a question.***
   2. This statement is not a research question; it describes a research problem.
   3. This statement is not a research question; it expresses the rationale for the significance of a research problem.
   4. This statement is not a research question; it is a hypothesis, which proposes a relationship between or among variables in a study.

TEST-TAKING TIP: The key word in the question stem is "question," and option 1 has the word "query" in the statement.

Content Area: *Research Question;* ***Cognitive Level:*** *Knowledge;* ***Question Type:*** *Multiple Choice*
CRITICAL THINKING FACILITATOR: Knowing the difference between the problem statement and research purpose will facilitate understanding of the research study and will be helpful later in the critical appraisal process. Identify the research question in a sample research study.

6. 1. Although this is a question that could be asked about the research problem, it is not appropriately articulated. The research question should ask about a relationship between or among variables. The question as expressed is not appropriate to guide a research inquiry.
2. This question asked might guide a scholarly discussion of research approaches and methodologies.
3. The title of the study identifies several variables, independent and dependent ones. The title implies a relationship between or among these variables. Therefore, a question about the relationship of the variables is most appropriate.
4. This question addresses an aspect of interventions, the independent variables. It is not the study's research question.

TEST-TAKING TIP: Think of an independent variable as an intervention, a program, an approach, or a treatment. There are two of these in the title. Think of the dependent variable as the outcome. Researchers want to investigate the relationship between or among these. Only option 3 is studying the relationship of these variables.

Content Area: *Research Question;* ***Cognitive Level:*** *Analysis;* ***Question Type:*** *Multiple Choice*
CRITICAL THINKING FACILITATOR: Look at two or more sample studies in the Appendix of your core textbook. Formulate an appropriate research question based on the title of the study.

7. 1. A study addressing a concern of nursing education and practice has the potential of generating new and useful information that can be used to improve education and practice outcomes.
2. Completion of a study with minimal time and effort is not related to the significance of the study to nursing. These factors might be desirable when doing a study, but they are unrealistic expectations. Studies take time and effort to conduct.
3. Findings of studies have the potential to build the knowledge base of the discipline and could be used in evidence-based practice to improve patient outcomes.
4. The experience and expertise of nurse researchers are relative to the feasibility of a study, but they are not criteria for significance. The experience and expertise of a nurse researcher would facilitate the identification of research problems which could be the bases of research that have the potential to make a contribution to the profession.
5. One of the purposes of nursing research is to build the knowledge base of the profession. A research study that builds on previous studies helps to refine the knowledge already generated by these.

TEST-TAKING TIP: The key word in the question is "significance." In nursing research, significance means that research findings have the potential to make contributions to nursing education, practice, and research. Even when findings lack statistical significance, significant contributions can be made in other aspects of the study, such as in the design and methodology.

Content Area: *Significance;* ***Cognitive Level:*** *Comprehension;* ***Question Type:*** *Multiple Response*
CRITICAL THINKING FACILITATOR: How do you know whether a study has the potential for making significant contributions to the discipline? Look at the introductory section of a research study. What kinds of information are described in the introductory paragraph that help determine the significance of the study?

8. relationship

TEST-TAKING TIP: A clue in the statement is the phrase "between two or more variables." Variables (concepts) are the building blocks of a theory. The relationships between and among variables, or concepts, facilitate understanding of the phenomenon that is the focus of the theory.

Content Area: *Hypothesis;* ***Cognitive Level:*** *Knowledge;* ***Question Type:*** *Fill-in-the-Blank*
CRITICAL THINKING FACILITATOR: An understanding of hypotheses facilitates understanding how theories are built and how they guide the research process, particularly in the analysis and interpretation of the data. Locate the hypothesis of a study that you have. What is the rationale for expressing a hypothesis at the beginning of the study?

9. 1. The hypothesis is appropriately worded. It articulates a proposed relationship between an independent variable and two dependent variables. It also includes the term "greater," which implies quantitative measurement.

2. The hypothesis is not worded correctly because the term "appropriate" does not imply measurement.
3. The hypothesis is not appropriately worded. The term "improve" cannot be quantified.
4. The statement is not a hypothesis. This statement is related to the methodology, specifically the implementation of the intervention or the independent variable.

TEST-TAKING TIP: Recall that a hypothesis is the statement of a relationship between or among variables. In quantitative research, the relationship has to be measurable. Only terms that denote quantity should be used in expressing a hypothesis.

Content Area: *Hypothesis;* ***Cognitive Level:*** *Application;* ***Question Type:*** *Multiple Choice*

CRITICAL THINKING FACILITATOR:
Look at a sample hypothesis in a study in the appendix of your core textbook. Is the relationship proposed quantifiable and measurable? Why?

10. 1. The hypothesis is not a simple one because it has two dependent variables and one independent variable.
2. The hypothesis has two dependent variables and one independent variable. Therefore, it is not a simple hypothesis.
3. The hypothesis is a simple one because it has one independent and one dependent variable.
4. The hypothesis has two dependent variables and one independent variable, and therefore it is not a simple one.

TEST-TAKING TIP: The key term in the question is "simple." "A simple hypothesis states the relationship between two variables" (Fain, 2009, p. 79).

Content Area: *Hypothesis;* ***Cognitive Level:*** *Application;* ***Question Type:*** *Multiple Choice*

CRITICAL THINKING FACILITATOR:
Look at a hypothesis of a quantitative study. How would you classify this hypothesis relative to the number of variables in the statement? This question would also facilitate understanding of dependent and independent variables (asked in a later question in this chapter).

11. 1. Patient-study vignettes are the independent variables, or interventions. These were given to one group (experimental group). This is the variable that is manipulated.
2. Clinical performance is the dependent variable. This is the variable the researcher is interested in describing, explaining, or predicting. The dependent variable is also called the outcome.
3. A simulated crisis was the situation used to observe how the research subjects (student registered nurse anesthetists) performed. It is not a variable of the study.
4. Written case studies and the lecture were the "variations" of the independent variable given to the other group of research subjects (control group).

TEST-TAKING TIP: The key term in the question is "dependent." "The dependent variable, also called the criterion or outcome variable, is the variable that is observed for change or reaction after the treatment is applied. The dependent variable is that which is under investigation; it is the variable that the researcher determines to be a result of conducting the study" (Fain, 2009, p. 86).

Content Area: *Dependent and Independent Variables;* ***Cognitive Level:*** *Application;* ***Question Type:*** *Multiple Choice*

CRITICAL THINKING FACILITATOR:
Look at the title of a study that is experimental or a randomized clinical trial or quasi-experimental. What is (are) the variable (s) of interest? Differentiate this from the independent variable.

12. 1. Bacteriuria is the dependent variable because it is the outcome or the variable of interest.
2. "Significantly decrease" is the phrase used to indicate the expected relationship as expressed in the hypothesis.
3. Nursing home residents are the research participants.
4. Fluid intake is the independent variable. Providing fluids for intake is the intervention or treatment given to subjects, and the researchers, in turn, observe the incidence of bacteriuria, the dependent variable.

TEST-TAKING TIP: The key term in the question is "independent." The independent variable is "the variable that is believed to cause or influence the dependent variable; in experimental research, the manipulated (treatment) variable" (Polit & Beck, 2014, p. 382).

Content Area: *Dependent and Independent Variables;* ***Cognitive Level:*** *Application;* ***Question Type:*** *Multiple Choice*

CRITICAL THINKING FACILITATOR:
Look at the title of a study that is experimental or quasi-experimental in design, and identify the independent variable. In the sample study, why is this variable the independent one? Take a clinical situation and formulate a hypothesis. Identify your dependent variable and independent variable.

13. two or more

TEST-TAKING TIP: Know the everyday meaning of "complex," which is consisting of various parts, such as an apartment complex with many buildings. The same could be applied to a complex hypothesis.

Content Area: *Dependent and Independent Variables in a Hypothesis;* ***Cognitive Level:*** *Knowledge;* ***Question Type:*** *Fill-in-the-Blank*

CRITICAL THINKING FACILITATOR: Look at some complex hypotheses in a sample experimental (randomized clinical trials) or quasi-experimental study. Identify the number of independent and dependent variables. For your sample clinical situation (in the Critical Thinking Facilitator in question 12), try to formulate a complex hypothesis.

14.
1. The hypothesis is a simple one because it has one independent variable and one dependent variable.
2. **The hypothesis is a complex one because it has more than one dependent variable (cognitive functioning, depressive symptoms, functional status, and quality of life).**
3. The hypothesis is a simple one because it has one independent variable and one dependent variable.
4. The hypothesis is a simple one because it has one independent variable and one dependent variable.

TEST-TAKING TIP: The key word is "complex," which means there are two or more independent or dependent variables in a hypothesis.

Content Area: *Dependent and Independent Variables in a Hypothesis;* ***Cognitive Level:*** *Application;* ***Question Type:*** *Multiple Choice*

CRITICAL THINKING FACILITATOR: Refine your ability to identify independent and dependent variables by looking at the incorrect options. Identify the variables in each hypothesis.

15.
1. Women with celiac disease are the research participants.
2. Psychological well-being is the dependent variable, or the focus, of the study.
3. **Patient education with an active method is the independent variable (or the treatment or intervention) that is manipulated.**
4. Women acting as controls are the research participants assigned to the control group.

TEST-TAKING TIP: The key word is "independent." Recall that the independent variable is the manipulated variable and that it can be an intervention, a treatment, or a program,

Content Area: *Dependent and Independent Variables in a Hypothesis;* ***Cognitive Level:*** *Application;* ***Question Type:*** *Multiple Choice*

CRITICAL THINKING FACILITATOR: By now you should be quite adept at identifying independent and dependent variables. At this point, read the section in a study that describes the intervention and how it is specifically manipulated. Familiarity with this process will facilitate understanding of intervention fidelity covered in a later chapter.

16.
1. This statement is a null hypothesis.
2. A directional hypothesis is described in this statement.
3. **This statement is the definition of a nondirectional hypothesis. The clue in the statement is the phrase "does not state."**
4. This statement is a basic definition of a hypothesis.

TEST-TAKING TIP: The key word is "nondirectional." The prefix *non-* means "absent." Therefore, in a nondirectional hypothesis, the direction of the relationship between the variables is absent or is not specified.

Content Area: *Dependent and Independent Variables in a Hypothesis;* ***Cognitive Level:*** *Knowledge;* ***Question Type:*** *Multiple Choice*

CRITICAL THINKING FACILITATOR: Recognizing a nondirectional hypothesis facilitates the identification and understanding of the other types of hypotheses. Additionally, knowledge of a nondirectional hypothesis facilitates understanding of other parts of the study, such as data analysis and the basis of future studies on the same topic.

17.
1. A hypothesis that uses the term "related to" simply suggests a relationship between variables.
2. **The hypothesis that uses the term "less than" suggests a relationship, and the direction is specified. "Less than" is at one end of a measurement continuum, and "greater than" is on the opposite end.**
3. **The hypothesis that uses the term "greater than" suggests a relationship, and the direction is specified. "Greater than" is at one end of a measurement continuum, and "less than" is at the other end.**
4. The phrase "not related to" is used in expressing the null hypothesis, which suggests that the variables do not have a relationship.
5. When the term "difference" is used in a hypothesis, the statement expresses an expected change, but the direction of the change is not specified.

TEST-TAKING TIP: The clue in the question is the word "direction." Imagine two variables existing on two perpendicular lines—one on the x-axis and the other on the y-axis. Initially, your thinking is that these two variables are unrelated (null hypothesis). Something is done (manipulation) to one variable (independent). As the other variable begins to change, you are not really sure where the change will go (nondirectional hypothesis). As you study the variables further and refine what you do to create the change, you can now predict the effect of the independent variable on the dependent variable. This is the concept of the directional hypothesis.

Content Area: *Hypothesis;* ***Cognitive Level:*** *Comprehension;* ***Question Type:*** *Multiple Response*
CRITICAL THINKING FACILITATOR: Identify a directional hypothesis in a sample study, and provide a rationale as to why this hypothesis is a directional one.

18. **1. The hypothesis is a nondirectional one because it only states that there is a relationship between the independent and dependent variables. The direction of the relationship is not specified. For instance, does the ability to think critically increase the probability of success on the NCLEX?**
2. The hypothesis is a directional one. The hypothesis specifies that following the intervention, the formal review class, the probability of success on the examination is greater.
3. The statement is a null hypothesis.
4. The statement is a directional hypothesis. The hypothesis is directional because it indicates the direction of the proposed relationship by the word "lower."

TEST-TAKING TIP: The clue in the question stem is the word "nondirectional." A nondirectional hypothesis suggests a relationship between variables, but the direction of the relationship is not specified.

Content Area: *Hypothesis;* ***Cognitive Level:*** *Application;* ***Question Type:*** *Multiple Choice*
CRITICAL THINKING FACILITATOR: Identify a nondirectional hypothesis in a study. Why was a nondirectional hypothesis proposed? Think of the levels of purpose of the study in answering this question.

19. **1. The hypothesis is a directional one. The term "strengthen" indicates a continuum of peer resistance skills; the other end would be "weaken."**
2. The hypothesis is a nondirectional one because all it expresses is the existence of a relationship.
3. The hypothesis is a nondirectional one because it does not specify the direction of the relationship between the variables.
4. The hypothesis does not specify the direction of the relationship; therefore, it is a nondirectional one.

TEST-TAKING TIP: The clue in the question stem is "directional," meaning that the hypothesis suggests what direction the change in the dependent variable is expected to take.

Content Area: *Hypothesis;* ***Cognitive Level:*** *Application;* ***Question Type:*** *Multiple Choice*
CRITICAL THINKING FACILITATOR: Identify a directional hypothesis in a study. Why did the researcher suggest a directional hypothesis? Recall the levels of purposes in research.

20. 1. The statement suggests a relationship between the variables, but it does not specify the direction. It is a nondirectional hypothesis.
2. The statement is a null hypothesis because it suggests that no relationship exists between the variables.
3. The statement suggests a relationship between the variables and specifies the direction. Therefore, this is a directional hypothesis.
4. The statement suggests a relationship between the variables but does not specify the direction of the relationship. Therefore, it is a nondirectional hypothesis.

TEST-TAKING TIP: The clue in the question stem is "null," which means "not existing."

Content Area: *Hypothesis;* ***Cognitive Level:*** *Application;* ***Question Type:*** *Multiple Choice*
CRITICAL THINKING FACILITATOR: Most reports of research studies do not include a null hypothesis (also known as the statistical hypothesis). For every hypothesis, it is understood that there is a corresponding null hypothesis. Look at some of the hypotheses you have already encountered and formulate the corresponding null hypothesis. Knowledge of the null hypothesis will be helpful in understanding type I and type II errors relative to data analysis and interpretation.

21. **1. The statement is a definition of an associative hypothesis.**
2. The statement is indicative of a directional hypothesis.
3. The statement is the definition of a testable hypothesis. The term

"measurable" indicates the proposed relationship can be quantitatively measured.
4. The statement is reflective of a nondirectional hypothesis. Only a relationship is proposed, but the nature of the relationship is not specified.

TEST-TAKING TIP: The clue in the question stem is the word "associative," derived from the word *association*, which means "a connection." Variables (concepts) that have an associative relationship coexist in the real world, and their association in a research study is explored without actively manipulating the independent variable. Examples of these types of variables that are not actively manipulated are attribute variables, including age, gender, religious affiliation, and socioeconomic levels, just to name a few.

Content Area: *Hypothesis;* ***Cognitive Level:*** *Comprehension;* ***Question Type:*** *Multiple Choice*
CRITICAL THINKING FACILITATOR: Apply your understanding of an associative hypothesis in looking at studies that are not experimental or quasi-experimental, in which the independent variable is not actively manipulated. Think of your own personal attributes and an outcome, such as success in a course or program, and formulate an associative hypothesis.

22. **1. This is an associative hypothesis because the three independent variables—age, gender, and ethnicity—are all attribute variables that already exist in the real world. They are not actively manipulated in the study.**
2. This is not an associative hypothesis. The statement suggests an independent variable (a cardiac exercise program) can be manipulated to cause an effect on the dependent variable (self-efficacy).
3. This is not an associative hypothesis. The statement suggests an independent variable (a formal, structured review course) can be manipulated to cause an effect on the dependent variable (performance level).
4. This is not an associative hypothesis. Course grade is the dependent variable that is expected to change as a result of the manipulation of the independent variable, taking practice examinations.

TEST-TAKING TIP: Apply your understanding of an associative hypothesis. Look for clues in each of the options. Options 2, 3, and 4 are hypothesis proposing a relationship between an independent variable that can be manipulated and a dependent variable. Option 1 is a hypothesis with attribute variables as independent variables. These exist as they are in the real world and are not manipulated.

Content Area: *Hypothesis;* ***Cognitive Level:*** *Application;* ***Question Type:*** *Multiple Choice*
CRITICAL THINKING FACILITATOR:
What types of studies have associative hypotheses? What are some examples of variables that can be used as independent variables as they exist in the real world but could have an effect on a dependent variable?

23. **cause and effect**

TEST-TAKING TIP: The key words in the statement are "independent and dependent variables." Recall the definitions of these from the introductory chapter on quantitative research. The independent variable is often referred to as the "cause," and the dependent variable is referred to as the "effect."

Content Area: *Hypothesis;* ***Cognitive Level:*** *Knowledge;* ***Question Type:*** *Fill-in-the-Blank*
CRITICAL THINKING FACILITATOR: The notion of cause and effect facilitates the understanding of a causal hypothesis. What are some clinical situations you can think of that involve causes and effects? Take the example of coughing and deep breathing as a postoperative measure. How would you measure the effect of this intervention?

24. 1. The hypothesis expressed is not a causal hypothesis because it does not relate two variables.
2. This statement is a nondirectional, associative hypothesis. The independent variables are not manipulated to cause an effect on the dependent variable, falls classification.
3. This statement is an associative hypothesis. Quality of work life (QWL) as the dependent variable was not "caused" by the nurses' intention to leave the organization (ITLorg), the independent variable. The independent variable was not manipulated to create an effect on the dependent variable.
4. This is a causal hypothesis. Care coordination is the independent variable administered to one group (experimental), and another group (control) did not get care coordination or got something else. Both groups are compared with regard to the dependent variable, health outcomes.

TEST-TAKING TIP: Recall the definition of a causal hypothesis and analyze the causal

relationship proposed by the statement. An independent variable, such as a treatment, approach, or intervention, is manipulated to cause an effect on another variable, the dependent one.

Content Area: *Hypothesis;* ***Cognitive Level:*** *Application;* ***Question Type:*** *Multiple Choice*
CRITICAL THINKING FACILITATOR: Identify a causal hypothesis in a sample study. Why is this hypothesis causal and not associative?

25. 1. **An important factor to consider in feasibility is whether ethical issues can be addressed appropriately. If the study has ethical issues that will compromise the rights of research participants, then the study is not feasible to conduct.**
2. **The researchers (and most importantly the principal investigator) must have the knowledge and skill to design and complete the research project. The experience of the researchers will facilitate all aspects of the project, ensure its timely completion, uphold ethical principles to protect research participants, and make a commitment to a project that will make significant contributions to evidence-based practice.**
3. The availability of extensive literature is not a factor to consider in determining the feasibility of the study. In fact, a dearth of literature validates the need for the study.
4. **Availability of resources is an important factor to consider in determining feasibility. Studies require material and human resources. Most research studies apply for funding to meet all types of expenditures.**
5. Potential influence on practice is not a feasibility factor. The contribution of a study to the profession is related to its significance, not its feasibility

TEST-TAKING TIP: The key word in the question stem is "feasibility." Feasibility asks, "Can this be done?" or "Is this possible to do?" In a research study, what is needed to get the project started and completed successfully? Have you ever heard of a feasibility survey?

Content Area: *Feasibility;* ***Cognitive Level:*** *Comprehension;* ***Question Type:*** *Multiple Response*
CRITICAL THINKING FACILITATOR: Think of a project that you completed in the past. What were your considerations before you embarked on this project? If you intend to achieve your goal, then you must consider feasibility.

26. 1. Availability of resources is not the specific feasibility factor addressed. Resources include space, equipment, and supplies.
2. **Researcher experience is the feasibility factor considered in this situation. The mentor would provide expert guidance to the novice researcher. Their working together ensures effective conduct and successful completion of the research project.**
3. Funding is not the feasibility factor addressed in this situation. Funding implies financial support for the research project to use for expenses such as remuneration for research assistants, stipends for research subjects, and consultation fees, just to name a few.
4. Potential influence on practice is not a consideration for feasibility; rather, it refers to the significance of the study.

TEST-TAKING TIP: The key words in the situation are "novice researcher" and "mentor." Whereas a novice is inexperienced, a mentor is someone who has a level of expertise and experience beyond the novice level.

Content Area: *Feasibility;* ***Cognitive Level:*** *Comprehension;* ***Question Type:*** *Multiple Choice*
CRITICAL THINKING FACILITATOR: If you identified the feasibility factors of your project in the Critical Thinking Facilitator in question 25, how did you address each factor to ensure the success of your project?

27. 1. Researcher experience has implications for the design and conduct of the research, but it is not the factor addressed in this situation.
2. Availability of subjects means that recruitment of research participants would yield adequate numbers of subjects who meet the criteria and are willing to participate.
3. Access to equipment is a feasibility consideration, but it is not the one addressed in this situation.
4. **Ethical considerations are major factors in considering feasibility. Potential risks to subjects such as discomfort, breach of privacy, or violation of participants' rights are major considerations.**

TEST-TAKING TIP: The key phrase in the situation is "ensured no harm." This refers to ethical guidelines in research.

Content Area: *Feasibility;* ***Cognitive Level:*** *Application;* ***Question Type:*** *Multiple Choice*
CRITICAL THINKING FACILITATOR: Recall the basic ethical principles in research. Pick

a sample study and identify an ethical principle of that study. What did the researcher do to address feasibility relative to this ethical aspect?

28. **1. This statement would be a correct rationale for deeming a study significant. Remember that new research builds on previous research to form the scientific base for the discipline.**

2. This statement would be a correct rationale for deeming a study significant. The overall goal of nursing research is to improve patient outcomes. Studies that can contribute to education and practice facilitate evidence-based practice and improve healthcare outcomes.

3. Enhancement of the expertise of the nurse researcher might be an end result, but this does not address significance of the study.

4. The National Institute for Nursing Research, Sigma Theta Tau International Honor Society of Nursing, the American Nurses Association, and other nursing organizations with research as one of their goals address research priorities to facilitate and support practitioners in providing quality care based on research outcomes. Therefore, a study that addresses these priorities would be considered a significant project.

5. A study that assures the protection of research subjects addresses the ethical aspects and not the significance of the study.

TEST-TAKING TIP: The key word in the question stem is "significant." A study is significant when it has the potential for making contributions to the practice of the discipline. Improvement of outcomes, whether in education, practice, or research, would make the study a significant one.

Content Area: *Critiquing Significance of the Research Problem;* ***Cognitive Level:*** *Application;* ***Question Type:*** *Multiple Response*

CRITICAL THINKING FACILITATOR:
Review the rationales that make a study and potential findings significant to education and practice of the discipline. Select a familiar study and determine its potential contribution to evidence-based practice.

29. 1. This question is not appropriate to ask in critically appraising a study's research problem. It asks about the study's ethical aspects.

2. This question is not appropriate to ask in critically appraising a study's research problem. It asks about the study's research hypothesis.

3. This question is appropriate when critiquing the study's research problem. It asks whether findings from studying this problem would make contributions to the discipline and to evidence-based practice.

4. This question is not appropriate to ask in critically appraising a study's research problem because it inquires about the design of the study.

TEST-TAKING TIP: The key word in the question stem is "significant." A study is significant when it has the potential for making contributions to the practice of the discipline. Improvement of outcomes, whether in education, practice, or research, would make the study a significant one.

Content Area: *Critiquing the Research Problem;* ***Cognitive Level:*** *Analysis;* ***Question Type:*** *Multiple Choice*

CRITICAL THINKING FACILITATOR:
What are the other appropriate questions to ask in appraising the research problem and problem statement of a study?

30. 1. This question is not a correct one. The hypothesis is not derived from the purpose of the study.

2. This question is not an accurate one to ask because the recruitment process of subjects is not addressed by a hypothesis.

3. This is the appropriate question to ask. A hypothesis is a statement of a relationship between variables.

4. The hypothesis does not articulate the significance of the topic to nursing or healthcare.

TEST-TAKING TIP: The key word in the question stem is "hypothesis." Recall the definition of the hypothesis and its difference from the other parts of the research study, including the research problem and problem statement.

Content Area: *Critiquing the Hypothesis;* ***Cognitive Level:*** *Analysis;* ***Question Type:*** *Multiple Choice*

CRITICAL THINKING FACILITATOR:
Look at one of the hypotheses in any study. Is it clearly expressed? Why or why not?

7 Searching for Relevant Literature

KEY WORDS

The following words include English vocabulary, nursing/medical terminology, concepts, principles, or information relevant to content specifically addressed in the chapter or associated with topics presented in it. English dictionaries, your nursing textbooks, and medical dictionaries such as *Taber's Cyclopedic Medical Dictionary* are resources that can be used to expand your knowledge and understanding of these words and related information.

Ancestry approach
Boolean operators
Citation
Complex search
Consistencies
Database
Gap
Generalizability
Inconsistencies
Monograph
Peer review
Relevant source
Search fields

QUESTIONS

Purposes of a Literature Review

1. Which of the following are purposes of a literature review? **Select all that apply.** A literature review
   1. predicts the outcomes of the study.
   2. assists in interpreting data.
   3. facilitates sample recruitment.
   4. helps shape the research question.
   5. sums up the current state of the problem.

Literature Review Processes and Terminology

2. One type of source that could be included in a literature review is a monograph. Which statement best describes a monograph? A monograph is
   1. the "documentation of the origin of the cited quote or idea and provides enough information for the readers to locate the original material" (Burns & Grove, 2010, p. 190).
   2. literature on a "specific topic, a record of conference proceedings, or a pamphlet, usually a one-time publication, and may be updated with a new edition" (p. 190).
   3. literature that includes "concept analyses, models, theories, and conceptual frameworks that support a selected research problem and purpose" (p. 190).
   4. literature that consists of research reports of published and unpublished research studies, including master's theses and doctoral dissertations.

3. A(n) __________ source is one that has a "direct bearing on the problem of concern." (Burns & Grove, 2010, p. 190).

4. Which of the following statements are true regarding bibliographical databases? **Select all that apply.**
   1. There are two types of bibliographical databases, the publisher's and the indexing databases.
   2. Databases consist of citations of works from only one discipline.
   3. Databases facilitate the quick retrieval and printing of information.
   4. Materials from library-held databases can be accessed via the Internet.
   5. RefWorks is an example of a database for the healthcare professions.

5. Which of the following is the most important advantage of searching the Internet for literature?
   1. The search can be quick and low in cost.
   2. Web sites are primary sources of research studies.
   3. Available documents have a high degree of accuracy.
   4. Retrieved data tend to be well organized.

6. What does it mean to "limit a search?" **Select all that apply.**
   1. Stipulate the number of articles one wants to view.
   2. Request only a specific type of literature.
   3. Specify the time range of the publications.
   4. Restrict the language of the publications.
   5. Search only those resources owned by the library.

7. Nocturia can be a disruptive problem among women. In a study on overactive bladder (OAB) and nocturia, researchers reported that "[s]ixty- three percent (N = 316 of 500) of nationally representative American women reported that not getting enough sleep throws off their sense of 'normalcy'" (Levkowicz, Whitmore, & Muller, 2011, p. 109). The information in parentheses above is a(n)
   1. hypothesis.
   2. position statement.
   3. citation.
   4. opinion.

8. In doing a literature search, the researcher uses key words. Which of the following statements are true regarding key words? **Select all that apply.**
   1. They can be "alternative terms (synonyms for concepts and variables)" (Burns & Grove, 2010, p. 211).
   2. They "are the major concepts or variables of a research problem or topic" (p. 211).
   3. They are citations that could provide information for locating references.
   4. They "combine two or more concepts or synonyms in one search" (p. 213).
   5. They "are the various categories of the information provided about an article by the bibliographic database" (p. 216).

9. Which of the following statements is true about a search field? A search field
   1. is a compilation of citations for an article.
   2. consists of the major concepts or variables of a research problem or topic.
   3. includes library sources for research reports.
   4. contains information about an article provided by the database.

10. A researcher wants to determine what studies have been done on life satisfaction among frail elderly adults and limits the search to literature in the past 5 years. What strategy will the researcher use?
    1. Limited review of the literature
    2. Mapping
    3. Ancestry approach
    4. Complex search approach

11. ________________, such as AND, OR, NOT, AND NOT, can be used to "expand or restrict a search" (Polit & Beck 2014, p. 120).

12. Which of the following statements is true regarding CINAHL? It is
   1. a primary source for biomedical literature.
   2. a database that can be accessed via PubMed.
   3. a database for nursing and allied health journals.
   4. a type of software that includes EndNote, RefWorks, and Zotero.

Critiquing Literature Reviews

13. A number of themes could be analyzed and synthesized in a literature review. What question can be asked when the generalizability or transferability of findings is analyzed and synthesized?
   1. "What gaps are there in the evidence?" (Polit & Beck, 2014, p. 125).
   2. "To what types of people or settings does the evidence apply?" (p. 125).
   3. "What methods have been used to address the question?" (p. 125).
   4. "What are the major methodological deficiencies and strengths?" (p. 125).

14. What are the characteristics of an informative and useful literature review? **Select all that apply.**
   1. Inconsistent results are omitted from the review.
   2. There is a summary that critically synthesizes the current evidence.
   3. There are multiple quotes and abstracts of different studies on the topic.
   4. There is a clustering of studies with comparable or similar findings.
   5. A clear need for the study is carefully articulated.

15. Which of the following statements are more likely to be included in a literature review? **Select all that apply.**
   1. A study by Yoon and Kim (2013) found that Korean nurses are at high risk for job-related stress and depressive symptoms.
   2. Levkowicz, Whitmore, & Muller (2011) contend that "The number of trips taken to the bathroom at night by women with nocturia may be more significant than acknowledged by healthcare providers and deserves more attention" (p. 106).
   3. It is a fact that diabetes in the U.S. population has reached epidemic proportions. Many patients with diabetes have been found to lack the knowledge and skills necessary to manage their illness.
   4. A cultural norm among persons with Hispanic backgrounds is respect for older family members. Elders from this culture are well respected and are viewed with esteem by the younger generation.
   5. "Anthony (1974) engaged in the study of children who seemed invulnerable or resilient to adverse life situations and discovered that certain children did well despite numerous risks and hardships" (Taylor & Hawkins, 2012, p. 2).

16. Which of the following questions is appropriate in critiquing a literature review?
   1. "Does the author paraphrase, or is there an overreliance on quotes from original sources?" (Polit & Beck, 2014, p. 127).
   2. "Does the report offer evidence of reliability of measures?" (p. 209).
   3. "Did the researchers use the best methods of capturing study phenomena?" (p. 193).
   4. "Does the report formally present a statement of purpose, research question, and/or hypothesis?" (p. 111).

17. In critiquing the literature section of a research study, what is usually made clear by the researcher at the conclusion of the review?
   1. There is an abundance of information on the topic.
   2. There is a dearth of literature on the topic.
   3. The significance and need for the study justify the investigation.
   4. There will be an attempt to prove the hypothesis as proposed.

18. In critiquing the review of the literature section of a research report, the reader identifies a gap in the body of knowledge about the topic. Which of the following statements reflects a gap?

1. "It is critical that programs are developed that help employees prevent and manage symptoms of job-related stress, thus enabling their long-term future success" (Yoon & Kim, 2013, p. 169).
2. "Daytime urinary frequency is the hallmark symptom of OAB, but how many times are women with OAB going to the bathroom during their waking hours, and how often are they getting up in the night?" (Levkowicz, Whitmore, & Muller, 2011, p. 107)
3. "If participants could not be reached following two attempts, the call was skipped and the next call was attempted at the scheduled date" (Hawkins, 2010, p. 221).
4. "Currently, there is only one study that has assessed medication adherence among older APS clients, but this study was not specific to older adults who are self-neglecting" (Grocki & Huffman, 2007; as cited in Turner et al., 2012, p. 742).

ANSWERS AND RATIONALES

The correct answer number and rationale for why it is the correct answer are given in **boldface blue type.** Rationales for why the other possible answer options are incorrect also are given, but they are not in boldface type.

1. 1. Based on the findings of other studies, a researcher might be able to propose an expected outcome (hypothesis), but there is no way to predict the outcome solely based on the literature review.
   2. The literature review would include studies that are relevant to the topic and variables of the current study. The researcher doing the current study could use findings of other studies and relate them to their current results. Statements relating the findings with previous works would be seen in the analysis of the data or discussion section (or both) of the published reports.
   3. Although the researcher conducting the literature review would have information about sampling from the reviewed studies, he or she cannot use the information in facilitating sample recruitment. The information gleaned from previous studies might help the current researchers avoid sampling errors.
   4. The literature review helps the researcher shape the current research question based on what has been done and what needs to be done by the proposed study.
   5. The current state of the topic or research problem can be analyzed by the researcher in the process of conceptualizing the study. What is known or not known about the topic could guide the researcher in shaping the question for the intended study.

   TEST-TAKING TIP: The key words are "literature review." Sometime in your academic programs, you have had to write a scholarly paper. Your topic might have come from a broad area, or it could have been very specific. In the conceptual phase of your project, you would have had to make a trip to the library or search the Internet for related material on the topic.

   Content Area: *Purposes of a Literature Review:* ***Cognitive Level:*** *Comprehension;* ***Question Type:*** *Multiple Response*
   CRITICAL THINKING FACILITATOR: Identify the section of a study that addresses the review of relevant literature. Note that some research reports do not have a separate section. Instead the literature review might be found in the introduction or background sections. Discern what this section means in relation to the topic. Does it provide a clear picture of where the topic is? Could you tell how the current study would fill the gap in the topic?

2. 1. The statement is a description of a citation.
   2. The statement describes a monograph. The clue in the option is "a one-time publication."
   3. The statement describes theoretical literature.
   4. The statement describes data-based literature.

   TEST-TAKING TIP: The key word in the question stem is "monograph." The prefix *mono-* means "one or single." Option 2 has the words "one-time publication."

   Content Area: *Literature Review Processes and Terminology;* ***Cognitive Level:*** *Knowledge;* ***Question Type:*** *Multiple Choice*
   CRITICAL THINKING FACILITATOR: Where have you encountered monographs? Why are monographs considered essential literature? Perhaps if you have a subscription to a journal, you might have gotten a special issue covering a single topic. Several nursing journals produce monographs on topics such as falls, pain, or pressure ulcers, just to name a few.

3. **relevant**

   TEST-TAKING TIP: The key words in the question stem are "direct bearing." ***Direct*** **means "first-hand," and the synonym for** ***bearing*** **is "relevance."**

   Content Area: *Literature Review Processes and Terminology;* ***Cognitive Level:*** *Knowledge;* ***Question Type:*** *Fill-in-the-Blank*
   CRITICAL THINKING FACILITATOR: Think of a potential topic or problem for research. What relevant areas would be part of the literature review? When the study has variables, what are potential studies related to each of the variables?

4. **1. The publishers' databases are "used by publishers to distribute their materials online" (Burns & Grove, 2010, p. 210). The indexing databases are "databases created after the publishers have made the material available" (p. 210).**
   2. This statement is not accurate. "A database may consist of citations relevant to a specific discipline or may be a broad collections of citations from a variety of disciplines" (p. 210).
   3. The statement is correct because databases make searching and retrieving information much easier.

4. The statement is correct. Faculty, staff, and students in academic settings can now look at their library's databases through the Internet. The user's computer must be networked with the institution's server. Requirements are a username and password.
5. RefWorks is not a database; it is reference-management software.

TEST-TAKING TIP: The key word in the question stem is "database." Identify what databases are used for. They are compilation of scholarly works organized for easy access and retrieval. Most databases would include works from several major disciplines related by a common focus such as health.

Content Area: *Literature Review Processes and Terminology;* ***Cognitive Level:*** *Knowledge;* ***Question Type:*** *Multiple Response*
CRITICAL THINKING FACILITATOR: What are some common databases you know? What is the overall link among the disciplines that are included in the database? How helpful are these databases in your work? How do you access these databases?

5. 1. Easy access and low cost relative to information are the most important advantages of using the Internet.
2. This statement is not accurate. Although there is an abundance of information, the best and primary sources of research information are professional databases, not the Internet.
3. This statement is not accurate. The mixture of information, both lay and professional, makes it difficult to judge the accuracy and validity of information. Research studies published in reputable journals are peer reviewed.
4. This statement is not accurate. The researcher has to use a system to organize retrieved data.

TEST-TAKING TIP: There are no key words in the question stem to help in arriving at the correct option. One has to think of the kinds of information that could be obtained through the Internet. Try to do a search on a topic and see how much information you can get. Judge the time and costs to you. What types of information do you get? What can you say about the accuracy of the information? What is the source of the information?

Content Area: *Literature Processes and Terminology;* ***Cognitive Level:*** *Analysis;* ***Question Type:*** *Multiple Choice*
CRITICAL THINKING FACILITATOR: Compare a literature search using CINAHL and Google. What kinds of material did you get for both searches? How would you go about validating the accuracy of the information you obtained? Which information would you use for a scholarly work?

6. 1. When one does a search, one uses keywords and completes the database's search fields. The number of "hits" relates to the broadness or narrowness of the search fields.
2. A way to limit a search is to stipulate the type of publication. For instance, one can stipulate only research studies that have been peer reviewed.
3. A way to limit the search is to specify the time range such as within the past 5 years.
4. One can also restrict the language. If you request literature only in English, then you will not get publications in Spanish or French.
5. One cannot require the search to come up with publications owned by the library. There is a way, however, to find out which publications are available in the library. For holdings not owned by the library, there is the interlibrary loan whereby the library can obtain the materials from another library.

TEST-TAKING TIP: The key word is "limit." If the search is getting too many hits, it is necessary to specify requirements for the search (i.e., narrow the search). Types of publications, language used, and time frame can be specified.

Content Area: *Literature Review Processes and Terminology;* ***Cognitive Level:*** *Analysis;* ***Question Type:*** *Multiple Response*
CRITICAL THINKING FACILITATOR: If you have ever done a search for literature for a paper, you have used the search field of a database. Recall how you narrowed your search so that you would only get the information directly relevant to your topic.

7. 1. A hypothesis states a relationship between two or more variables.
2. A position statement expresses someone's perspectives on an issue or topic.
3. A citation is information used to locate a reference.
4. An opinion is a subjective judgment about something. It may or may not be based on a sound rationale.

TEST-TAKING TIP: Derived from the verb *cite*, *citation* means to refer to something for verification. A statement with information for the reader to verify or check the source of the statement is a citation. Citations guide readers with the necessary information to locate literature used as evidence.

Content Area: *Literature Review Processes and Terminology;* ***Cognitive Level:*** *Analysis;* ***Question Type:*** *Multiple Choice*

CRITICAL THINKING FACILITATOR: Why are citations important to include in scholarly works? When you get one publication on a topic, how do you get to other resources, particularly those used by the author whose work you are using? One publication leads you to several more and so on. Say you see statements about a research instrument in a research report. The researcher would cite sources to support her or his statements about the instrument. Those citations can be used to obtain more information. Authors have an obligation to provide accurate and complete citations.

8. **1. Synonyms for concepts and variables can be used as key words when doing literature searches.**
2. Key words can also be the major concepts or variables of the study.
3. Key words are not citations. Citations include information that guide in retrieving information relative to a topic.
4. Two or more synonyms or concepts in one search are called a complex search.
5. Search fields include the information about an article provided by the database.

TEST-TAKING TIP: Know the meaning of key words that would trigger a search. Key words are the major words in a title, and knowing these would help one in identifying the main idea(s) in published works.

Content Area: *Literature Review Processes and Terminology;* ***Cognitive Level:*** *Comprehension;* ***Question Type:*** *Multiple Response*

CRITICAL THINKING FACILITATOR: Look at several titles of research studies. If you were to search the literature, what are the key words you would use? If you were writing a paper about an experience, what words would you use so that your title conveys the main idea to the readers?

9. 1. A reference list is a compilation of citations for an article or publication.
2. The major concepts or variables used for a literature search are the key words.
3. Library sources include all the resources of the library, including bibliographic databases.
4. The search field has the information provided by the database. The search field allows one to customize the search.

TEST-TAKING TIP: The key word is "search field." A search field would need to have choices for the searcher to guide in limiting the search. For instance, the search field would allow one to select the type of publication, time frame of the publication, language of the publication, and so on.

Content Area: *Literature Review Processes and Terminology;* ***Cognitive Level:*** *Comprehension;* ***Question Type:*** *Multiple Choice*

CRITICAL THINKING FACILITATOR: Recall a time when you had to search for literature on a particular topic. You were able to specify the type of publication you wanted (research or nonresearch articles), time frame (within the past 5 years), in a specific language (English only). What would happen if you failed to specify what you wanted? You would get a large number of publications (many hits), and many of them would not be helpful.

10. 1. A limited review of the literature can be done by limiting the search, but the approach is not specific.
2. Mapping is a search strategy that "allows you to search for topics using your own key words, rather the exact subject heading used in the database" (Polit & Beck, 2014, p. 119).
3. The ancestry approach is a search strategy "in which citations from relevant studies are used to track down earlier research on which the studies are based" (p. 119).
4. A complex search "combines two or more concepts or synonyms in one search" (p. 119).

TEST-TAKING TIP: The key phrase in the question stem is "in the past 5 years." This means that the search moves back 5 years earlier. When someone asks you to create a genogram, you move backward to trace your beginnings, your ancestry, including your parents, grandparents, great grandparents, and so on.

Content Area: *Literature Review Processes and Terminology;* ***Cognitive Level:*** *Comprehension;* ***Question Type:*** *Multiple Choice*

CRITICAL THINKING FACILITATOR: If you did a literature review on a topic and limited the search to the past 5 years, would the state of the topic be the same as if your search went 10 years back? Probably not, and it shouldn't be! One of the reasons researchers have a program of research is to build and develop their research interest. Their updated findings are essential in evidence-based practice. Think of well-known researchers and how they started and where they are now in their work.

11. **Boolean operators**

TEST-TAKING TIP: Recall any introductions to library research you may have had, also recall any tricks you learned if you have done a literature search.

Content Area: *Literature Review Processes and Terminology;* ***Cognitive Level:*** *Knowledge;* ***Question Type:*** *Fill-in-the-Blank*

CRITICAL THINKING FACILITATOR: A research course opens many new doors for students who acquire a "new set of glasses" to see the world. You also acquire new skills or refine old ones such as library skills. In your search for information, you will come across terms such as *Boolean operators* and others. How has your vocabulary changed now that you are speaking the language of research?

12. 1. The primary source for biomedical literature is Medline.
 2. Medline can be accessed via PubMed.
 3. CINAHL is the database for nursing and allied health disciplines.
 4. EndNote, RefWorks, and Zotero are reference-management systems.

TEST-TAKING TIP: Know that CINAHL is an acronym. If you know that it stands for Cumulative Index for Nursing and Allied Health Literature, then it would be easy to select the correct option.

Content Area: *Literature Review Processes and Terminology;* ***Cognitive Level:*** *Knowledge;* ***Question Type:*** *Multiple Choice*

CRITICAL THINKING FACILITATOR: When you hear unfamiliar words spoken by others, what do you usually do? Ask for a definition or example? Look them up later? Ignore them? For instance, many people use the acronym AIDS. But how many people really know what it stands for? If you are someone who has a sense of curiosity, you would look it up and discover that it is more than just four letters of the alphabet. So, too, with CINAHL; it is a huge database that opens a big door to knowledge or at least supports your quest for it.

13. 1. The question asks about substantive themes in a literature review.
 2. The question is appropriate to ask in analyzing and synthesizing the generalizability or transferability of research findings.
 3. The question asks about methodologic themes in a literature review.
 4. The question asks about methodologic themes in a literature review.

TEST-TAKING TIP: The key words in the question stem are "generalizability" and "transferability." "Generalizability is the degree to which the research methods justify the inference that the findings are true for a broader group than study participants; in particular, the inference that the findings can be generalized from the sample to the population" (Polit & Beck, 2014, p. 381). "Transferability is the extent to which qualitative findings can be transferred to other setting or groups; analogous to generalizability" (p. 393).

Content Area: *Critiquing the Literature Review;* ***Cognitive Level:*** *Analysis;* ***Question Type:*** *Multiple Choice*

CRITICAL THINKING FACILITATOR: Review the purposes of a literature review. Match these with the types of analysis of themes (substantive, methodologic, and generalizability or transferability) one would do. Some of the questions might be similar to the questions for a critique. Remember, though, that you are looking at the entire review of the literature within the context of the new study.

14. 1. The statement is incorrect. Studies with inconsistent results are usually clustered together, and the literature reviewer analyzes the inconsistencies in light of other studies. These studies are definitely not excluded from the review.
 2. A helpful literature review has a summary that presents the synthesized state of current evidence on the topic. This summary is enlightening in understanding the need for the current study and its potential contribution to the discipline (its significance).
 3. The literature review would include salient information about the reviewed studies, but multiple quotes and abstracts are not included, nor are they necessary.
 4. Studies with comparable or similar findings are clustered, and just like the studies with inconsistent results, they are analyzed within the context of the topic and the current state of the evidence.
 5. A clear need for the current study is articulated and becomes evident as one reads the review of the literature section of a research report.

TEST-TAKING TIP: The key words in the question stem are "informative" and "useful." The most important purpose of a literature review is that it tells the reader the state of the art of the topic (what has been done and the current state of the topic). The review also shows the current researcher what direction to take and what needs to be done.

Content Area: *Critiquing the Literature Review;* ***Cognitive Level:*** *Analysis;* ***Question Type:*** *Multiple Response*

CRITICAL THINKING FACILITATOR: Look at one of the studies in the appendix of your core textbook and read the literature review section. Can you identify any studies that have inconsistent findings? What about those with consistent findings? Were gaps identified by the researcher? With the information on inconsistent and consistent findings and gaps, are you able to articulate the need for the study and what the researcher might want to do?

15. 1. **The statement describes a research finding that is appropriate to include in a review of the literature.**
2. **The statement by the researchers is an appropriate statement to include in a literature review.**
3. The statement indicates important information, but it lacks the link with research evidence that is the focus of the literature review. The statement might be more appropriate as background information.
4. The statement lacks the research link to consider it as part of the current evidence for the research topic.
5. **The statement indicates a research finding and is appropriate to include in a review of the literature.**

TEST-TAKING TIP: The key phrase in the question stem is "more likely to be included." You know that the review of literature includes research evidence. Look at the options that indicate statements of findings from research studies.

Content Area: *Critiquing the Literature Review;* ***Cognitive Level:*** *Analysis;* ***Question Type:*** *Multiple Response*

CRITICAL THINKING FACILITATOR: What would help in identifying appropriate statements that belong in a literature review for a research study? Read a literature review of any study and look at the statements made by the researcher in presenting the information. Where did the statements come from? Look at the citation(s) following the statement and check out the references for the authors and the complete citations. The citations lead you to more information.

16. 1. **The question is appropriate in critiquing the literature review of a research report. The key word in the question is "sources," meaning the literature on the topic.**
2. The question is appropriate to ask when critiquing the quality of research instruments (i.e., their reliability and validity).
3. The question is appropriate to ask when critiquing the data collection methods of a research study. The key words in this option are "capturing the study phenomena."
4. The question is appropriate to ask when critiquing the research question, purpose, and hypothesis of a study. Question, purpose, and hypothesis are in the words included in the option.

TEST-TAKING TIP: Look carefully at each option and identify a clue. Option 1 has the word "sources." ***Sources*** **would refer to literature.**

Content Area: *Critiquing the Literature Review;* ***Cognitive Level:*** *Analysis;* ***Question Type:*** *Multiple Choice*

CRITICAL THINKING FACILITATOR: What are the appropriate questions to ask when critiquing the literature review of a research report? What are your expectations based on what you know about the purposes of the review? Make a list of these questions and compare them with the questions suggested by the authors of your research textbook.

17. 1. The current evidence of a topic is usually discussed at the beginning or in the body of the literature review.
2. The dearth of evidence on the research topic is usually described at the beginning of the research report such as in the introduction or background.
3. **The review of the literature concludes with a statement articulating the significance and need for the study along with the purpose(s) for the investigation. This is appropriate at the end of the literature review, after the researcher has laid down the foundation for the current study.**
4. A hypothesis might be part of the last section of the literature review, but this is not always the case. Through the hypothesis, the researcher shows the relationship (strong or weak) between or among the variables of the study.

TEST-TAKING TIP: The key phrase in the question stem is "at the conclusion of the review." This phrase indicates a summary or a closing perspective. After discussing the current evidence on the topic, the researcher justifies the need and potential significance of the current study to the discipline.

Content Area: *Critiquing the Literature Review;* ***Cognitive Level:*** *Analysis;* ***Question Type:*** *Multiple Choice*

CRITICAL THINKING FACILITATOR: Look at a sample research study. Locate the literature review sections. If there is no separate section, read the background section. Look at the paragraph just above the methods. This is usually the summary or the closing statement about the literature review.

Are you able to identify the statements describing the need for the study and its significance?

18. 1. The statement explains the need for the study.
2. The statement articulates the concern with the topic of interest.
3. The statement describes an aspect of methodology or a procedural aspect.
4. **The statement describes a gap in the knowledge and evidence regarding the topic. The scarcity of evidence provides the rationale and the need for the study.**

TEST-TAKING TIP: The key word in the question stem is "gap," which means an opening or empty space. When there is a dearth of evidence in a topic, then a gap exists. The role of research is to fill those gaps in evidence or knowledge.

Content Area: *Critiquing the Literature Review;* ***Cognitive Level:*** *Analysis;* ***Question Type:*** *Multiple Choice*

CRITICAL THINKING FACILITATOR: Look at a quantitative study and read over the literature review or the background section. Identify gaps in the current evidence. Be alert for a statement such as: "Although a number of studies have shown a relationship among XYZ variables, none has looked at ___________." Another statement to watch for would be something like this: "Two studies have looked at XYZ variables and have found a strong relationship with ________, but none has considered _________ (another variable) among ____________ (the sample)." Gaps in evidence might also relate to the types of subjects (rural vs. urban dwellers) and settings (hospital vs. community).

8 Describing Theories and Conceptual Frameworks and Models

KEY WORDS

The following words include English vocabulary, nursing/medical terminology, concepts, principles, or information relevant to content specifically addressed in the chapter or associated with topics presented in it. English dictionaries, your nursing textbooks, and medical dictionaries such as *Taber's Cyclopedic Medical Dictionary* are resources that can be used to expand your knowledge and understanding of these words and related information.

Concepts
Constructs
Models
Frameworks
Research program
Theory
Variables

QUESTIONS

Concepts in Research

1. Which of the following differentiates a concept from a variable? Unlike a variable, a concept
   1. "implies that the term is defined so that it is measurable and suggests that numerical values of the term are able to vary from one instance to another" (Burns & Grove, 2011, p. 230).
   2. "is an occurrence or a circumstance that is observed, something that impresses the observer as extraordinary, or a thing that appears to and is constructed by the mind" (p. 544).
   3. "is a term that abstractly describes and names an object, idea, or phenomenon, thus providing it with a separate identity or meaning" (p. 230).
   4. "is an area of concern in which there is a gap in the knowledge base needed for nursing practice" (p. 547).
2. Which of the following are concepts? **Select all that apply.**
   1. Hierarchy of human needs
   2. Self-efficacy
   3. Resilience
   4. Health promotion model
   5. Health

Theories in Research and Evidence-Based Practice

3. A theory is defined as "an integrated set of defined concepts and statements that present a view of a phenomenon and can be used to __describe__, __explain__, __predict__ and __control__ that phenomenon" (Burns & Grove, 2011, p. 228).

4. Why are theories important to research and evidence-based practice? **Select all that apply. Theories**
1. "Explain phenomena important to clinical practice" (Burns & Grove, 2011, p. 227).
2. Serve as "initial inspiration for developing a study" (p. 227).
3. Provide "insight or understanding of a situation or an event as a whole that usually cannot be logically explained" (p. 540).
4. Are the "meaning of research conclusions for the body of knowledge, theory, and practice" (p. 540).
5. Facilitate "the interpretation of research findings" (p. 227).

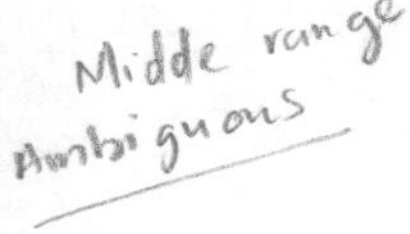

5. Which of the following statements is true about middle-range theories of nursing? Middle-range theories
1. "attempt to explain broad areas and include numerous concepts that are not well defined and that have ambiguous and unclear relationships" (Fain, 2009, p. 67).
2. include Orem's Self-Care Deficit Theory.
3. include the germ theory and principles of infection.
4. "focus on answering particular practice questions and often specify factors such as patients' health conditions, family situations, and nursing actions" (Tomey & Alligood, 2006; as cited in Burns & Grove, 2011, p. 235).

6. Marek et al.'s (2013) study looked at older adults' enhanced self-management of medications. They proposed that "care coordination and use of technology are two mechanisms to support older adults" (p. 269). Identify the basic concepts in the two statements that would serve as study variables. **Select all that apply.**
1. Self-management of medications
2. Care coordination
3. Two mechanisms
4. Older adults
5. Use of technology

7. __Practice theory__ are more specific than middle-range theories because they propose specific approaches to particular nursing situations.

8. Which of the following statements from a study indicates the researcher's use of intervention theory?
1. "On the basis of life-course theory and social determinants of health, we proposed that low-income women bring with them enduring burdens of socio-economic disadvantage that often affect their health" (Walker, Sterling, Guy, & Mahometa, 2013, p. 234).
2. "The purpose of the study is to investigate potential ambiguities of the National Quality Forum definition of falls and to explore the impact of fall classification at the individual, unit, or hospital level" (Simon, Klaus, Gajewski, & Dunton, 2013, p. 74).
3. "The independent contribution of fatigue to depression, satisfaction with ability, and perceived health impairment in RA [rheumatoid arthritis] patients was determined" (Franklin & Harrell, 2013, p. 404).
4. "Adolescents can use peer resistance skills to avoid being pressured into risky behavior, such as early sexual behavior. Avatar-based reality technology offers a novel way to help build these skills" (Norris, Hughes, Hecht, Peragallo, & Nickerson, 2013, p. 25).

9. **Study Title:** Lai, H. L., Li, Y. M., & Lee, L. H. (2011). The effects of music intervention with nursing presence and recorded music on psycho-physiological indices of cancer patient caregivers. What type of theory would these researchers use in this study? **Select all that apply.**
   1. Grand theory
   2. Intervention theory
   3. Scientific theory
   4. Middle-range theory
   5. Borrowed theory

Conceptual Models and Frameworks

10. Conceptual models are unlike theories in several ways. Select all that apply. A conceptual model
    1. "broadly explains a phenomenon of interest" (Burns & Grove, 2011, p. 228).
    2. consists of "defined concepts and statements that present a view of a phenomenon" (p. 228).
    3. reflects the researcher's philosophical perspectives.
    4. can be used as an umbrella for a study.
    5. do not include assumptions about the phenomenon.

11. Which of the following ways would best facilitate knowledge building for evidence-based practice?
    1. Presentation of the model in a conference, convention, and other professional meetings
    2. Publication of the development of the model in peer-reviewed scholarly publications
    3. Publication of a monograph by the developer of the model
    4. Conducting research studies related to the conceptual model by scholars

Qualitative Research and Theory

12. Which statement is true regarding qualitative research? Qualitative research studies
    1. deduce their hypothesis from a theory developed from a number of studies.
    2. "identify the critical concepts and processes that characterize a phenomenon" (Burns & Grove, 2011, p. 245).
    3. merge a number of conceptual frameworks and theories to support the study hypothesis.
    4. "often examine multiple factors to understand a phenomenon not previously well studied" (p. 242).

Critiquing the Framework of a Study

13. Which of the following statements would be used to critique the framework of a study?
    1. "Do hypotheses (if any) flow from a theory or previous research?" (Polit & Beck, 2014, p. 111).
    2. "If there is an intervention, are intervention components consistent with the theory?" (p. 143).
    3. "Are relevant landmark studies described?" (Burns & Grove, 2011, p. 202).
    4. "How might the research contribute to nursing practice, administration, education, or policy?" (Polit & Beck, 2014, p. 111).

ANSWERS AND RATIONALES

The correct answer number and rationale for why it is the correct answer are given in **boldface blue type.** Rationales for why the other possible answer options are incorrect also are given, but they are not in boldface type.

1. 1. This statement is the definition of a variable. A clue in the option is the word "vary."
2. This statement is the definition of a phenomenon.
3. **This statement is the definition of a concept; a concept is only a name given to something.**
4. This statement is the definition of a research problem. Although there might several concepts in a research problem, the research problem expresses what is needed for the investigation.

TEST-TAKING TIP: The key word in the question stem is "concept," which means an idea. When someone has an idea, it is just the beginning of something. Although the idea could have a name to identify it, the originator of the idea has not fully described or developed the idea. Further developments in the concept are needed before it can be used. Therefore, concepts are building blocks to theories.

Content Area: *Concepts in Research;* ***Cognitive Level:*** *Comprehension;* ***Question Type:*** *Multiple Choice*
CRITICAL THINKING FACILITATOR: If concepts are ideas, then think of all the concepts you know. You would fill up a small notebook. Take a concept you know and differentiate it from a variable.

2. 1. The hierarchy of human needs is a theory proposed by Abraham Maslow.
2. **Self-efficacy is a concept. It is abstract, and it is simply a name for something.**
3. **Resilience is also a concept that has been identified and has no specific description.**
4. The health promotion model is a theory proposed by Nola Pender.
5. **Health is a concept because it is simply a name for something.**

TEST-TAKING TIP: Because the question asks for concepts, look at the options that are single terms; these are concepts. Remember that concepts are abstract, and when one encounters a concept, one can identify it only by a name. The incorrect options have more than one word, so they must refer to other things, not concepts.

Content Area: *Concepts in Research;* ***Cognitive Level:*** *Application;* ***Question Type:*** *Multiple Response*

CRITICAL THINKING FACILITATOR:
Think of concepts as the building blocks of theories. Take a very well-known theory such as Maslow's hierarchy of human needs. Need is one concept in the theory. Other concepts emerged as the theorist developed the theory.

3. **describe, explain, predict, and control**

TEST-TAKING TIP: Review the purposes of a theory. Take a well-known theory, such as Selye's theory of stress, and think of how that theory would serve its different purposes.

Content Area: *Theory in Research;* ***Cognitive Level:*** *Knowledge;* ***Question Type:*** *Fill-in-the-Blank*
CRITICAL THINKING FACILITATOR: Look at a sample research study and locate the section identified as theory or theoretical framework. Read the information provided by the researcher about the theory. Then decide which purpose of the theory the information in the study serves.

4. 1. **Theories consist of concepts as building blocks, and the relationships of the concepts are expressed as hypotheses. Hypotheses, as proposed statements, are also used to explain and predict research outcomes.**
2. **"When an idea for a study emerges, researchers have a theory about what the study outcomes will be and why. This theory may not be formally stated or even written, but it is nonetheless an initial theory that stimulates ideas for a study" (Burns & Grove, 2011, p. 227).**
3. This statement is not reflective of theories. The statement is a definition of intuition.
4. This statement is a definition of the research study's implications for nursing.
5. **A theory consists of statements about how concepts interrelate. "A study tests the accuracy of theoretical ideas. In explaining the study findings, the researcher will interpret those findings in relation to the theory" (Burns & Grove, 2009; Smith & Liehr, 2008; as cited in Burns & Grove, 2011, p. 227).**

TEST-TAKING TIP: Think of theories as guidelines for discovering, creating, thinking, and doing. Each of these acts is inherent in the research process from inception to dissemination and eventually integration into evidence-based practice.

Content Area: *Theory in Research;* ***Cognitive Level:*** *Comprehension;* ***Question Type:*** *Multiple Response*

CRITICAL THINKING FACILITATOR: Look at two or more steps in a quantitative study. Can you identify the use of theory in these steps?

5\. 1. This statement is a definition of grand theories. "Because these theories are not grounded in empirical data, they are not useful as guides for nursing practice" (Fain, 2009, p. 67).
2. Orem's theory is an example of a grand theory.
3. The germ theory and principles of infection is a borrowed theory and not a nursing theory.
4. **This statement describes a middle-range nursing theory. Middle-range theories "look at a piece of reality and contain clearly defined variables in which the nature and direction of relationships are specified" (Fain, 2009, p. 67).**

TEST-TAKING TIP: Nursing is a practice discipline. It relies on research that improves care delivery. Middle-range theories focus on phenomena that are relevant to practice.

Content Area: *Theory in Research;* ***Cognitive Level:*** *Comprehension;* ***Question Type:*** *Multiple Choice*
CRITICAL THINKING FACILITATOR: Think of different clinical situations that interest you. A search of the literature would most likely yield a middle-range theory that can be used as a framework to study one of these situations. Most research textbooks have a table of these theories. Familiarize yourself with these.

6\. 1. **Self-management of medications is an initial concept of interest with the researchers' knowledge of the many issues relating to older adults' management of chronic illnesses including medication regimens. This concept would probably be the *variable* of interest or the dependent variable in the study.**
2. **Care coordination is another initial concept deemed important as a strategy to facilitate management of a medication regimen. Because this is identified as a strategy, this would serve as an independent variable.**
3. "Two mechanisms" is a concept, but it is not specific enough to serve as a variable.
4. Older adults are the potential target population.
5. **Use of technology is another initial concept deemed important as a strategy to facilitate management of a medication regimen. Because this is a strategy, it would serve as an independent variable.**

TEST-TAKING TIP: The key words in the question stem are "concepts" and "variables." In a research study, concepts become the variables of the study. The term *variable* "implies that the term is defined so that it is measurable and suggests the numerical values of the term are able to vary ('variable') from one instance to another" (Burns & Grove, 2011, p. 230).

Content Area: *Theory in Research;* ***Cognitive Level:*** *Analysis;* ***Question Type:*** *Multiple Response*
CRITICAL THINKING FACILITATOR: Look at a sample quantitative study and identify the concepts or variables of the study.

7\. **Practice theory**

TEST-TAKING TIP: The key phrase in the question is "propose specific approaches." Recall that an independent variable can be an approach, a program, a strategy, a treatment, or an intervention. A study with an intervention as the independent variable would use practice theory as a theoretical framework.

Content Area: *Theory in Research;* ***Cognitive Level:*** *Analysis;* ***Question Type:*** *Fill-in-the-Blank*
CRITICAL THINKING FACILITATOR: Look at studies that are experimental or quasi-experimental in design. (Hint: The abstract tells you the study's design.) These types of studies have an independent variable that is actively manipulated. What theory was used as a framework for the studies? How were elements of the theory integrated into the intervention?

8\. 1. This statement from the study does not indicate that a practice theory was used. The independent variables are social attributes that cannot be manipulated.
2. This statement indicates that the study was not an interventional one; therefore, the use of a practice theory is not appropriate. Additionally, the design of the study is nonexperimental, and no manipulation of an independent variable would be done.
3. This statement indicates that the theory for the study is not a practice theory. The independent variable is not an approach, a program, a strategy, or a treatment.
4. **This statement clearly indicates that this study used a practice theory because the independent variable will be manipulated. A strategy or program is implemented to determine its effects on a dependent variable.**

TEST-TAKING TIP: The clue in the question stem is "intervention." An intervention is a

"treatment or independent variable that is manipulated during the conduct of study to produce an effect on the dependent or outcome variables" (Burns & Grove, 2011, p. 540). Only option 4 has an intervention, peer resistance skills, mentioned in the research statement.

Content Area: *Theory in Research;* ***Cognitive Level:*** *Analysis;* ***Question Type:*** *Multiple Choice*

CRITICAL THINKING FACILITATOR: Review independent variables, specifically those that are used in experimental and quasi-experimental studies. Why are these studies also identified as intervention studies?

9. 1. A grand theory would not be appropriate. Grand theories are complex and broad in scope. Because these theories "are not grounded in empirical data, they are not as useful as guides for nursing practice" (Fain, 2009, p. 67).
2. **An intervention or practice theory would be appropriate to use because the independent variables are music intervention with nursing presence and recorded music.**
3. **A scientific theory would also be appropriate because the variables of interest (dependent variables or outcomes) are physiological ones, including heart and respiratory rates.**
4. Middle-range theories are more specific. However, there might not be one that could be used to study physiological variables.
5. **A borrowed theory might be appropriate to use. A physiological theory can be a borrowed theory as well.**

TEST-TAKING TIP: A clue in the study's title is "physiological indices." This indicates that some of the variables of interest are physiological. Examples of physiological variables are height, weight, blood pressure, temperature, pulse, respiration, and others. Studies with these variables use physiological or scientific theories.

Content Area: *Theory and Models in Research;* ***Cognitive Level:*** *Analysis;* ***Question Type:*** *Multiple Response*

CRITICAL THINKING FACILITATOR: Review other types of theories that can be used in nursing and healthcare research. Nursing has many different aspects, and the use of knowledge from other disciplines ensures a better understanding of humans that are the focus of nursing.

10. 1. **This statement is true of a conceptual model. The clue words are "broadly explains."**
2. This statement partially describes a theory.
3. **The philosophical perspectives of the researcher are part of the conceptual model.**
4. **A conceptual model can be used as the umbrella for the study because it includes the theories, assumptions, and philosophical perspectives of the researcher.**
5. This statement is not applicable to a conceptual model. Assumptions and philosophical perspectives of the developer of the model are integrated into the model.

TEST-TAKING TIP: The meaning of a theory is easier to grasp than that of a conceptual model. A conceptual model begins and evolves out of the thinking of the person developing it. Therefore, the emerging model includes the person's philosophical beliefs and assumptions about the phenomenon that is the focus of the model. Theories are built from concepts, and the relationships between and among concepts are established through empirical research. This work on a theory allows for the description, explanation, prediction, and control of the phenomenon.

Content Area: *Conceptual Models and Frameworks;* ***Cognitive Level:*** *Comprehension;* ***Question Type:*** *Multiple Response*

CRITICAL THINKING FACILITATOR: Locate a research study that identifies a conceptual model or framework. Note that there might be several interrelated models as well as a theory used in one study. How did the conceptual model guide the study?

11. 1. Presentation of the model would familiarize attendees of the meetings with the model.
2. The further development of the model by the developer would orient the professional community to new ideas and insights.
3. A monograph on the model published by the developer would further disseminate information about the model.
4. **A program of research using the model would build knowledge about the model. Research studies based on the model would test propositions of the model. Researchers could also form a network to share their findings and facilitate the development of theoretical ideas (Burns & Grove, 2011). These activities would, in time, make significant contributions to evidence-based practice.**

TEST-TAKING TIP: A clue in the question stem is "research." Recall that one of the aims of research is to build the knowledge base of a particular discipline. Only option 4 is a research-related activity.

Content Area: *Research Tradition;* ***Cognitive Level:*** *Comprehension;* ***Question Type:*** *Multiple Choice*
CRITICAL THINKING FACILITATOR: One example of a program of research is by Dr. Elaine Larson, whose work spans more than 35 years. Her frameworks for her studies are physiological, with her initial studies focusing on handwashing. A consultant for the Centers for Disease Control and Prevention, Dr. Larson now conducts multisite studies, and her work is the basis of evidence-based practice on infection control. Other notable researchers with research programs can be accessed on the NINR website. You can also look at the references of a research study to find multiple citations by a single author or group of authors. These multiple citations indicate programs of research.

12. 1. This statement refers to quantitative studies, not qualitative ones. Qualitative studies are inductive in their approach to research.
2. **This statement is true of qualitative studies. Data are analyzed by identifying themes or codes that will later be identified as concepts.**
3. This is not an accurate statement about qualitative studies. Many qualitative studies do not start with a theory. The theory emerges from the analysis of the data in these studies.
4. This statement is not accurate regarding qualitative studies. The statement refers to a descriptive study.

TEST-TAKING TIP: Recall your basic understanding of qualitative research. Qualitative research generates descriptive data. Qualitative studies do not have hypotheses, which are deduced from theory. You also know that the inductive approach is used in qualitative studies.

Content Area: *Qualitative Research and Theory;* ***Cognitive Level:*** *Application;* ***Question Type:*** *Multiple Choice*
CRITICAL THINKING FACILITATOR: Think of Kübler-Ross's model on death and dying. How do you think Kübler-Ross identified the five stages? Others use her model in looking at the process of a loss. Use the five stages and describe what a person experiences at each stage.

13. 1. This question is appropriate to ask when critiquing the study's hypothesis.
2. **This question is appropriate to ask when critiquing the theory of the study. The intervention should be guided by practice theory. "Practice theories are designed to theoretically propose specific approaches to particular nursing practice situations" (Burns & Grove, 2011, p. 237).**
3. This question is appropriate when critiquing the study's review of the literature.
4. This question is appropriate when critiquing the study's research problems, questions, and hypothesis.

TEST-TAKING TIP: Look at each answer option and try to determine what part of a study the question is addressing. Eliminate the incorrect options. Option 1 has hypothesis in the question. Option 3 asks about landmark studies, so this has to do with literature. Finally, option 4 has the word "contribute," which refers to the significance of the problem.

Content Area: *Critiquing a Study's Theory;* ***Cognitive Level:*** *Analysis;* ***Question Type:*** *Multiple Choice*
CRITICAL THINKING FACILITATOR: What are other questions that could be asked in critiquing a study's theory or conceptual framework? Review the purposes of theories and conceptual frameworks before answering the question.

9 Evaluating Quantitative Research Designs

KEY WORDS

The following words include English vocabulary, nursing/medical terminology, concepts, principles, or information relevant to content specifically addressed in the chapter or associated with topics presented in it. English dictionaries, your nursing textbooks, and medical dictionaries such as *Taber's Cyclopedic Medical Dictionary* are resources that can be used to expand your knowledge and understanding of these words and related information.

Attrition
Bias
Causality
Correlation
Control
Cross section
Experimental design
Extraneous variable
Homogeneous and heterogeneous samples
Longitudinal
Manipulation
Quasi-experimental
Power analysis
Random assignment
Random selection
Research design
Retrospective

QUESTIONS

Research Design Concepts

1. Which of the following statements is true regarding research design? Research design
   1. "deals with abstractions (concepts) that are assembled because of their relevance to a common theme" (Polit & Beck, 2014, p. 133).
   2. "visually represent[s] relationships among phenomena, and [is] used in both qualitative and quantitative research" (p. 134).
   3. "is the vehicle for testing research questions and hypotheses" (LoBiondo-Wood, 2010, p. 159).
   4. "is a logical, orderly, and objective means of generating and testing ideas" (LoBiondo-Wood & Haber, 2010, p. 586).

2. What questions are appropriate to ask in determining the design of a study? **Select all that apply.**
   1. How large should the sample be?
   2. Will there be an intervention?
   3. Where will the study take place?
   4. How will controls be imposed?
   5. Who will be the research participants?

3. A concept relevant to design is causality which means that "things have causes, and causes lead to effects" (Burns & Grove, 2011, p. 253). Which of the following are needed to establish causality? **Select all that apply.**
   1. The purpose of the study is to describe the phenomenon.
   2. The dependent variable (effect) occurred after the independent variable (cause).
   3. A proposed relationship between the variables must be evident at the start of the study.
   4. No other variable explains the outcome or the dependent variable.
   5. The independent variable (cause) and the dependent variable (effect) must have an association.

4. Which of the following research study titles implies causality?
   1. Davidson, K. M., & Rourke, L. (2012). Surveying the orientation learning needs of clinical nursing instructors. *International Journal of Nursing Education Scholarship, 9* (1), 1-11.
   2. Hawkins, S. Y. (2010). Improving glycemic control in older adults using a video-phone motivational diabetes self-management intervention. *Research and Theory for Nursing Practice: An International Journal, 24* (4), 217-232.
   3. Naab, F., Brown, R., & Heidrich, S. (2013). Psychosocial health of infertile Ghanaian women and their infertility beliefs. *Journal of Nursing Scholarship, 45* (2), 132-140.
   4. Yoon, S. L., & Kim, J. H. (2013). Job-related stress, emotional labor, and depressive symptoms among Korean nurses. *Journal of Nursing Scholarship, 45* (2), 169-176.

5. "Bias in a study distorts the findings from what the results would have been without the bias" (Burns & Grove, 2011, p. 254). Which situation would produce bias in a study?
   1. The research assistants were all trained on the implementation of the intervention protocols and were regularly checked by the principal investigator.
   2. The research participants were volunteers in the community who have experienced some type of violence perpetuated by nonmembers of the community.
   3. The researchers randomly selected the participants based on eligibility criteria and then randomly assigned them to the experimental or control groups.
   4. All research instruments adopted for use have an acceptable degree of reliability and validity established in multiple studies.

Experimental and Quasi-Experimental Designs

6. What are the requirements of a true experimental design? **Select all that apply.**
   1. There must be an intervention that is actively manipulated.
   2. Sample size must be adequate as per power analysis.
   3. The researcher imposes controls over the research situation.
   4. Random assignment must be implemented.
   5. The research question must be clearly articulated.

7. Which of the following statements describe manipulation?
   1. An intervention is given to one group and withheld from another group.
   2. The researcher assigned research subjects to the control or experimental group.
   3. Data collectors were trained and regularly supervised by the researcher.
   4. Only persons who met the eligibility criteria were selected as the sample.

8. Which of the following situations indicates the best control over the data collection process?
   1. "A convenience sample of uncontrolled diabetic adults aged 60 years and older who were interested in improving their blood glucose control was recruited for this study" (Hawkins, 2010, p. 217).
   2. "Participants assigned to the headphone group were asked to wear the foam-lined headphone and rest with their eyes closed for 30 minutes. Music was not played for this group" (Han et al., 2010, p. 981).
   3. "The nurse practitioners were master's-prepared family nurse practitioners who had a minimum of 6 months of training using videophones to deliver healthacre and had recently taken an MI [motivational interviewing] self-instructional course" (Hawkins, 2010, p. 220).
   4. "A total of 137 patients receiving mechanical ventilation were randomly assigned to [the] music-listening group, headphone group, or control group" (Han et al., 2010, p. 978).

9. **Research Statements**: The researchers sought to study the effects of yoga on mood and quality of life in Chinese women undergoing heroine detoxification. "Participants in the intervention groups were divided equally into two groups (21 and 20 per class), who attended the yoga class at different times but were guided by the yoga instructor" (Zhuang, An, & Zhao, 2013, p. 261). "Patients in the control group received routine hospital care without exercise guidance or practice" (p. 262). What controls are evident in the statements? **Select all that apply.** In discriptive studies there is
   1. manipulation of the independent variable.
   2. random selection of research participants.
   3. specific eligibility criteria for participation.
   4. use of a comparison group.
   5. variation of the intervention for the control group.

10. What are some of the critical steps necessary to conduct a true experiment or a randomized clinical trial (RCT)? **Select all that apply.**
    1. The researcher presents a comprehensive review of the literature.
    2. An appropriate sample is recruited from the population.
    3. Essential baseline information is collected from the sample.
    4. Subjects are assigned randomly to experimental or control groups.
    5. The researcher selects appropriate statistical methods to analyze the data.

11. Which statement describes the control group in an experimental study?
    1. This group of research participants has been consciously selected by the researcher.
    2. This group of research subjects is not exposed to the intervention or receives an alternate intervention in an experimental study.
    3. This group of research participants exhibits a diverse set of characteristics relevant to the phenomenon being studied.
    4. This group of research participants is randomly assigned to a group that will receive the experimental intervention or treatment.

12. Which of the following element must be present in a quasi-experimental study?
    1. Control of extraneous variables
    2. Random assignment of research participants
    3. Manipulation of the independent variable
    4. Directional hypothesis

13. The control group in an experimental study might get the ______, which is a "pseudointervention" presumed to have no therapeutic value. This pseudointervention is also called the attention control condition (the control group gets attention, but not the intervention's active ingredients)" (Polit & Beck, 2014, p. 155).

14. Which of the following is the major advantage of experimental designs?
1. They exclude those variables that cannot be manipulated because of ethical reasons.
2. Controls must be imposed on all extraneous variables.
3. Experimental designs cannot study human characteristics that are "not amenable to interventions" (Polit & Beck, 2014, p. 156).
4. They are the strongest in implying causal relationships.

15. Which of the following sequential steps can be identified as the classic experimental design?
1. A sample is selected from the population, subjects are randomized into experimental and control groups, intervention is conducted, postintervention data are collected from each group, and comparisons are made.
2. A sample is recruited from volunteers, subjects are assigned to experimental and control groups, intervention is conducted, and postintervention data are collected.
3. A sample is selected from the population, subjects are assigned to experimental and control groups, intervention is conducted, and postintervention data are collected.
4. A sample is selected from the population, baseline data are collected, subjects are randomized into experimental and control groups, intervention is conducted, and postintervention data are collected from each group.

Nonexperimental Designs

16. Which of the statements is true regarding nonexperimental studies?
1. Nonexperimental studies do not make significant contributions to the knowledge base of a discipline.
2. These studies can be used when the researcher wants to identify causality.
3. In these studies, the independent variable cannot be actively manipulated.
4. In the level of evidence, nonexperimental studies are at the lowest, weakest level.

17. Which of the following study titles suggests a nonexperimental study?
1. Nwankwo, T., Yoon, S. S., Burt, V., & Gu, Q. (2013). Hypertension among adults in the United States: National Health and Nutrition Survey, 2011-2012. *National Center for Health Statistics Brief, no. 133.*
2. Laguna-Parras, J. M., Jerez-Rojas, M. R., García-Fernández, F. P., Carrasco-Rodríguez, M. D., & Nogales-Vargas-Machuca, I. (2013). Effectiveness of "sleep enhancement" nursing intention in hospitalized mental health patients. *Journal of Advanced Nursing, 69* (6), 1279-1288.
3. Kaplan, B. G., Abraham, C., & Gary, R. (2012). Effects of participation vs. observation of a simulation experience on testing outcomes: Implications for logistical planning for a school of nursing. *International Journal of Nursing Education Scholarship, 9* (1), 1-15.
4. Zhuang, S. M., An, S. H., & Zhao, Y. (2013). Yoga effects on mood and quality of life in Chinese women undergoing heroine detoxification. *Nursing Research, 62* (4), 260-268.

18. What statements are true regarding descriptive studies? **Select all that apply.**
1. May "contain two variables; others may contain multiple variables" (Burns & Grove, 2011, p. 256)
2. Have as a purpose "to provide a picture of a situation as it naturally happens" (p. 256)
3. Attempt to control bias through sample selection and size, use of reliable and valid instruments, and appropriate data collection procedures
4. Designate which variables are independent and which are dependent
5. Randomly select their samples from the target population

19. Kwok, Fethney, and White (2012) looked at the mammographic screening practices among Chinese-Australian women. What is the appropriate design of this study?
    1. Correlation
    2. Descriptive
    3. Longitudinal
    4. Quasi-experimental

20. Which statement is true about correlation studies? Correlation studies
    1. allow the researcher to infer causality.
    2. include an independent variable that can be manipulated.
    3. can show that a change in one variable can be related to a change in another.
    4. use random selection and assignment to groups.

21. Which of the following information suggests a correlational study?
    1. Hackney, Hall, Echt, and Wolf (2013) looked at the efficacy of an adapted tango program in improving balance and gait of the oldest old with visual impairment.
    2. Lansiquot, Tullai-McGuinness, and Madigan (2012) studied the turnover intention among hospital-based registered nurses in the Eastern Caribbean.
    3. Friese and Manojlovich (2012) examined nurse–physician relationships in ambulatory oncology settings.
    4. Stanley and Pollard (2013) investigated the relationship among knowledge, attitudes, and self-efficacy of nurses in the management of pediatric pain.

22. What is the major advantage of correlational studies? In correlation studies,
    1. results provide a high level of evidence for evidence-based practice.
    2. large amounts of data can be collected on a particular problem.
    3. only a small number of research participants are required.
    4. the researcher can begin to infer causal relationships between or among variables.

23. Which of the following statements are true regarding retrospective studies? **Select all that apply.**
    1. They are a subcategory of correlational studies.
    2. They look at a present outcome and predict what caused it.
    3. They use samples that are more representative of the population.
    4. They look at a current outcome linked to a potential cause that occurred in the past.
    5. They can effectively control confounding variables.

24. Which of the following research questions could be answered effectively by using a retrospective design?
    1. What factors have influenced falls among elderly residents in a long-term care facility in the past 5 years?
    2. What is the relationship among age, gender, and level of nursing preparation of registered nurses on their attitudes toward older people?
    3. What is the relationship between a mentorship program and student performance in the first clinical nursing course in a baccalaureate program in nursing?
    4. What are the characteristics of registered nurse caregivers of elderly parents?

25. **Research Study:** Phillips, Esterman, Smith, and Kenny (2013) identified predictors of successful transition from undergraduate student to registered nurse and whether pre-registration paid employment choice impacted that transition. In this cross-sectional study, the researchers collected data from 392 registered nurses who were grouped according to their chosen work type (hospital/retail, enrolled nurse, other healthcare worker, and nonworker) and transition scores were identified. What aspects of the study indicate that it was a correlational, cross-sectional study? **Select all that apply.**
    1. Data were collected only one time from all subjects in the study.
    2. Subjects were randomly selected from the target population.
    3. Each subject came from a category of registered nurses.
    4. There were several independent variables that were actively manipulated.
    5. The underlying purpose of the study was to explore relationships among variables that can be related to transition.

26. Which statement is true regarding longitudinal studies?
1. The researcher collects data once on all the subjects in all the groups.
2. The study is done when the researcher is interested in changes of the same subjects over time.
3. The researcher wants to observe differences among subjects on a number of variables.
4. Longitudinal studies examine the lived experience of participants regardless of time.

27. Which of the following studies has a longitudinal design?
1. Flynn, Liang, Dickson, Xie, and Suh (2012) looked at the relationships among characteristics of the nursing practice environment, nurse staffing levels, nurses' error interception practices, and rates of nonintercepted medication errors in acute care hospitals.
2. Othman, Kiviniemi, Wu, and Lally (2012) determined the influence of demographic factors, knowledge, and beliefs on Jordanian women's intention to undergo mammography screening.
3. Hasson and Gustavsson (2010) monitored the development of sleep quality in nurses starting from the last semester at the university, with three subsequent annual follow-ups after the nurses had entered working life.
4. Kao and An (2012) studied the effects of acculturation and mutuality on family loyalty among Mexican-American caregivers of elders.

28. Attrition________ is the major concern when doing a longitudinal study.

Critiquing a Study Design

29. The first thing to do to critically appraise a study's design is to
1. determine the variables to be studied.
2. find out the specific design used.
3. identify the level of purpose addressed.
4. decide the level of research evidence.

30. Which of the following questions is an appropriate one to ask in critically appraising an experimental study?
1. Will the study contribute significant findings to nursing and healthcare?
2. Did the design clearly identify the relationship among the variables?
3. What measures were taken to control extraneous variables?
4. Did the design minimize risks for the study participants?

ANSWERS AND RATIONALES

The correct answer number and rationale for why it is the correct answer are given in **boldface blue type**. Rationales for why the other possible answer options are incorrect also are given, but they are not in boldface type.

1. 1. The statement is true of a conceptual model, not a research design. Note the phrase "abstractions that are assembled," which is indicative of a model.

2. The statement is true of a schematic model, not a research design. "Schema" means a diagram. Note the words "visually represent" in the statement.

3. The statement is true of research design. The design used by the researcher guides the types of research questions asked and determines what statements regarding concepts or variables can be proposed.

4. The statement is true of the scientific approach, commonly known as the problem-solving approach.

TEST-TAKING TIP: The key word is "design." A design is a plan and serves as a guide for making decisions about the study. The design selected would have to be appropriate to the purpose of the study. Think of how the design of a house determines what it looks like. A ranch-type house is built on one floor, and the configuration of the rooms is different than a Tudor, Victorian, or Cape Cod–type house.

Content Area: *Research Design Concepts;* ***Cognitive Level:*** *Comprehension;* ***Question Type:*** *Multiple Choice*
CRITICAL THINKING FACILITATOR: Think of where you use design. For instance, the design for a party dress is different from the design of an outfit for playing sports. The purpose of each outfit is different; therefore, they will look different and function differently.

2. 1. In quantitative studies, the size of the sample has relevance to statistical significance not to the design of the study. In qualitative studies, sample size is not a relevant concept.

2. This is an appropriate question to ask to determine the study's design. Experimental and quasi-experimental designs have an intervention. Nonexperimental designs and qualitative designs do not use interventions.

3. This is an appropriate question to ask. Research settings must be appropriate to the type of study. Quantitative studies use environments where control can be imposed. On the other hand, qualitative studies are conducted in naturalistic settings where control is not an issue.

4. This is an appropriate question to ask. Experimental designs impose the most controls compared with quasi-experimental and nonexperimental designs.

5. This is not an appropriate question to ask when determining design. The question is related to sample selection.

TEST-TAKING TIP: What are the elements that distinguish experimental designs from nonexperimental ones? Recall that experimental designs seek to test "cause and effect." Therefore, experimental designs need to have more controls and rigor.

Experimental designs are also the most advanced of all research designs. Using these designs, the researcher must have an intervention, conduct the study in an environment where controls can be imposed, and have other controls in place for all aspects of the study.

Content Area: *Research Design Concepts;* ***Cognitive Level:*** *Application;* ***Question Type:*** *Multiple Response*
CRITICAL THINKING FACILITATOR: Review the elements of an experimental study. Because this is a quantitative study, what research paradigm is guiding the researcher? Review the assumptions and beliefs of this paradigm to fully understand why certain measures have to be in place for these types of studies.

3. 1. A study that aims to describe the variables does not imply causality. Description is an identification of factors that might influence the phenomenon.

2. An independent variable—usually an intervention, treatment, or approach—must be implemented first before determining its impact or effect on the dependent variable or the outcome.

3. The proposed relationship between or among variables is the hypothesis that might suggest causality, but it is not needed to establish causality.

4. An independent variable proposed to cause an effect on a dependent variable is the overall purpose of an experimental study with causality as an underlying implication. Therefore, the researcher imposes all types of control so that this particular independent variable would be the only explanation for the outcome. All other variables, called extraneous variables, are controlled.

5. **There must be an association between the independent and dependent variables. Many preliminary studies (descriptive, correlation, quasi-experimental) are done to build the case for causality in future experimental designs that require the most rigor.**

TEST-TAKING TIP: The key words in the statement before the question are "causes" and "effects." The options that imply cause and effect include those that have an independent variable (cause) and a dependent variable (effect) and their association and those that address extraneous variables.

Content Area: *Research Design Concepts;* ***Cognitive Level:*** *Comprehension;* ***Question Type:*** *Multiple Response*
CRITICAL THINKING FACILITATOR: What are some "cause-and-effect" situations you know from your clinical experience? Is shearing a "cause" of pressure ulcers? Is a review course a "cause" of success in the NCLEX-RN?

4. 1. The title of the study does not imply causality. There is only one concept, or phenomenon, of interest, learning needs of clinical nursing instructors. Also, the word "surveying" indicates a study that has description as its purpose.

2. **The title suggests either an experimental or quasi-experimental in design. Both designs imply causality. There is an independent variable, videophone motivational diabetes self-management intervention. The word "intervention" is a clue that the researchers will manipulate this independent variable (cause) and see its effects on the dependent variable, which is glycemic control.**

3. The study title does not suggest causality because the researchers are interested in looking at the relationship between two variables. There is no independent variable that is actively manipulated to cause an effect on a dependent variable. The possible design of this study might be a correlation. Correlational studies do not imply causality and are done to establish a relationship.

4. The researchers are interested in determining the relationships among the three variables. The study does not have an independent variable that can be manipulated. The study is most likely a descriptive study. Causality is not implied in descriptive studies.

TEST-TAKING TIP: The key word in the question is "causality." Therefore, the title of the study should name at least two variables, one of which can be actively manipulated. Recall that an independent variable that can be manipulated could be an intervention, a program, treatment, or approach. Only option 2 has this independent variable.

Content Area: *Research Design Concepts;* ***Cognitive Level:*** *Analysis;* ***Question Type:*** *Multiple Choice*
CRITICAL THINKING FACILITATOR: Look at one or two of the studies in your core textbook and determine from the title which one could imply causality.

5. 1. The situation is indicative of imposing controls on extraneous variables that could produce bias. Consistency in data collection is ensured through training and periodic monitoring of research assistants.

2. **The situation has a high probability of producing bias. Volunteers were not screened, and no criteria were established to recruit a sample. The heterogeneity of the volunteers could provide many possible extraneous variables that could then lead to bias.**

3. The random selection and assignment process are safeguards in reducing or eliminating bias. Experimental designs must use these processes to weed out any extraneous variables. Because experimental designs imply causality, it is important to have rigor and control in order to avoid bias.

4. Control of bias is ensured when research instruments have a high degree of reliability (consistency) and validity (accuracy).

TEST-TAKING TIP: The key word in the question is "bias," which means prejudice. Prejudice implies unfair treatment. Only option #2 has evidence of bias because the subjects were volunteers, and there was no mention of how they were selected or what criteria were used to select them. There is no assurance that the sample was homogeneous with regards to certain characteristics. Heterogeneous characteristics in a sample would produce bias in a study.

Content Area: *Research Design Concepts;* ***Cognitive Level:*** *Application;* ***Question Type:*** *Multiple Choice*
CRITICAL THINKING FACILITATOR: What measures are taken to ensure that control is imposed on sample selection? For instance, if the subjects are not the same age, what bias would age have on the study variables?

6. 1. **"A precisely defined independent variable and researcher-controlled manipulation of the intervention or the independent variable" (Burns & Grove, 2011, p. 270) are essential requirements.**

2. Adequacy of the sample is a requirement for statistical significance. A requirement for the sample is that eligibility criteria must be clearly identified.
3. All possible controls to reduce or eliminate bias are elements of a true experimental design that implies causality.
4. Random assignment means that subjects have an equal probability of being assigned to the experimental or control groups. This process eliminates bias.
5. A clearly articulated research question is not an element in a true experimental design. A clearly articulated question communicates the topic of interest to the research consumer and is a requirement for any study regardless of design.

TEST-TAKING TIP: The key words in the question are "experimental designs." Recall that these designs test cause and effect (causality). Options that imply control over the research situation (an intervention that is manipulated, controls, and random process) are the correct options.

Content Area: *Experimental and Quasi-Experimental Designs;* ***Cognitive Level:*** *Comprehension;* ***Question Type:*** *Multiple Response*
CRITICAL THINKING FACILITATOR: It is worthwhile to understand the elements of an experimental design. Identify these elements in a study from your core textbook that used an experimental design. (Identifying these elements is not as difficult as you may think.)

7. **1. The statement is correct in defining manipulation.**
2. The statement is a definition of random assignment.
3. The statement describes a method of controlling extraneous variables to eliminate bias.
4. The statement describes sample selection.

TEST-TAKING TIP: The key word in the question is "manipulation," from the word *manipulate*, which means to alter. Only option 1 expresses an "alteration," and it is the only option with the word "intervention" that is synonymous with the independent variable.

Content Area: *Experimental and Quasi-Experimental Designs;* ***Cognitive Level:*** *Comprehension;* ***Question Type:*** *Multiple Response*
CRITICAL THINKING FACILITATOR: The question requires you to distinguish the independent from the dependent variable. Identify an experimental study from your core textbook and look at how the independent variable was manipulated in the study.

8. 1. The statement does not address control. The statement describes the type of sample for the study.
2. The statement describes manipulation in which a control or comparison group gets a different intervention from the experimental group. Although manipulation of the independent variable is a form of control, the statement indicates control over the intervention and not the data collection process.
3. The statement describes control over the data collection process. The statement describes the educational and experiential credentials of the nurse practitioners who are research assistants involved in data collection.
4. The statement describes the process of assigning the research participants into the different groups. The statement does not address control in the data collection process.

TEST-TAKING TIP: The key phrase in the question is "control over the data collection process." Persons qualify as research assistants because of educational and experiential backgrounds. Control over the data collection process includes using research assistants who have undergone training and can implement the research protocols in an accurate and efficient manner.

Content Area: *Experimental and Quasi-Experimental Designs;* ***Cognitive Level:*** *Analysis;* ***Question Type:*** *Multiple Choice*
CRITICAL THINKING FACILITATOR: What if research assistants lack the appropriate credentials and training to implement the experimental intervention? Would research subjects exhibit the same outcomes?

9. **1. Manipulation, a form of control, is evident in the statement. The intervention group is the experimental group, and subjects received the intervention, which is yoga with guidance.**
2. Random selection is not evident in the statement.
3. Eligibility criteria were not mentioned or specified. No information is evident in the statement about the characteristics of the sample. To impose controls, researchers select participants who must meet eligibility criteria. This process produces a homogeneous sample, thereby eliminating characteristics that could serve as extraneous variables.
4. The use of a comparison group or control group is a form of imposing control on the study. The control group does not receive the intervention given to the

experimental group, or the control group might get a different intervention.

5. **The control condition is specified in the statement by the words "usual care." The condition indicates that the control group did not get the same intervention as the experimental group.**

TEST-TAKING TIP: The key words, phrases, and clauses in the research statements are "effects," "intervention groups," "who attended the yoga class at different times but were guided by the yoga instructor," "control group," and "received routine hospital care without exercise guidance." The word "effects" indicates that the study is testing causality; therefore, there should be manipulation of an independent variable and a comparison group or control group that gets a modification of the independent variable.

Content Area: *Experimental and Quasi-Experimental Designs;* ***Cognitive Level:*** *Analysis;* ***Question Type:*** *Multiple Response*

CRITICAL THINKING FACILITATOR: Using your knowledge of controls, identify controls in an experimental study just by reading the abstract of the study.

10. 1. Although a comprehensive literature review is extremely important in a true experiment to present the current status of the topic, a literature review is not considered a critical step in a true experiment.

2. **The sample in an experimental study has to meet specified eligibility criteria to create a homogeneous group. Consideration is made regarding factors or situations that could act as extraneous variables. For instance, if age will influence the dependent variable, then all subjects must fulfill the age criteria. An appropriate sample is randomly selected.**
3. **Baseline information from research participants would ensure that data collected after the intervention can be attributed to the intervention (independent variable) and not to another variable. The baseline information serves as a basis for comparison of changes in the dependent variable. For instance, a subject's weight before the implementation of the intervention, weight reduction program, would be information collected before the study. Preintervention weight is compared with postintervention weight. Therefore, collection of baseline information is a critical step.**
4. **Random assignment to groups ensures that each subject has an equal probability of assignment to the experimental or the control group. This is considered a critical step and is one of the most important control measures in an experimental study.**
5. Selection of statistical method is related to the type of data, the hypothesis, and the variables in the study. Although it is an important step, it is not considered a critical one.

TEST-TAKING TIP: The key word in the question is "critical." One meaning of critical is precise. The true experimental study is the "gold standard" for all studies. The design must have all the critical elements so that findings have the strongest inference for cause and effect.

Content Area: *Experimental and Quasi-Experimental Designs;* ***Cognitive Level:*** *Comprehension;* ***Question Type:*** *Multiple Response*

CRITICAL THINKING FACILITATOR: All research studies need certain elements to achieve the purpose for the study. Create a grid of all types of studies—descriptive, correlation, quasi-experimental, and experimental. Compare and contrast the elements needed for each.

11. 1. The statement describes a purposive sample that is used in a qualitative study.

2. **The statement describes the control group. In an experimental study, the group that receives the intervention is the experimental group, and the control group does not receive the intervention or gets a different one. Then both groups are measured on the outcome, and comparisons are made between the two groups.**
3. The statement describes a sample that might be appropriate in a qualitative study. For instance, a study on the lived experience (phenomenology) of having had an above-knee amputation would recruit persons with this experience. The main focus of the study is the experience and not the other characteristics of the person.
4. The statement describes the experimental group.

TEST-TAKING TIP: The key words in the question are "control group." You are familiar with the concept of control in laboratory blood work. Take clotting times, which are needed when a patient is taking an anticoagulant. The "control" time for clotting is used as the basis of

comparison for the clotting times of a patient after he or she has taken the anticoagulant for a certain amount of time. The effect of the anticoagulant is judged based on the difference of the patient's clotting time after administration of the medication compared with the control. For this reason, the control group is also known as the comparison group.

Content Area: *Experimental and Quasi-Experimental Designs;* ***Cognitive Level:*** *Knowledge;* ***Question Type:*** *Multiple Choice*

CRITICAL THINKING FACILITATOR: Knowing the basic information about the control group and its purpose will facilitate in understanding the statistical analysis when a researcher is describing group differences and whether these are statistically significant or not.

12. 1. There is some control over extraneous variables in a quasi-experimental design, but this is not a critical element in this design. Therefore, the quasi-experimental designs do not have the strong inference for cause and effect that experimental designs do.
2. There is often no random assignment to control and experimental groups in a quasi-experimental study.
3. Manipulation of the independent variable is a must in a quasi-experimental study. Derived from the word "experiment," experimental implies doing something to create an effect.
4. A directional hypothesis is not just an element in quasi-experimental studies. It is also an element in other types of studies, including correlation and experimental studies.

TEST-TAKING TIP: The key word in the question is "quasi-experimental." The word "quasi" means similar but not quite the same. A quasi-experimental study has some elements of the experimental study, but certain elements of the experimental design are missing. Because the quasi-experimental study also has a purpose of testing cause and effect, it has to have the most important element to infer causality, the manipulation of an independent variable (cause) to determine its effect on a dependent variable. Not all elements of control required in an experimental study are fulfilled in a quasi-experimental study.

Content Area: *Experimental and Quasi-Experimental Designs;* ***Cognitive Level:*** *Comprehension;* ***Question Type:*** *Multiple Choice*

CRITICAL THINKING FACILITATOR: The question facilitates understanding of the difference between quasi-experimental and experimental studies. Compare a quasi-experimental study and an experimental study. You know that both must have manipulation of the independent variable. What elements are missing in the quasi-experimental study you examined?

13. placebo

TEST-TAKING TIP: The key word in the statement is "pseudointervention." The prefix "pseudo-" means false. Therefore, a pseudointervention might look and sound like the real thing, but in essence, it does not have the ingredients of the real thing. You have heard of placebos in relation to medications. The same idea applies here.

Content Area: *Experimental and Quasi-Experimental Designs;* ***Cognitive Level:*** *Knowledge;* ***Question Type:*** *Multiple Choice*

CRITICAL THINKING FACILITATOR: The placebo is only one modification of an independent variable. What are the other ways the independent variable is modified for the control group?

14. 1. Experimental designs require manipulation of the independent variables. Variables that cannot be manipulated have to be studied by using other designs. This is a limitation of experimental designs.
2. This is not an advantage; rather, it is a requirement of experimental designs.
3. Human characteristics are also variables that cannot be studied using experimental designs. Age, gender, and ethnicity are characteristics that cannot be actively manipulated.
4. This statement is the major advantage of experimental designs. The rigor and controls imposed produce results that can have strong inference for cause and effect.

TEST-TAKING TIP: Evidence-based practice requires practitioners to base care delivery on approaches that have been tested using rigorous methods. How would a nurse involved in ostomy practice know what types of supplies and equipment are best in "causing" the desired "effects" for the patient population of the facility? The answer: Critical appraisal of evidence from experimental studies.

Content Area: *Experimental and Quasi-Experimental Designs;* ***Cognitive Level:*** *Comprehension;* ***Question Type:*** *Multiple Choice*

CRITICAL THINKING FACILITATOR: Determine the level of experimental studies in the hierarchy of evidence. Why are these studies at this level compared to descriptive and correlation studies?

15. 1. The design is not the classic experimental design. No baseline data were collected. This design is called the after-only experimental design.
2. The design is not experimental because the sample is from volunteers who might or might not have met the eligibility criteria. Also, there is no random assignment to groups.
3. The design is not the classic experimental one because subjects were not randomly assigned to the control or experimental group.
4. **The sequential steps are typical of the classic experimental design. Random selection, collection of baseline data, random assignment to groups, a control and an experimental group, and postintervention data are all the required steps of the classic experimental design.**

TEST-TAKING TIP: Apply your knowledge of the elements of a true experimental study. Incorporate these as you list the steps for any study.

Content Area: *Experimental and Quasi-Experimental Designs;* ***Cognitive Level:*** *Application;* ***Question Type:*** *Multiple Choice*
CRITICAL THINKING FACILITATOR: Look at options 1, 2, and 3. Each of these options has a problem with establishing causality. Identify the problem each has.

16. 1. The statement is an erroneous one. Nonexperimental studies can make significant contributions to the knowledge base of the discipline. Many variables cannot be studied using an experimental design. Although weaker in establishing cause-and-effect implications, nonexperimental studies have clinical usefulness. Nonexperimental studies are the basic foundation upon which evidence-based practice is built.
2. The statement is a false one. To imply causality, the study design must be experimental because the requirements of an experimental design address extraneous variables that produce bias in a study.
3. **The statement is true regarding nonexperimental studies. Nonexperimental studies look at variables that are not amenable to manipulation or at variables that cannot be manipulated because of ethical reasons.**
4. The statement is untrue. Nonexperimental studies are not at the bottom of the level of research evidence. Reports of committees and opinions of respected authorities are the weakest forms of evidence (Burns & Grove, 2011).

TEST-TAKING TIP: The key word in the question is "nonexperimental." If experimental studies need active manipulation of the independent variable, then nonexperimental studies involve no active manipulation. The prefix "non-" means an absence of.

Content Area: *Nonexperimental Designs;* ***Cognitive Level:*** *Knowledge;* ***Question Type:*** *Multiple Choice*
CRITICAL THINKING FACILITATOR: Use your knowledge of nonexperimental studies and create a comparison grid of the different types.

17. 1. **The title indicates that the study is a nonexperimental one. There is no independent variable to be manipulated. Also, the title is very specific, indicating that the study is a survey. Survey research is "non-experimental research that obtains information about people's activities, beliefs, preferences, and attitudes via direct questioning" (Polit & Beck, 2014, p. 393).**
2. The title indicates that the study is either an experimental or a quasi-experimental one. There is an independent variable to be manipulated, sleep enhancement intervention. Furthermore, the title also includes the word "effectiveness," which implies a cause-and-effect relationship between variables.
3. The title indicates that the study is either quasi-experimental or experimental in design. The independent variable, some type of teaching approach, will be manipulated. One group will participate, and another group will observe. Both groups will then be observed for the outcome, or the dependent variable. Another clue in the option is the word "effects," which implies a cause-and-effect relationship between variables.
4. The title suggests either a quasi-experimental or experimental study in which yoga is the independent variable to be manipulated to determine its effects on quality of life, the dependent variable.

TEST-TAKING TIP: The key word in the question is "nonexperimental." Look at each title. Option 1 is the only title that

does not name both an independent variable and a dependent variable. No independent and dependent variables means no manipulation.

Content Area: *Nonexperimental Designs;* ***Cognitive Level:*** *Analysis;* ***Question Type:*** *Multiple Choice*
CRITICAL THINKING FACILITATOR:
Take this opportunity to identify the reasons why nonexperimental studies are important to nursing. Think of clinical situations that can be studied using a nonexperimental design.

18. **1. The statement is true of descriptive studies. For example using a descriptive design, a researcher could examine the characteristics of students admitted into a nursing program and create a profile of these students.**
2. The statement is true because descriptive studies collect information to establish knowledge about a particular situation. For instance, looking at the types of patients requiring home care nursing might be the focus of a study by a hospital that wants to establish a home care department.
3. Descriptive studies do have some controls over the research context. Information learned from descriptive studies is beneficial for later studies. Researchers build their program of research by beginning with descriptive studies.
4. This is not a true statement about descriptive studies. The purpose of descriptive studies is to collect information about a situation, not to propose a cause-and-effect relationship.
5. This not a true statement about descriptive studies. Although there are some specific procedures for obtaining a sample, researchers doing a descriptive study do not use a random process.

TEST-TAKING TIP: The key word in the question is "descriptive." Derived from the verb "describe," it means to portray something. Descriptive research "typically has as its main objective the accurate portrayal of people's characteristics or circumstances and/or the frequency with which certain phenomena occur" (Polit & Beck, 2014, p. 379).

Content Area: *Nonexperimental Designs;* ***Cognitive Level:*** *Comprehension;* ***Question Type:*** *Multiple Response*
CRITICAL THINKING FACILITATOR:
Take a look at a descriptive study in your core textbook and identify its purpose. Why is its purpose different from the purpose of an experimental study?

19. 1. The title does not suggest a correlational study. A correlational study "explores the interrelationships among variables of interest without researcher intervention" (Polit & Beck, 2014, p. 378).
2. The title of the study suggests a descriptive study. A descriptive study's purpose is "to provide a picture of a situation as it naturally occurs" (Burns & Grove, 2011, p. 256). The interests of the researchers are simply to ascertain the women's mammographic practices. "No manipulation of variables is involved in a descriptive study" (p. 256).
3. The title of the study does not imply that the study was longitudinal. Trends were not the focus of the study. Most research titles would include the word "longitudinal" if it was applicable to the study.
4. The title does not suggest that the study was a quasi-experimental one. There are no variables to be manipulated. A quasi-experimental study looks at a cause-and-effect relationship.

TEST-TAKING TIP: A key word in the question is "practices." The researcher simply wants to identify or describe practices. Looking at relationships or cause and effect is not evident in the title of the study. Therefore, the appropriate design would be a descriptive one.

Content Area: *Nonexperimental Designs;* ***Cognitive Level:*** *Application;* ***Question Type:*** *Multiple Choice*
CRITICAL THINKING FACILITATOR:
What are some examples of nursing phenomena that can be studied using a descriptive design?

20. 1. Correlational studies have a weaker design than quasi-experimental and experimental designs. Causality is not implied by correlation studies.
2. Although there is an independent variable, it is one that is not actively manipulated like the independent variable in an experimental or quasi-experimental study. The lack of controls over sample selection and assignment would produce bias in the study and would allow extraneous variables to influence the outcome, or the dependent variable. The researcher cannot attribute the outcome to the independent variable that was not manipulated in the study.
3. Correlational studies can look at the relationships between and among variables. However, this in no way implies causality. For instance, consider the

relationship between gender and pain response. Gender cannot be actively manipulated. Although there is a relationship between these two variables, the relationship is not a causal one.

4. Random selection and random assignment are not processes consistent with correlational studies. These processes are requirements of an experimental study.

TEST-TAKING TIP: A key word in the question is "correlation." Derived from "correlate," it means mutually related. So in a correlational study, the variables relate to each other. The relationship could be negative or positive. A cause-and-effect situation is not implied.

Content Area: *Nonexperimental Designs;* ***Cognitive Level:*** *Comprehension;* ***Question Type:*** *Multiple Choice*

CRITICAL THINKING FACILITATOR:
Correlational studies are also known as relationship studies. Think of clinical situations when a correlation study might be appropriate.

21.
1. The title suggests either a quasi-experimental or experimental design. There is an independent variable, adapted tango program, that can be manipulated, and outcomes, which are balance and gait.
2. The title suggests a descriptive study. The researchers will collect information about turnover intention. There are no independent and dependent variables.
3. The title suggests a descriptive study. There are no independent or dependent variables. The researchers are not even looking at relationships among variables. There is only a situation, nurse–physician relationship, that researchers are seeking to describe.
4. **The title suggests a correlational study. There are several independent variables that are nonmanipulable and an outcome, management of pediatric pain. The researchers are interested in discovering a relationship among the variables. Causality is not evident in the title.**

TEST-TAKING TIP: A key word in the question is "correlation." Recall that the purpose of a correlation is to demonstrate a relationship between or among variables. In a correlational study, the independent variable is one that is not actively manipulated. Only option 4 meets this criterion. Options 1, 2, and 3 all have independent variables that can be actively manipulated.

Content Area: *Nonexperimental Designs;* ***Cognitive Level:*** *Application;* ***Question Type:*** *Multiple Choice*

CRITICAL THINKING FACILITATOR:
Identify a correlation study in your core textbook and provide a rationale as to why this was an appropriate design.

22.
1. Correlational studies do not provide a high level of evidence for evidence-based practice. They are considered beginning studies, and there are few controls imposed, so they are weak in implying cause and effect.
2. **The statement expresses an advantage of correlational studies. A researcher could collect large amounts of information about a particular problem such as attrition rates in a baccalaureate program. Later, the problem could be correlated with something such as personal issues. Correlational studies can provide bases for future studies.**
3. The statement is not an advantage of correlational studies. Large samples are needed for correlational studies.
4. The statement is not an advantage of correlational studies because the purpose of these studies is to examine possible relationships and not imply causality. Correlational studies do not have the rigor and elements in the design to imply causality.

TEST-TAKING TIP: Recall the reasons why experimental designs are not always appropriate to use. One reason is that some variables, such as human characteristics, cannot be actively manipulated. This reason makes nonexperimental designs, such as correlational, more appropriate even though the inference for causality is weaker. Using a weaker design still provides significant information about a phenomenon. An important perspective to have is that "it is better to know something about a situation than to know nothing about it at all."

Content Area: *Nonexperimental Designs;* ***Cognitive Level:*** *Application;* ***Question Type:*** *Multiple Choice*

CRITICAL THINKING FACILITATOR:
Think of all the different phenomena in nursing and healthcare that cannot be manipulated. For instance, what do nurses use to predict risk for falls or pressure ulcer development? The answers come from descriptive and correlational studies. These become the building blocks for interventions that can then be tested using experimental designs.

23.
1. **The statement is true regarding correlational studies. Retrospective studies look at possible relationships between**

or among variables. What differentiates retrospective studies from other types of correlation studies is that the outcome has already occurred, and the researcher "goes back in the past" to determine what possible factors have "caused" it.

2. The statement is only partially true. Retrospective studies do look at present outcomes, but these studies do not make predictions.
3. Correlational studies use big samples, but these are not necessarily representative of the population because random selection is not used. Therefore, there might be bias in sample selection, and research subjects may differ in their characteristics. These differences can serve as potential extraneous variables.
4. **The statement is true of retrospective studies. The outcome has already occurred, and the researcher "goes back" to determine what situations may have caused the outcome. For instance, a health-related infection (outcome) is observed in several patients. The nurse epidemiologist looks back to see what possible factors have led to the infection.**
5. Retrospective studies lack many controls in the research situation. Because the process in these studies entails looking at past events, the researcher has virtually no control of those events. Therefore, extraneous variables can be expected in using these types of designs.

TEST-TAKING TIP: The key word in the question is "retrospective." The prefix "retro-" means to go backwards. Retrospective studies have a dependent variable, or an outcome, that has already manifested itself. The researcher then goes to past events to determine potential causes. For instance, a wound has not healed in a timely manner. Then a researcher would trace past events that have led to the situation (e.g., poor nutrition, low immunity, poor environmental conditions, nonadherence to the therapeutic regimen).

Content Area: *Nonexperimental Designs;* ***Cognitive Level:*** *Comprehension;* ***Question Type:*** *Multiple Response*

CRITICAL THINKING FACILITATOR: Let's say you are currently involved in a negative situation. Thinking about how the situation started, you might say, "I should have done this instead of that." You have just identified a potential cause and what you could have done to prevent the current situation. A retrospective study follows this same process. Think of a situation that has already occurred. Then go back and identify what could have caused it.

24. 1. **A retrospective design is appropriate. The question suggests looking at a present outcome (e.g., falls in elderly adults) and what potential factors or situations have "caused" them. The question suggests looking back 5 years.**
2. The question suggests looking at the attitudes (dependent variable) and the influence of three independent variables (all are not manipulated). A relationship is sought by the researcher. A correlational design is appropriate to answer the question.
3. A retrospective design is not appropriate to use because the question needs to be answered by using an experimental or quasi-experimental design. There is an intervention, or an independent variable (mentorship program), that can be manipulated.
4. The retrospective design is not appropriate to use to answer the question. The question can be answered effectively by using a descriptive study.

TEST-TAKING TIP: The key word in the question is "retrospective." Look for something in the statement that points to the past. Only option 1 has a reference to the past: "in the past 5 years."

Content Area: *Nonexperimental Designs;* ***Cognitive Level:*** *Application;* ***Question Type:*** *Multiple Choice*

CRITICAL THINKING FACILITATOR: Why are retrospective studies important in nursing? What other phenomena in the clinical or academic settings can be studied by using a retrospective design?

25. 1. **A characteristic of cross-sectional studies is the one-time data collection. This is an advantage of these studies and makes them cost effective.**
2. The statement is not a true one. The subjects are not randomly selected but are rather taken from a cross section of registered nurses according to categories selected by the researcher.
3. **The statement is true. The total number of subjects represents a cross section of all types of registered nurses according to type of preregistration work.**
4. There are a number of variables in the study, but these cannot be identified as independent variables because they are not amenable to manipulation.
5. **The statement is true of this correlation, cross-sectional study. The purpose of**

this cross-sectional study was to explore possible relationship and not to test causality.

TEST-TAKING TIP: The key words in the question are "correlational" and "cross section." Recall the description of a correlation study. Then add "cross section," which means to divide the sample into groups according to some criteria. In this study, the groups were "cross sectioned" according to type of chosen work.

Content Area: *Nonexperimental Designs;* ***Cognitive Level:*** *Analysis;* ***Question Type:*** *Multiple Response*

CRITICAL THINKING FACILITATOR:
What is the purpose of adding a cross-sectional design onto a correlational study? Find a study with a cross-sectional design and determine what characteristic was used to cross section the sample.

26. 1. A longitudinal study has multiple data collection periods. Data are collected from the same subjects over time.
2. The statement is true. Changes over time and trends can be observed because the subjects are observed multiple times over a long period of time. Each subject is compared to herself or himself over the course of the study, which could span many years. For this reason, longitudinal studies can be very costly.
3. The statement is not true regarding longitudinal studies. Subjects are not compared with each other. In longitudinal studies, each subject is compared with herself or himself.
4. The statement is not true regarding longitudinal studies. Phenomenological studies are qualitative approaches that focus on the lived experience. Time is not relevant in this study.

TEST-TAKING TIP: The key word in the question is "longitudinal." Longitudinal studies are "designed to collect data at more than one point in time" (Polit & Beck, 2014, p. 384).

Content Area: *Nonexperimental Designs;* ***Cognitive Level:*** *Comprehension;* ***Question Type:*** *Multiple Choice*

CRITICAL THINKING FACILITATOR:
What topics should be studied using a longitudinal design? What is the purpose of the researcher when a topic is examined longitudinally? For more insights into a longitudinal study, look at the Nurses' Health Study II on the Internet.

27. 1. The study information does not indicate that the study had a longitudinal design. Multiple data collection periods that are characteristic of longitudinal studies are not expressed in the statement.
2. The information does not suggest any longitudinal aspects. The information implies one data collection period.
3. The information indicates a longitudinal design. The phrase "with three subsequent annual follow-ups" indicates additional data collection periods, an essential element in longitudinal studies.
4. The information indicates the study is a correlation. Acculturation and mutuality are the independent variables that were not manipulated, and family loyalty is the dependent variable.

TEST-TAKING TIP: The key word in the question is "longitudinal." Recall the definition of a longitudinal study. Critical elements in longitudinal studies are the multiple data collection points. Only option 3 indicates more than one data collection time.

Content Area: *Nonexperimental Designs;* ***Cognitive Level:*** *Analysis;* ***Question Type:*** *Multiple Choice*

CRITICAL THINKING FACILITATOR:
When does a study have two designs with a longitudinal design as one of them (i.e., experimental or longitudinal)?

28. Attrition, or mortality, of the sample

TEST-TAKING TIP: What is the major difference of longitudinal designs from the other types of design? Answer: Multiple data collection periods on the same subjects. Think of a study that might last 20 years. Will there be the same number of subjects in the next data collection period? Subjects relocate to other states or countries, die, or become disinterested. They are lost from the study.

Content Area: *Nonexperimental Designs;* ***Cognitive Level:*** *Knowledge;* ***Question Type:*** *Fill-in-the-Blank*

CRITICAL THINKING FACILITATOR:
How does attrition affect a longitudinal study? What measures do the investigators take to address attrition?

29. 1. Determining the variables to be studied is not the first step in appraising the study's design. The variables to be studied are identified from the research question and not from the design of the study.
2. The specific design of the study is selected after the purpose and research question are formulated. The design serves as the blueprint for answering the research question.

3. This is the first step in appraising the design of a study. If the purpose of the study is to identify and describe a phenomenon, then a descriptive design is used. If the purpose is to establish a relationship between and among variables, then the design is correlation. If the purpose is to imply causality, then the design would be quasi-experimental or experimental. The same goes for qualitative studies because the purpose of the study guides the selection of the design.

4. Deciding on the level of research evidence is not the first step in appraising the study's design. The level of research evidence is important in appraising the significance of the study.

TEST-TAKING TIP: The clue in the question is "first." All aspects of a study depend on the purpose of the study. For instance, if the purpose of the study is to test cause and effect, then the design needs to be quasi-experimental or experimental. If the purpose is to gather facts about a certain phenomenon, then a descriptive design is warranted.

Content Area: *Critiquing a Study's Design;* ***Cognitive Level:*** *Analysis;* ***Question Type:*** *Multiple Choice*

CRITICAL THINKING FACILITATOR: Think of other appropriate questions to ask in critically appraising the design of a study.

30. 1. The question is not appropriate to ask in critiquing an experimental design. The question should be asked when critiquing the research question.

2. The question is not appropriate in appraising the design because it is the hypothesis that identifies the relationship between the variables.

3. The question is appropriate to ask when critiquing an experimental design. Recall that it is the most rigorous of all the designs because of the inference to causality. Experimental designs, more than any other design, impose control measures over all aspects of the research situation. Lack of control produces bias from extraneous variables and thus weakens the case for causality.

4. The question is not appropriate in appraising the design. The question is asked in relation to the ethical and legal aspects of a study. Any design would have concerns over the ethical and legal issues.

TEST-TAKING TIP: The clue in the question is "experimental design." Recall that an experimental design imposes the most controls over the research context. What is the purpose of control? Answer: To eliminate or account for extraneous variables.

Content Area: *Critiquing an Experimental Study;* ***Cognitive Level:*** *Analysis;* ***Question Type:*** *Multiple Choice*

CRITICAL THINKING FACILITATOR: Think of other appropriate questions to ask in critiquing a study with an experimental design.

10 Evaluating Other Types of Studies and Integrative Processes

KEY WORDS

The following words include English vocabulary, nursing/medical terminology, concepts, principles, or information relevant to content specifically addressed in the chapter or associated with topics presented in it. English dictionaries, your nursing textbooks, and medical dictionaries such as *Taber's Cyclopedic Medical Dictionary* are resources that can be used to expand your knowledge and understanding of these words and related information.

Clinical trial
Cost analysis
Effectiveness
Efficacy
Evaluation
Meta-analysis
Metasynthesis
Methodologic studies
Outcome
Safety
Secondary analysis
Systematic reviews
Tolerance

QUESTIONS

Other Types of Research Studies

1. Clinical trials are studies that assess clinical interventions. In which phase of a clinical trial does the researcher test the efficacy of an intervention?
   1. Phase I
   2. Phase II
   3. Phase III
   4. Phase IV

2. Which of the following studies is an example of a clinical trial?
   1. "The purpose of the study was to evaluate the effectiveness of musical intervention on preoperative anxiety and vital signs in patients undergoing day surgery" (Ni, Tsai, Lee, Kao, & Chen, 2011, p. 620).
   2. Stanley and Pollard (2013) "examined the level of knowledge of pediatric pain management, the attitudes of nurses, and the level of self-efficacy of pediatric nurses in acute care" (p. 165).
   3. "The purpose of the study was to describe the views and beliefs that Black nurses hold regarding several conceptual areas of genetic research and testing" (Powell-Young & Spruill, 2013, p. 151).
   4. Through an online questionnaire, Molanari, Jaiswal, and Hollinger-Forrest (2011) looked at the relationship among lifestyle preferences, perceptions of educational preparedness for rural generalist role, and the intent to move.

3. **Research Study Information:** Edwards and Siebert (2010) did a study "to analyze the outcome of a BrCRA [breast cancer risk assessment] program developed to enhance NPs' [nurse practitioners'] knowledge of risk assessment and use of empiric risk assessment models." What type of study is suggested by the information?
   1. Descriptive
   2. Randomized clinical trial
   3. Correlation
   4. Evaluation

4. **Research Study Information:** Bobay, Yakusheva, and Weiss (2010) "examined the impact of unit-level nurse staffing on unplanned readmissions and emergency department (ED) visits within 30 days after discharge from 16 medical-surgical units." One aim of the study was to "investigate the predictive relationship between nurse staffing and unplanned related post-discharge utilization ED visits and readmissions for reason directly related to the index admission or co-morbidities" (pp. 68-69). What is the focus of this evaluation research based on the statements?
   1. Tolerance analysis
   2. Cost analysis
   3. Safety analysis
   4. Impact analysis

5. ______________________, a "subset of health services research, comprises efforts to understand the end results of particular health care practices and to assess the effectiveness of health care services" (Polit & Beck, 2014, p. 347).

6. Which of the following research information indicates the study was an outcomes study?
   1. "The Healthy Bones Program effectively uses NPs to meet the goals of the program. The NP was able to assist in identifying patients at risk and ordered DXA exams appropriately. The increased cost associated with obtaining more DXA scans and having additional patients on antiosteoporosis medications was more than offset by the cost-savings associated with the reduction see in hip and other fragility fractures" (Greene & Dell, 2010, pp. 328-229).
   2. "More research is needed to examine whether telephone surveys or personal interviews would result in higher response rates in this population and if the preference for paper surveys over Internet surveys is generalizable to other rural and urban older adults populations" (Edelman, Yang, Guymon, & Olson, 2013, p. 286).
   3. "This research suggests the need for future research to examine how psychological openness can be increased among older adults and African American men, with the goal of increasing treatment-seeking behaviors" (Ward, Wiltshire, Detry, & Brown, 2013, p. 193).
   4. "There were several important strengths that enhance the findings in this study. This study contributes to a substantial body of knowledge that has developed from each research guided by the disablement process. It is timely to study PF [personal function] in older adults given the shifting demographics and known prevalence of FM [fibromyalgia]" (Toma, Houck, Wagniki, Messecar, & Jones, 2013, p. 22).

7. Which of the following statements are true regarding surveys? **Select all that apply.**
   Surveys
   1. yield quantitative data that could be collected cross sectionally or longitudinally.
   2. can show the relationship(s) among the variables of interest.
   3. are appropriate to use for all types of populations.
   4. yield high-quality data when done by personal interviews.
   5. can be low cost when using self-administered questionnaires.

8. Which of the following study titles suggests the use of a survey?
   1. Cho, S. H., Yee, J. Y., Mark, B. A., & Yun, S. C. (2012). Turnover of new graduate nurses in their first job using survival analysis.
   2. Moreland, S. S., Lemieux, M. L., & Myers, A. (2012). End-of-life care and the use of simulation in a baccalaureate nursing program.
   3. Whisenant, D. P., & Woodring, B. (2012). Improving attitudes and knowledge toward organ donation among nursing students.
   4. Franklin, A. L., & Harrell, T. H. (2013). Impact of fatigue on psychological outcomes in adults living with rheumatoid arthritis.

9. **Research Study Information:** Riegel et al. (2010) did a study of 29 persons with confirmed diagnoses of chronic heart failure of at least 6 months' duration. Research subjects were asked to self-detect shortness of breath when given a simulated shortness of breath test. The subjects' perception of shortness of breath was compared with gold standard ratings of each subject's shortness of breath made by trained registered nurses. Researchers did in-depth interviews of each subject to determine her or his ability to interpret symptoms. What type of study is evident in the information given?
   1. Randomized clinical trial
   2. Correlational study
   3. Mixed methods study
   4. Survey method study

10. Which of the following is an appropriate rationale for using a mixed methods approach in research? Mixed methods in research
    1. enhance all measures to control extraneous variables.
    2. provide a more cost-effective approach to the study.
    3. give researchers more confidence in study findings.
    4. strengthen the proposed causal relationships between or among variables.

11. **Research Study Information:** "The aim of the study was to examine the differences related to gender among informal caregivers serving older disabled individuals" (Del-Pino, Frias-Osuna, Palomino-Moral, & Ramon Martinez-Riera, 2012, p. 349). The researchers used the data from the most recent national cross-sectional survey to do the study. What type of study is suggested by the research information?
    1. Correlational study
    2. Survey study
    3. Secondary analysis study
    4. Retrospective study

12. Which of the following statements is true regarding methodologic researchers? Methodologic researchers
    1. must follow all the steps of the quantitative research process.
    2. are interested in examining the relationship between independent and dependent variables.
    3. deal with measurement instruments or measurement techniques.
    4. look only at the work of others in the same profession or discipline.

13. Which of the following information is indicative that the study is a methodologic one? The researchers:
   1. Investigated the effect of a visual art–based friendly environment on nursing home residents' satisfaction with their living environment (Chang, Lu, Lin, & Chen, 2013).
   2. "Tested a full model of the antecedents to and consequences of various forms of workplace aggression, considering psychosocial factors, for hospital nursing staff" (Demir & Rodwell, 2012, p. 376).
   3. "Examined the influence of parental marital status, parent-child sexual communication, parent-child closeness on HIV-related knowledge, safe-sex intentions, and behaviors of late adolescent urban African American males" (Harris, Sutherland, & Hutchinson, 2013, p. 141).
   4. Used the health belief model to examine the beliefs of women, which were then used to develop and validate a questionnaire about cervical cancer and the Pap test (Urrutia & Hall, 2013).

Integrative Processes for Evidence-Based Practice

14. Which of the following statements is true of metasynthesis, meta-analysis, and secondary analysis? These three processes
   1. involve only studies that have an experimental design.
   2. require researchers to have a program of research.
   3. do not require collection of new data.
   4. require studies published from peer-reviewed journals

15. What is the purpose of meta-analysis studies? Meta-analysis studies
   1. "provide information of the existence of an effect but also allow for the estimate of the magnitude of relationships among variables" (Polit & Beck, 2014, p. 356).
   2. "integrate the research evidence to sum up what is known and what is not known" (Polit & Beck, 2014, p. 116) about a research phenomenon.
   3. produce grand narratives from the integration and comparison of findings from qualitative studies (Polit & Beck, 2014).
   4. provide an "evaluation of the effects of a program or intervention on outcomes of interest, net of other factors influencing those outcomes" (p. 382).

16. **Research Information:** A literature search was conducted on electronic information systems. Included studies were those that were uncontrolled and controlled randomized clinical trials and were reported in English, Portuguese, or Spanish. Only five of the 496 studies reviewed were included in the report (Vieira, Bachion, Mota, & Munari, 2013). What is the integrative process reflected in the information?
   1. Meta-analysis
   2. Metasynthesis
   3. Review of the literature
   4. Systematic review

17. What are the requirements of a systematic review? **Select all that apply.**
   1. Do comprehensive literature searches.
   2. Use rigorous inclusion and exclusion criteria.
   3. Collect new data on existing samples.
   4. Include both qualitative and quantitative studies.
   5. Report on the most current and valid research on intervention effectiveness.

ANSWERS AND RATIONALES

The correct answer number and rationale for why it is the correct answer are given in **boldface blue type.** Rationales for why the other possible answer options are incorrect also are given, but they are not in boldface type.

1. 1. Safety, tolerance, and dose for the intervention are the foci in phase I.
   2. In phase II of a clinical trial, researchers are concerned with any side effects and ways to refine the intervention.
   3. **Phase III studies have as their objective the development of evidence about the treatment's efficacy. Efficacy addresses "whether the innovation is more efficacious than usual care or another alternative" (Polit & Beck, 2014, p. 347).**
   4. Phase IV of a clinical trial "involves studies of the effectiveness of an intervention in the general population" (p. 345).

   TEST-TAKING TIP: The key word is "efficacy," which means the ability to produce useful results. The phase that produces useful results has to be beyond developing the intervention and refining it (phases I and II), but before testing the intervention's effectiveness, which is phase IV.

   ***Content Area:** Other Types of Research Studies;* ***Cognitive Level:** Knowledge;* ***Question Type:** Multiple Choice*

   CRITICAL THINKING FACILITATOR: Compare the phases of a clinical trial and the process of developing and testing a new consumer product. Phase I of product development would include a description of the product's components. In phase II, researchers test readiness of the product and identify what can be done to improve it by looking at the different components. In phase III, researchers are ready to see if the product works better than previous versions or others in its class. In phase IV, researchers implement or release the product because they know it works.

2. 1. **This statement indicates that the study would qualify as a clinical trial. The study has an independent variable (intervention) and two dependent variables. Additionally, the researchers are interested in the effectiveness of the intervention, which indicates phase IV of a clinical trial.**
   2. This statement indicates that the study was not a clinical trial because the independent variables cannot be actively manipulated. A correlation was more appropriate.
   3. This statement indicates that the study was not a clinical trial. A descriptive study was more appropriate because the researchers were interested in description. There are no independent and dependent variables, and a relationship was not sought.
   4. This statement indicates that the study was not a clinical trial. There are no independent and dependent variables. A correlational design was more appropriate.

   TEST-TAKING TIP: The key words in the statement are "clinical trial." A clinical trial is a study designed to assess the safety, efficacy, and effectiveness of a new clinical intervention" (Polit & Beck, 2014, p. 376).

   ***Content Area:** Other Types of Research Studies;* ***Cognitive Level:** Application;* ***Question Type:** Multiple Choice*

   CRITICAL THINKING FACILITATOR: Think of designing the clinical trial for a new medication to lower cholesterol levels. Plan the four phases of that clinical trial.

3. 1. The study is not a descriptive one. Descriptive research "typically has as its main objective the portrayal of people's characteristics or circumstances and/or the frequency with which certain phenomena occur" (Polit & Beck, 2014, p. 379).
   2. The study is not a randomized clinical trial (RCT). An RCT is a full experimental test of an intervention involving random assignment to treatment groups; often an RCT is phase III of a full clinical trial (p. 390).
   3. The study is not a correlation. Correlational research "explores the interrelationships among variables of interest without researcher intervention" (p. 378).
   4. **The study is an evaluation of the outcomes of a program to enhance knowledge. Evaluation research is "aimed at learning how well a program, practice, or policy is working" (p. 380).**

   TEST-TAKING TIP: The key words in the information are "outcome" and "program." These terms imply evaluation.

   ***Content Area:** Other Types of Research Studies;* ***Cognitive Level:** Analysis;* ***Question Type:** Multiple Choice*

   CRITICAL THINKING FACILITATOR: Why are evaluation studies important in evidence-based practice?

4. 1. Tolerance is not the focus of the study. Tolerance is a concern in phase I of a clinical trial.
   2. **Cost analysis is the focus of the study. Cost analysis, as a component of evaluation research, "assesses whether the program's benefits outweigh its monetary costs" (Polit & Beck, 2014, p. 345).**
   3. Safety analysis is a concern in phase I of a clinical trial.
   4. Impact analysis is a component of evaluation research; it is concerned with the influence or effects of the program "over and above the effects of usual care" (Polit & Beck, 2014, p. 345).

   TEST-TAKING TIP: The key words in the information are "nurse staffing." The concern in the study is whether increasing the number of nurses on a unit reduces subsequent ED visits or readmissions. The cost of additional staff is balanced against the cost of readmissions and ED visits.

   Content Area: *Other Types of Research Studies;* ***Cognitive Level:*** *Analysis;* ***Question Type:*** *Multiple Choice*

   CRITICAL THINKING FACILITATOR: How does a nurse manager get administration to "buy into" a new program for improving care delivery?

5. **Outcomes research**

   TEST-TAKING TIP: The key words in the statement are "subset of health services research." The goal of nursing research is improvement of patient care outcomes. Although the word "effectiveness" might also refer to evaluation research, the statement specifically addresses health services, not just interventions.

   Content Area: *Other Types of Research Studies;* ***Cognitive Level:*** *Knowledge;* ***Question Type:*** *Fill-in-the-Blank*

   CRITICAL THINKING FACILITATOR: What are some examples of nursing care practices that could be investigated as outcomes research?

6. 1. **The information from the study indicates that the study was an outcomes one. The information mentions specifically a program and the results, or "outcomes," because of this program.**
   2. The information from the study does not indicate that the study was an outcomes one. The information addressed the recommendation of the researchers for future studies and was most likely found in the discussion section of the research report.
   3. The information from the study does not indicate that study was an outcomes one. The statements from the report expressed the researchers' recommendation for future studies on the topic.
   4. The information from the study does not indicate that the study was an outcomes one. The statements expressed the strengths of the study and were most likely found under the discussion section of the report.

   TEST-TAKING TIP: The key word in the question is "outcomes." Recall that outcomes research is about aspects of healthcare services and results seen in healthcare.

   Content Area: *Other Types of Research Studies;* ***Cognitive Level:*** *Analysis;* ***Question Type:*** *Multiple Choice*

   CRITICAL THINKING FACILITATOR: Think of a health service or other program you are familiar with. Identify what types of analyses you would do to evaluate the service or program.

7. 1. **This statement is correct about surveys.**
   2. This statement is not true regarding surveys. Surveys "obtain information about people's activities, beliefs, preferences, and attitudes via direct questioning" (Polit & Beck, 2014, p. 381). Surveys do not look at relationships between variables.
   3. Surveys, particularly those done using self-administered instruments, are not appropriate to use for some populations such as older adults and children.
   4. **This statement is true about surveys. Although personal interviews are costly to conduct, the response rates are high because the respondent has a personal interaction with the researcher or data collector.**
   5. **Surveys using self-administered questionnaires have low costs because they can be posted online or mailed in bulk. The low response rates to self-administered surveys are a disadvantage.**

   TEST-TAKING TIP: The key word in the question is "survey." One meaning of the term is "overview." With an overview, one collects much data but lacks depth. A survey can be cross sectioned to categorize data. A survey may also have multiple data collection periods to determine changes over time.

   Content Area: *Other Types of Research Studies;* ***Cognitive Level:*** *Knowledge;* ***Question Type:*** *Multiple Response*

CRITICAL THINKING FACILITATOR: What information might you gain from a survey of the faculty of a school of nursing? You could cross section the survey to look at age, gender, and educational credentials. You would have a great deal of data about the faculty, but the data would not be in depth. Even so, a survey could be very useful in many practical ways such as in recruitment initiatives.

8. 1. **The study's title suggests data that are descriptive such as rates of turnover, characteristics of nurses, areas of employment, and so on. The data cannot be used for any other type of advanced analysis.**
   2. The title suggests a study that could be quasi-experimental or experimental in design because there is an independent variable that can be actively manipulated to see its effect on a dependent variable.
   3. The title suggests a study that could be quasi-experimental or experimental in design. There is an independent variable, an intervention, that can be actively manipulated to see its effect on a dependent variable.
   4. The study's title does not suggest a survey. There is an independent variable that cannot be manipulated. The title suggests a correlational study.

   TEST-TAKING TIP: Apply what you already know about surveys. A key word in option 1 is "turnover." If you were to complete the term and say "turnover rates," that would give you a clue to the answer. Rates, or frequency, of occurrence are the foci of surveys. Options 2, 3, and 4 have variables, and a survey is not appropriate to use in those cases.

   Content Area: *Other Types of Research Studies;* ***Cognitive Level:*** *Application;* ***Question Type:*** *Multiple Choice*

   CRITICAL THINKING FACILITATOR: What kinds of study situations would a survey be appropriate for? Choose one situation. How could the data from the study be used?

9. 1. The information is not indicative of a randomized clinical trial. There is no independent variable that was manipulated to see its effects on a dependent variable. Other requirements of the randomized clinical trial are not evident in the information.
   2. The information is not indicative of a correlational study. There is no independent or dependent variable.
   3. **The information indicates two methods of research. The first is a quantitative one, in which subjects were asked to report specific data. The research participants could have been asked whether they detected shortness of breath or not. The second method was a qualitative one, in which research participants had to describe their ability to detect shortness of breath.**
   4. A survey could have been one of the data collection methods used, but this option is incomplete because only one method is stated.

   TEST-TAKING TIP: Separate the information in the question into four statements. Look at statements 2 and 4. Statement 2 indicates subjects being asked a close-ended question. Statement 4 indicates subjects being asked to describe their ability. Think of the type of data collected from each question, and you will come up with both quantitative and qualitative methods (a mix of the two).

   Content Area: *Other Types of Research Studies;* ***Cognitive Level:*** *Analysis;* ***Question Type:*** *Multiple Choice*

   CRITICAL THINKING FACILITATOR: What are some clinical situations that can be studied by using a mixed methods design?

10. 1. The rationale is not a correct one because only quantitative approaches are concerned with extraneous variables.
    2. A mixed methods design could be more costly because of two or more data collection times. One data collection would focus on collecting the data for the quantitative aspect and the other for the qualitative part.
    3. **This is the correct rationale for doing a mixed methods design. Quantitative data could be confirmed or verified by the qualitative statements (descriptions) of research participants.**
    4. This is not always a correct rationale because a mixed methods design might include those designs that do not test causality such as descriptive or correlation studies.

    TEST-TAKING TIP: The key word in the question is "mixed." What is one good reason why you mix two things together? Answer: To make the results better than they would be from either thing alone.

Content Area: *Other Types of Research Studies;* ***Cognitive Level:*** *Comprehension;* ***Question Type:*** *Multiple Choice*

CRITICAL THINKING FACILITATOR:
What are the other rationales for using mixed methods in looking at nursing phenomena?

11. 1. The study information does not suggest a correlational study because there is no independent variable to be correlated with a dependent variable.
2. The first statement might suggest a survey as the method to collect primary data. However, the second statement indicates using existing data from another study that the researchers analyzed, and this information is not covered by the survey.
3. **The information indicates that primary data were not collected by the researchers but analyzed a second time. Therefore, this is a secondary analysis. It uses existing data, and the current researchers did not collect new data.**
4. A retrospective study is not suggested by the information. A retrospective study is a type of correlation study that looks at past events as possible "causes" of an outcome that currently exists.

TEST-TAKING TIP: The clue is in the second statement. The statement indicates use of data from another study.

Content Area: *Other Types of Research Studies;* ***Cognitive Level:*** *Analysis;* ***Question Type:*** *Multiple Choice*

CRITICAL THINKING FACILITATOR:
What are the purposes of doing secondary analysis? Think of the massive data collected by the U.S. Census.

12. 1. This statement is not true about methodologic research. LoBiondo-Wood and Haber (2010) identify the following steps in methodologic studies:
   a. Defining the construct or concept or behavior to be measured
   b. Formulating the tool's items
   c. Developing instructions for users and respondents
   d. Testing the tool's reliability and validity (p. 208)
2. This statement is not true regarding methodologic researchers because their focus is on research instrument development and refinement.
3. **This statement is true of methodologic researchers. Their studies "address the development, validation, and evaluation of research tools or methods" (Polit & Beck, 2014, p. 349).**
4. This statement is not true of methodologic researchers because they also look at the work of other disciplines.

TEST-TAKING TIP: The key word is "methodologic," which is derived from the term "method," which means a systematic procedure. Only option 3 has something to do with methods.

Content Area: *Other Types of Research Studies;* ***Cognitive Level:*** *Comprehension;* ***Question Type:*** *Multiple Choice*

CRITICAL THINKING FACILITATOR:
Why are methodologic studies important in research and evidence-based practice?

13. 1. The information suggests that the study is either quasi-experimental or experimental. There is an independent variable that was actively manipulated to determine its effects on a dependent variable.
2. The information suggests that the study is a correlation. The independent variables were not manipulated. The purpose of the study is to determine relationships among the variables and not to test causality.
3. The information suggests that the study is a correlation. The independent variables are characteristics of parent–child relationships. The researchers looked at the possible relationship of these characteristics to HIV-related knowledge, safe sex intentions, and behaviors.
4. **The study is a methodologic one. A clue in the statement is "questionnaire," which is a type of research instrument.**

TEST-TAKING TIP: Examine each answer option and eliminate those that do not contain words pertaining to research tools or instruments.

Content Area: *Other Types of Research Studies;* ***Cognitive Level:*** *Application;* ***Question Type:*** *Multiple Choice*

CRITICAL THINKING FACILITATOR:
Look at the references cited in a research study and see whether you can identify some methodologic studies. The titles will give you very strong clues.

14. 1. The statement is not common to all three processes. Secondary analysis might use data from large surveys but not from experimental studies.
2. The statement is not common to all three processes. Many researchers have a program of research focusing on one or two

phenomena. However, those who do meta-analysis, metasynthesis, and secondary analysis do not always have a specific program of research.

3. **The statement is common to metasynthesis, meta-analysis, and secondary analysis. Existing data, not new data, from primary sources are analyzed.**
4. The statement is not true of all three processes. Studies included in meta-analysis, metasynthesis, and secondary analysis are not always from peer-reviewed sources.

TEST-TAKING TIP: All three processes go beyond an initial study. Therefore, to do any one of these processes, one does not have to collect data.

Content Area: *Integrative Processes for Evidence-Based Practice;* ***Cognitive Level:*** *Analysis;* ***Question Type:*** *Multiple Choice*

CRITICAL THINKING FACILITATOR:
Look at samples of a systematic review, meta-analysis, and metasynthesis and determine their commonalities and differences.

15. 1. **This statement is true of meta-analysis studies. Meta-analysis studies combine the findings from multiple studies and provide the high degree of confidence in conclusions about the relationship between or among variables.**
2. This statement describes the review of the literature that is done as part of the conceptual phase of a quantitative study.
3. This statement is true of metasynthesis.
4. This statement is true of impact analysis, which is a focus of an evaluation study.

TEST-TAKING TIP: The key word in the question is "meta-analysis." Meta-analyses use the data from randomized clinical trials that test for causality among variables. Option 1 provides a clue in the word "effects," which pertains to the dependent variable in an experimental study.

Content Area: *Integrative Processes for Evidence-Based Practice;* ***Cognitive Level:*** *Knowledge;* ***Question Type:*** *Multiple Choice*

CRITICAL THINKING FACILITATOR:
Differentiate metasynthesis from meta-analysis. Where are meta-analysis and metasynthesis in the hierarchy of evidence?

16. 1. A meta-analysis is a "research method that takes the results of multiple studies in a specific area and synthesizes the findings to make conclusions regarding the area of focus" (Polit & Beck, 2014, p. 581).
2. A metasynthesis "integrates qualitative research findings on a topic and is based on comparative analysis and interpretive statements" (p. 581).
3. A review of the literature is an "extensive, systematic, and critical review of the most important published scholarly literature on a particular topic" (p. 585).
4. **A systematic review is a "review that methodically integrates research evidence about a specific research question using careful sampling and data collection procedures that are spelled out in advance in a protocol" (p. 355).**

TEST-TAKING TIP: The key term in the question is "systematic review." Apply your knowledge of the definition of a systematic review and its level in the hierarchy of evidence. Then look at the research information line by line and decide whether the statement reflects aspects of a systematic review.

Content Area: *Integrative Processes for Evidence-Based Practice;* ***Cognitive Level:*** *Analysis;* ***Question Type:*** *Multiple Choice*

CRITICAL THINKING FACILITATOR:
Look at a study with systematic review included in the title. Then look at a table with the report that summarizes the studies according to the criteria set forth by the researchers doing the systematic review.

17. 1. **Systematic reviews use all available databases to search for appropriate studies.**
2. **To conclude with a high degree of confidence that the studies for evidence-based practice are valid, researchers create rigorous criteria to select and analyze the studies.**
3. No new data are collected. The systematic review uses data from the selected studies for the analysis.
4. Only quantitative studies would be included in a review.
5. **To provide data for evidence-based practice, the researchers doing a systematic review must include the most current and valid interventions.**

TEST-TAKING TIP: The key term in the question is "systematic review." Think of the purposes of a systematic review to select the requirement for this type of study.

Content Area: *Integrative Processes for Evidence-Based Practice;* ***Cognitive Level:*** *Knowledge;* ***Question Type:*** *Multiple Choice*

CRITICAL THINKING FACILITATOR: If you have an opportunity to look at another systematic review, look for the features in the report that distinguish this type of study from others.

11 Considering the Characteristics of a Good Design

KEY WORDS

The following words include English vocabulary, nursing/medical terminology, concepts, principles, or information relevant to content specifically addressed in the chapter or associated with topics presented in it. English dictionaries, your nursing textbooks, and medical dictionaries such as *Taber's Cyclopedic Medical Dictionary* are resources that can be used to expand your knowledge and understanding of these words and related information.

Attrition
External validity
Generalizability
History
Instrumentation
Internal validity
Intervention fidelity
Maturation
Measurement effects
Reactivity
Selection bias

QUESTIONS

Controls in Research

1. Which of the following are control strategies in the research situation? **Select all that apply.**
   1. Using consistent data collection procedures
   2. Selecting participants with homogenous characteristics
   3. Manipulating the intervention (independent variable)
   4. Anticipating issues with the outcome (dependent variable)
   5. Ensuring that ethical and legal guidelines are implemented

2. What is the purpose of imposing controls over the research situation? Researchers want to
   1. get significant findings and prove their proposed hypothesis.
   2. have confidence that the dependent variable was truly influenced by the independent variable.
   3. protect the subjects' rights, especially anonymity and confidentiality of information.
   4. ensure positive contributions to the body of evidence on the topic.

3. An academic educator administered an instrument on critical thinking to all the students in the class after implementing a semester-long program on critical thinking. How would age and previous college experience influence the outcome? These characteristics will
   1. influence the design of the intervention.
   2. serve as extraneous variables in the situation.
   3. pose difficulties in administering the instrument.
   4. facilitate analysis of the data.

Intervention Fidelity and Controls

4. What does it mean when intervention fidelity is evident in a study?
1. The researchers have faithfully complied with all the required ethical and legal measures to protect the rights of research participants.
2. Controls have been set in place to administer the intervention or the independent variable to the specified research participants.
3. The intervention was carefully designed so that it is administered in the same manner and condition each time to every research participant.
4. The researchers have carefully selected which research participants will get the intervention and which participants will not get it.

5. Which of the following statements is true regarding matching as a control strategy? Matching
1. results in a sample whose members share similar characteristics.
2. "involves consciously forming comparable groups" (Polit & Beck, 2014, p. 165).
3. randomly assigns research participants to experimental or control groups.
4. entails "keeping data collectors unaware of group allocation" (p. 164).

6. **Research Study Information:** Han et al. (2010) looked at the effects of music intervention on physiological stress response and anxiety level of mechanically ventilated patients in China. The researchers indicated that "a total of 137 patients receiving mechanical ventilation were randomly assigned to either music listening group, headphone group, or control group" (p. 978). What type of control is described in the situation?
1. Matching of research participants
2. Manipulation of the independent variable
3. Randomization of the sample
4. Blinding of the data collectors

7. A strategy to control confounding variables is through homogeneity. Which of the following situations demonstrates homogeneity?
1. "Inclusion criteria were the registered nurses (RNs) who provided direct patient care and had been employed for more than 3 months, which is the probationary period" (Yoon & Kim, 2013, p. 168).
2. "Nearly 1 in 4 (n = 34 of 149) or 23% of OAB [overactive bladder] respondents with nocturia felt somewhat or extremely dissatisfied with the current treatment of their symptoms" (Levkowicz, Whitmore, & Muller, 2011, p. 109).
3. In a study of self-efficacy and resilience among baccalaureate nursing students, Taylor and Reyes (2012) used 295 students who completed one or both administrations of the self-efficacy and resilience tools.
4. Hawkins' (2010) study on improving glycemic control in adults with diabetes had a sample size of "66 (34 in the experimental group and 32 in the attention control group)" (p. 219).

8. Blinding is a strategy to control confounding variables. Which of the following studies implemented this?
1. In a randomized clinical trial, Zhuan, An, and Zhao (2013) placed the allocation outcome in opaque envelopes. The research assistant who did this was excluded from recruiting subjects and did not know the identity of the subjects.
2. Norris et al. (2013) explained that research assistants completed training before the data collection period. The research assistants had no affiliations with the school that was used as the site for the study.
3. Taylor and Reyes (2012) reported that "the study was conducted over a relatively short period and may not be reflective of the changes in self-efficacy and resilience over an entire program of nursing study" (p. 9).
4. Levkowicz, Whitmore, and Muller (2011) explained that "an e-mail invitation was used and quotas were set to ensure reliable and accurate representation of the U.S. female population 40-65 years of age" (p. 107).

9. **Research Study Information:** Han et al. (2010) studied the "effects of music intervention on physiological stress response and anxiety level of mechanically ventilated patients in China" (p. 978). Which of the following statements indicates manipulation of the independent variable in the study?
   1. "Patients in the music intervention group will exhibit a greater mean difference in state anxiety level (C-SAI) than [patients in the] two comparison groups" (p. 980).
   2. "The purpose of the study was to identify the effects of music listening on the physiological responses and anxiety levels of patients receiving mechanical ventilation while in ICU [intensive care unit]" (p. 980).
   3. Subjects in the experimental group had a 30-minute session of listening to music. The placebo group did not listen to music but had headphones on. The control group had neither music nor headphones.
   4. "The environment for all three groups was enhanced to promote rest by closing the blinds, dimming the lights and posting a 'Please Do Not Disturb' sign" (p. 980).

Internal Validity

10. Which statement is true regarding internal validity? Internal validity is the
    1. "ability of a design or analysis strategy to detect true relationships that exist among variables" (Polit & Beck, 2014, p. 388).
    2. "extent to which it can be inferred that the independent variable is truly causing the outcome" (p. 167).
    3. extent to which "inferences about relationships found for study participants might hold true for different people, conditions, and settings" (Polit & Beck, 2014, p. 169).
    4. "process of holding constant confounding influences on the dependent variable (the outcome) under study" (p. 377).

Threats to Internal Validity

11. **Hypothetical Research Study.** The chief executive officer for nursing affairs at a tertiary facility wants to determine the relationship between her leadership style and the job satisfaction of the nursing staff. During the course of the study, a celebrity became a patient at the facility. When she was discharged, she spoke very positively on a popular television talk show about the care she received. What threat to the study's internal validity is described?
    1. Selection effects
    2. Maturation
    3. History
    4. Attrition

12. A threat to internal validity called ____________ results from loss of subjects in the experimental or control groups.

13. Which of the following situations involving instrumentation would pose a threat to internal validity?
    1. The reliability coefficients of the instruments are slightly above 0.70.
    2. There are several types of instruments to collect data.
    3. Data collectors were not similarly trained by the researcher.
    4. The same instrument was used to measure the outcomes in the different groups.

External Validity

14. Which of the following statements are true regarding external validity? **Select all that apply.**
    1. It is a major concern in implementing evidence-based practice (EBP).
    2. It asks whether processes that occur over time influence the outcome.
    3. It deals with the generalizability of findings to other people.
    4. It is concerned with concurrent events that could influence the study.
    5. It has demands that could conflict with those of internal validity.

15. **Research Study Information:** Yang et al. (2012) indicated that in their study, "findings cannot be generalized since only individuals who had undergone spinal surgery were selected. It is not clear whether these findings would be clinically relevant to patients undergoing different types of surgery, such as open heart or open abdominal surgery" (pp. 8-9). What do these statements indicate? The researchers were
    1. identifying a threat to internal validity.
    2. acknowledging a threat to external validity.
    3. describing a difficulty with sample selection.
    4. explaining a potential area of concern for future studies.

Threats to External Validity

16. Liou et al. (2013) used a pretest and a posttest quasi-experimental design in their study on innovative strategies for teaching nursing research. What is the possible threat to external validity in this study?
    1. Measurement effects
    2. Selection bias
    3. Attrition
    4. Maturation

17. Which of the following questions demonstrates a concern for external validity?
    1. What situations might have influenced the study outcome?
    2. Was the sample truly representative of the target population?
    3. Did the same number of subjects remain in the groups throughout the study?
    4. Were the intervention protocols implemented in a consistent manner?

18. Which of the following statements is true regarding reactivity? Reactivity
    1. "means critical self-reflection about one's own biases, preferences, and preconceptions" (Polit & Beck, 2014, p. 390).
    2. is considered a threat to the study's internal validity.
    3. is a "measurement distortion arising from the participants' awareness of being observed or, more generally, from the effect of the measurements procedures itself" (p. 390).
    4. "is the measurement error resulting from the tendency of some individuals to respond to items in characteristic ways (e.g., always agreeing), independently of item content" (p. 391).

19. Which statement explains why issues relating to external validity are more difficult to control?
    1. "Subjects who remain in the study are not similar to those who dropped out" (LoBiondo-Wood, 2010, p. 169).
    2. "The researcher is assuming that other populations are similar to the one being tested" (p. 170).
    3. The intervention (independent variable) was not implemented in a consistent way to all participants (Polit & Beck, 2014).
    4. There was a lack of control over events that might have influenced the outcome.

Critiquing Validity of Research Findings

20. What question would be appropriate to ask in critiquing the validity of the findings of a study?
    1. "Given the research question and characteristics of the participants, did the researcher use the best method of capturing study phenomena?" (Polit & Beck, 2014, p. 193).
    2. What measures did the researcher take to prevent the influence of confounding variables on the study outcome?
    3. Were the literature sources comprehensive enough to provide guidelines for shaping the research questions?
    4. Is the need for the study and its potential contribution to EBP clearly articulated by the researcher?

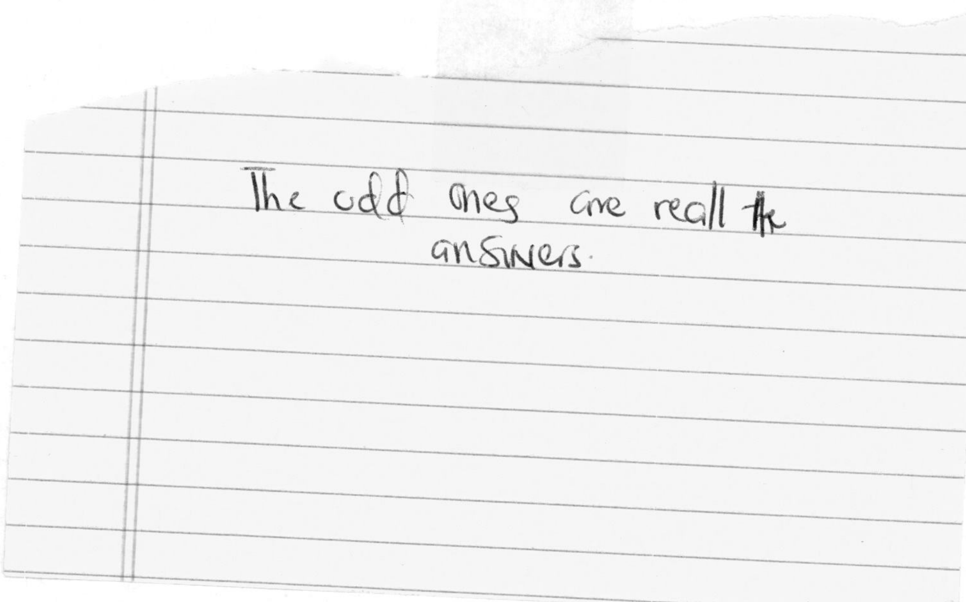

ANSWERS AND RATIONALES

The correct answer number and rationale for why it is the correct answer are given in **boldface blue type.** Rationales for why the other possible answer options are incorrect also are given, but they are not in boldface type.

1. **1. Data collection procedures should be implemented in a consistent manner. Any inconsistency could affect the response of the research participant. Data collectors must also be trained and checked regularly to ensure that they are implementing the intervention protocols consistently.**

2. A homogenous sample should be used by recruiting research participants using inclusion and exclusion criteria. "The researcher's subjects should demonstrate homogeneity or similarity with respect to the extraneous variables relevant to the particular study" (LoBiondo-Wood, 2010, p. 163).

3. Manipulation means "the provision of some experimental treatment, in one or varying degrees, to some of the subjects in the study" (LoBiondo-Wood & Haber, 2010, p. 581). In other words, the differences between groups of subjects can be ascertained if the intervention was given to one group and withheld or given a different one to another group of subjects.

4. The outcome is the dependent variable. This is the variable of interest, and nothing is done to it except measure or observe it.

5. Ethical and legal guidelines are implemented to protect the rights of research participants.

TEST-TAKING TIP: The key word in the question stem is "control," which means to impose or regulate. In research, control means to exert efforts to eliminate anything that could contaminate the study.

Content Area: *Controls in Research;* ***Cognitive Level:*** *Analysis;* ***Question Type:*** *Multiple Response*

CRITICAL THINKING FACILITATOR: What do you do when you want a situation to be free from outside influences? You weed them out. For instance, you are striving to get a high grade on an examination. You identify all possible influencing factors and impose controls over these. If your study space is not conducive to studying, you change it. If you have other activities that interfere with your studying, you put them on hold. What if you want to do a procedure efficiently? What controls would you impose so that you achieve your goal?

2. 1. Researchers propose a hypothesis that suggests a relationship between or among variables. There is no assurance that the findings will be significant. Hypotheses are not proven; they are supported. Hypotheses indicate the existence or strength of the relationships between and among variables.

2. This is the purpose of imposing controls in the research context. Researchers would want to reduce or eliminate anything unrelated to the intervention that could influence the outcome.

3. This statement addresses the ethical and legal responsibilities of the researchers to their research participants.

4. Every research study has a goal of contributing to EBP. Even when studies do not have significant findings, something is gained by the researchers and the profession. Improvements in methodologies, research instruments, research protocols, new knowledge, and the experience of the researchers are a few of the contributions of these research studies.

TEST-TAKING TIP: The key word in the question stem is "control." Researchers would want to implement strategies that assure them that whatever intervention they introduce would have an impact on the dependent variable.

Content Area: *Controls in Research;* ***Cognitive Level:*** *Comprehension;* ***Question Type:*** *Multiple Choice*

CRITICAL THINKING FACILITATOR: Let's say you are going to implement a program to improve patients' adherence to their therapeutic regimens. Why would it be useful to consider all the factors that could influence your desired outcome? Considering these factors could help you deal with barriers to learning or the approach you will be using, such as language issues or cultural beliefs

3. 1. Age and previous college experience will not influence the design of the intervention.

2. Age and previous college experience are extraneous variables. An extraneous variable is a "variable that confounds the relationship between the independent and dependent variables and that needs to be controlled either in the research design or through statistical procedures" (Polit & Beck, 2014, p. 380).

3. Difficulties in administering the instrument are related to the instrument itself and not related to age and previous college experience of the research participants.

4. Age and previous college experience are not relevant factors in data analysis.

TEST-TAKING TIP: The academic educator wants to determine the effect of a program (independent variable) on critical thinking (dependent variable). If the educator did not impose controls on the situation, then something other than the program could affect the outcome. These "something elses" are called extraneous variables.

Content Area: *Controls in Research;* ***Cognitive Level:*** *Analysis;* ***Question Type:*** *Multiple Choice*

CRITICAL THINKING FACILITATOR: Look at a quantitative study. What are some possible extraneous variables? Look at the inclusion criteria for sample selection. Why do you think there is a need for these? Taking one of the criteria, think: If this were not controlled, what would be the effect on the dependent variable?

4. 1. The statement describes commitment to the ethical and legal aspects of a study.
2. The statement describes the process of administering the intervention to the experimental group.
3. **The statement describes intervention fidelity.**
4. The statement describes the process of implementing the independent variable to the experimental group and withholding it from or administering something different to the control group.

TEST-TAKING TIP: The key word in the question stem is "fidelity," which means exactness. Option 3 with the phrases "carefully designed" and "in the same manner and condition each time" fulfills the conditions of intervention fidelity.

Content Area: *Controls in Research;* ***Cognitive Level:*** *Analysis;* ***Question Type:*** *Multiple Choice*

CRITICAL THINKING FACILITATOR: Consult an experimental study in the appendix of your core textbook. Locate the procedures section, where the researcher discusses the intervention protocols. Does the description indicate whether the intervention was implemented in a consistent manner? Also look for a statement on the role of assistants relative to the intervention.

5. 1. The statement describes the concept of homogeneity as a strategy to control extraneous variables.
2. **The statement describes matching.**
3. The statement describes randomization.
4. The statement describes blinding.

TEST-TAKING TIP: The key word in the question stem is "matching." In research, matching is an active process, and it entails identifying characteristics shared by subjects such as age, education, gender, residence, or other qualities deemed important by the researcher. The researcher then makes sure there is an equal assignment of subjects with these characteristics to each group.

Content Area: *Controls in Research;* ***Cognitive Level:*** *Comprehension;* ***Question Type:*** *Multiple Choice*

CRITICAL THINKING FACILITATOR: To understand further the concept of matching, think of a group of friends planning to play a basketball game. What do they do to make it a fair game? They might put one tall friend on each team. Then they might take two shorter friends and put one on each team. If they have two very good players, they put one on each team. They have just done matching to make the teams as equal as possible. One team would not have the "edge" because it has both tall players or both very good players.

6. 1. Matching is not the control strategy described in the statement from the study.
2. Manipulation of the independent variable means that the intervention (the independent variable) was administered to the experimental group and withheld from the control group. The control group could also get a variation of the intervention or a totally different one in the process of manipulation.
3. **Randomization is a "sampling selection in which each person or element in a population has an equal chance of being selected to either the experimental or the control group" (LoBiondo-Wood & Haber, 2010, p. 584).**
4. Blinding is not the strategy described in the statement from the study.

TEST-TAKING TIP: The key phrase in the situation is "randomly assigned." "Random" means by chance and not deliberate. It is believed that randomization "controls all possible sources of extraneous variables, without any conscious decision about which variables need to be controlled" (Polit & Beck, 2014, p. 165).

Content Area: *Controls in Research;* ***Cognitive Level:*** *Comprehension;* ***Question Type:*** *Multiple Choice*

CRITICAL THINKING FACILITATOR: Look at a study that used random assignment to groups. This information can be found under the methods section. What do the researchers say about why they chose random assignment? What advantages were seen when this process was used in the study?

7. **1. Homogeneity of the sample is described in the statement. Key words in the option are "inclusion criteria" that indicate specific characteristics that must be met before a potential research participant could be considered.**
   2. The statement from a study presents statistics regarding the problem, overactive bladder. The statement is unrelated to control strategies.
   3. The statement from a study describes an aspect of data collection and does not imply control.
   4. The statement from a study describes the number of research participants in each group. The statement does not imply control.

   TEST-TAKING TIP: The key word in the question stem is "homogeneity." It is derived from the verb "homogenize," which means to make something the same or similar. Option 1 also has the clue words "inclusion criteria." This means that whoever is selected has to meet a set of characteristics specified by the researchers.

   Content Area: *Controls in Research;* ***Cognitive Level:*** *Analysis;* ***Question Type:*** *Multiple Choice*
   CRITICAL THINKING FACILITATOR: Look at a study and locate the section that describes the recruitment of research participants. You will note that for potential participants to qualify, specific characteristics are stipulated. Relate the criteria to the research question. Take one criterion and try to provide a rationale for making it part of the inclusion criteria. What would happen if this criterion was not included?

8. **1. The process described in the statement from the study is called blinding.**
   2. The process described relates to another control strategy that entails training data collectors to ensure consistency of data collection. The second statement relates to ethical and legal guidelines and not to control.
   3. The statement explains a limitation of the study and relates to external validity and not to control.
   4. The statement indicates information relative to the recruitment of an adequate and appropriate sample.

   TEST-TAKING TIP: The key word in the question stem is "blinding." In research, it means not knowing or obscuring. Not knowing group participants' assignments prevents data collectors from treating the subjects differently. The blinding process ensures consistent implementation of the intervention, that is, no preferential or prejudicial treatment.

   Content Area: *Controls in Research;* ***Cognitive Level:*** *Analysis;* ***Question Type:*** *Multiple Choice*
   CRITICAL THINKING FACILITATOR: The process of blinding is not unique to research. For example, professional journals require blind reviews of manuscripts for potential publication; the reviewers do not know who wrote the manuscript being reviewed. Why is blinding important for professional publications? What purpose does it serve?

9. 1. The statement is a directional hypothesis. A hypothesis is a "prediction about the relationship between one or more variables" (LoBiondo-Wood & Haber, 2010, p. 579).
   2. The statement presents the purpose of the study. A purpose is "that which encompasses the aims or objectives the investigator hopes to achieve with the research, not the question to be answered" (584).
   3. The statement describes manipulation of the independent variable. Music is the independent variable that was administered to the experimental group. The other groups, placebo and control, had a variation of the independent variable.
   4. The statement describes a part of the protocol during the data collection process.

   TEST-TAKING TIP: The key word in the question stem is "manipulation," derived from the verb "manipulate," which means to change or alter. If you had an intervention and gave it to some but changed it for others, would you expect a difference in the outcome? Option 3 indicates that one group got an intervention but that something was changed for the other groups.

   Content Area: *Controls in Research;* ***Cognitive Level:*** *Analysis;* ***Question Type:*** *Multiple Choice*
   CRITICAL THINKING FACILITATOR: In long-term care facilities, there are many elderly residents with a high risk for pressure ulcer development. Let's say you create a program to decrease their risk. How would you go about determining the effect of your program? How would you know it works? Who would get it? In this scenario, you cannot compare your program with no pressure ulcer prevention because that would cause harm to the patients who receive no treatment. So what can you use for comparison?

10. 1. The statement describes the concept of power in a study.
    2. The statement is a definition of internal validity.
    3. The statement is a definition of external validity. Note the statement refers to something outside the study.

4. The statement is a definition of control of the research context.

TEST-TAKING TIP: The key words in the question stem are "internal validity." "Internal" pertains to situations within the study. "Validity" means based on evidence. When something is internally valid, it is based on evidence arrived at from within the study.

Content Area: *Internal Validity;* ***Cognitive Level:*** *Comprehension;* ***Question Type:*** *Multiple Choice*

CRITICAL THINKING FACILITATOR: Look at a quantitative study. What makes the study internally valid? What are some internal aspects of the study? A review of the phases and steps in a quantitative study will help you with this.

11\. 1. A threat to external validity is selection effects that occur "when the researchers cannot attain an ideal sample population" (Polit & Beck, 2014, p. 171).
2. Maturation is a threat to internal validity, and it refers "to the developmental, biological, or psychological processes that operate within an individual as a function of time and are external to the events of the investigation" (p. 167).
3. **History is a threat to internal validity and is "another specific event that may have an effect on the dependent variable. It may occur inside or outside the experimental setting" (p. 167).**
4. Attrition, also known as mortality, is a threat to internal validity. It is defined as the "loss of study subjects from the first data-collection point (pre-test) on the second data-collection point (post-test). If the subjects who remain in the study are not similar to those who dropped out, the results could be affected" (p. 169).

TEST-TAKING TIP: The key phrase in the described situation is "the course of the study." This indicates an event occurring while the study is in progress. This event might influence the outcome, job satisfaction of the nursing staff, because of possible exposure to or knowledge of the television interview of the celebrity.

Content Area: *Threats to Internal Validity;* ***Cognitive Level:*** *Analysis;* ***Question Type:*** *Multiple Choice*

CRITICAL THINKING FACILITATOR: Look at a quantitative study. Read the procedure section of this study. During the course of this study, what events could have influenced the outcome of the study? Think about this familiar situation: Nursing students are asked to evaluate courses and faculty. If grades on an examination were announced the day before the evaluations were due, how might this affect results of the evaluation?

12\. **attrition**

TEST-TAKING TIP: The key word in the question stem is "loss."

Content Area: *Threats to Internal Validity;* ***Cognitive Level:*** *Knowledge;* ***Question Type:*** *Fill-in-the-Blank*

CRITICAL THINKING FACILITATOR: It is important to understand the terminology used in research. In reviewing the section of your textbook on internal and external validity, identify the page that lists key words in the chapter. Read over the definitions of these terms and look out for them as you read. You will find reading subsequent chapters easier when you are familiar with the terminology.

13\. 1. The statement is about reliability, which is a quality characteristic of a research instrument; the coefficient indicates its degree of reliability. Most psychometricians (instrument developers) would agree that a coefficient of 0.70 is considered acceptable. A reliable instrument does not pose a threat.
2. It is not unusual to use several types of instruments in a study. The requirements are that they are reliable and valid.
3. **Data collectors assist researchers in obtaining data from research subjects. Lack of consistency in the data collection protocols might result in different outcomes. Recognizing this as a threat to internal validity, investigators not only train data collectors but also monitor and check these data collectors.**
4. Using the same measurement instrument is a required protocol in data collection. What is made different between or among the groups is the intervention, the independent variable. The independent variable is manipulated as a control strategy to determine the outcomes in the experimental and control groups.

TEST-TAKING TIP: The key word in the question stem is "instrumentation." Instruments are the data collection tools in research, and often these are administered by research assistants or data collectors. Therefore, the concept of instrumentation includes the who and the how relative to administration.

Content Area: *Threats to Internal Validity;* ***Cognitive Level:*** *Application;* ***Question Type:*** *Multiple Choice*

CRITICAL THINKING FACILITATOR: To help you better understand how instrumentation might affect internal validity, think about what would happen if two data collectors in the same study do not follow the same protocols for administering the instrument. What if one data collector sets a different time limit on subjects? What if one data collector has subjects write their responses and the other writes what the subjects tell him? How might these situations affect internal validity?

14. 1. **External validity is a major concern in EBP. Research studies must demonstrate internal and external validity. EBP is "the use of best evidence in making patient care decisions, and such evidence typically comes from research conducted by nurses and other health care professionals" (Polit & Beck, 2014, p. 2).**
2. Processes that occur over time refer to maturation, a threat to internal validity.
3. **Generalizability, or applicability of findings to other people, refers to external validity.**
4. Events that are concurrent with the research study and are threats to internal validity are known as history.
5. **The statement is applicable in looking at both internal and external validity. When a researcher exerts controls over all the threats to internal validity, he or she creates an almost "pure" situation that could lack relevance when findings are applied to the outside world, where situations are rarely pure.**

TEST-TAKING TIP: Focus on the true statements or try to eliminate those statements that are not relevant. In most textbooks, the discussion of internal validity precedes that of external validity. In this instance, you can get to the correct options by smart elimination of the false statements based on what you already know.

Content Area: *External Validity;* ***Cognitive Level:*** *Comprehension;* ***Question Type:*** *Multiple Response*
CRITICAL THINKING FACILITATOR: Create a table listing threats to external validity. Look over a study with an experimental design or a randomized clinical trial. For each threat to external validity you find, comment on how these were addressed by the researcher(s).

15. 1. The statement from the research study is not identifying a threat to internal validity. The second statement in the situation gives a clue that the researchers are describing a threat to *external* validity. Note the word "different" in the statement.
2. **The statement is acknowledging a threat to external validity. Recall that external validity is concerned with generalizability, or transferability, of research findings to other populations, settings, or situations. Note the first statement of the situation.**
3. The statement is not relevant to the situation described by the researchers. This might be an accessibility issue.
4. Describing a potential area of concern for future studies is relevant to the recommendations of the current researchers.

TEST-TAKING TIP: Read the situation carefully. Note key words such as "cannot be generalized" and "different types of surgery." These indicate concerns of applying findings to other people and situations.

Content Area: *External Validity;* ***Cognitive Level:*** *Analysis;* ***Question Type:*** *Multiple Choice*
CRITICAL THINKING FACILITATOR: Locate the discussion or recommendation section of a study. What are some of the statements made regarding the study's limitations? To what extent is the study generalizable?

16. 1. **The study used a pretest that could pose a threat to external validity; such a threat is known as a measurement effect. The "administration of a pre-test in a study affects the generalizability of the findings to other populations" (LoBiondo-Wood, 2010, p. 172). The concept of generalizability is relevant to external validity.**
2. Selection bias is a threat to internal validity. It results when a representative sample was not recruited.
3. Attrition, or mortality, is the loss of research participants. Although attrition is also a threat to internal validity, it is not the threat indicated in the question.
4. Maturation is another threat to internal validity, but it is not the one indicated in the statement. Maturation has to do with "developmental, biological, or psychological processes that operate within an individual as a function of time and are external to the events of the investigation" (LoBiondo-Wood, 2010, p. 167).

TEST-TAKING TIP: The key words in the question stem are "pretest" and "posttest." A pretest might give the research participants an "edge" to the

questions or statements on an instrument. This edge would affect the outcome measured in the post-test. If the study findings are to be generalized to other populations (external to the study), could these findings be considered valid?

Content Area: *Threats to External Validity;* ***Cognitive Level:*** *Analysis;* ***Question Type:*** *Multiple Choice*

CRITICAL THINKING FACILITATOR: If study findings are to be applied to other populations and settings, what must be considered? For example, let's say you were asked to demonstrate a particular skill (pretest). After this, you were taught a way to do it (intervention). When you do the skill after the teaching (posttest), will you do it better than someone who only got the teaching and then had to demonstrate the skill (posttest only)? Will your performance data be valid when applied to other nursing students who only get the teaching and then have to perform the skill?

17. 1. Situations that might influence the outcome (dependent variable) are threats to internal validity, which asks whether the independent variable truly causes the dependent variable, or the outcome.
2. **The question is indicative of a concern for external validity. External validity concerns "inferences about whether relationships found for study participants might hold true for different people, conditions, and settings. If the sample is representative of the population, generalizability of results to the population is enhanced" (Polit & Beck, 2014, p. 169).**
3. The question is a concern for internal validity. The threat addressed by the question is called mortality, or attrition.
4. The question is a concern for internal validity. The threat relates to instrumentation that includes concern for the data collectors.

TEST-TAKING TIP: Keep in mind that external validity addresses applicability of findings to other populations and settings. Research findings from a nonrepresentative sample would have limited applicability to the outside world.

Content Area: *External Validity;* ***Cognitive Level:*** *Application;* ***Question Type:*** *Multiple Choice*

CRITICAL THINKING FACILITATOR: Create a table comparing the threats to internal and external validity. How does each affect the outcome of the study? Look at a sample randomized clinical trial.. Compare identified threats with internal and external validity.

18. 1. The statement describes reflexivity.
2. Reactivity is a threat to the study's external validity, not internal validity.
3. **The statement describes reactivity.**
4. The statement refers to response set bias, a concept relevant to data collection.

TEST-TAKING TIP: "To react" means to respond. Therefore, reactivity has something to do with responding to something. In this instance, the response is made not because of the intervention (independent variable) but because research participants know they are expected to respond knowing they are in a study.

Content Area: *External Validity;* ***Cognitive Level:*** *Comprehension;* ***Question Type:*** *Multiple Choice*

CRITICAL THINKING FACILITATOR: Take an instance when you practiced a skill several times and then had to demonstrate it to your clinical instructor. You did it well with few minor errors. Then several weeks later, you do the same skill and do not demonstrate the same level of competency compared with the time your clinical instructor was testing you. Did you show competency just because your clinical instructor was testing you?

19. 1. The statement refers to a threat to internal validity called attrition.
2. **External validity addresses generalizability of findings to other people, settings, and situations. If the study population is different from the targeted population, then generalizability is in question. The assumption must be addressed by recruiting a more representative population.**
3. The statement does not address the question. The question refers to a threat to internal validity, instrumentation.
4. The statement refers to a threat to internal validity, history.

TEST-TAKING TIP: Look carefully at each of the options. Option 1 points to attrition as the issue, and this relates to internal validity. Option 3 points to the intervention, and this concerns internal validity. Option 4 asserts lack of control on events, or history. So, that leaves option 2 that addresses other populations, indicating generalizability, a concern in external validity.

Content Area: *External Validity;* ***Cognitive Level:*** *Analysis;* ***Question Type:*** *Multiple Choice*

CRITICAL THINKING FACILITATOR: Compare the strategies used to control threats to internal validity and external validity. Why do researchers attempt to control threats to internal validity versus external validity?

20. 1. The question is appropriate to ask when critiquing the study's data collection methods.

2. **This is the appropriate question to ask. A clue in the question stem is "confounding variables," which could affect the validity of the research findings.**

3. The question is appropriate to ask when critiquing the literature review of a study.

4. The question is appropriate to ask when critiquing the literature review of a study.

TEST-TAKING TIP: Look carefully at each of the options, and try to apply what you already know. Option 1 asks about capturing the phenomenon, and this points to data collection. Option 3 asks about sources, which indicates review of the literature. Option 4 asks about the need for the study and contributions. This also addresses the literature review. That leaves option 2. The question asks about confounding variables, and from your basic knowledge of control, you can deduce that this has to do with validity of findings.

Content Area: *Critiquing Control in Research Studies;* ***Cognitive Level:*** *Application;* ***Question Type:*** *Multiple Choice*

CRITICAL THINKING FACILITATOR:
What are other questions could you ask when determining the validity of research findings?

Determining Sampling Plans

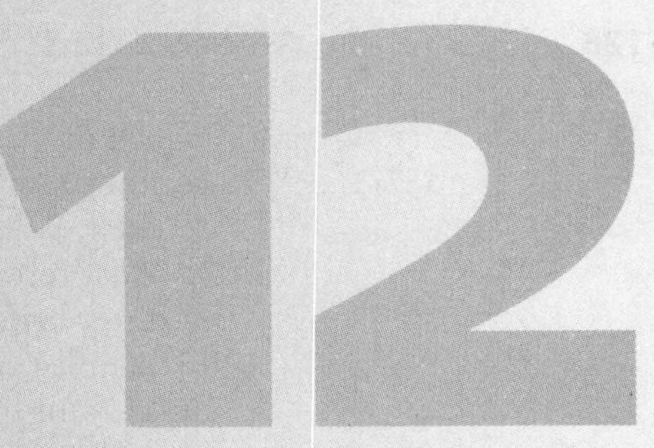

KEY WORDS

The following words include English vocabulary, nursing/medical terminology, concepts, principles, or information relevant to content specifically addressed in the chapter or associated with topics presented in it. English dictionaries, your nursing textbooks, and medical dictionaries such as *Taber's Cyclopedic Medical Dictionary* are resources that can be used to expand your knowledge and understanding of these words and related information.

Accessible population
Cluster sampling
Convenience sampling
Data saturation
Eligibility criteria
Exclusion criteria
Power analysis
Purposive sampling
Quota sampling
Random assignment
Random selection
Representativeness
Sampling bias
Snowball sampling
Stratified random sampling
Representativeness
Target population

QUESTIONS

Basic Sampling Terminology

1. Which of the following is a target population?
   1. Baccalaureate students 20 to 30 years of age
   2. All registered nurses in New York State
   3. Registered nurses with associate degrees
   4. Nurse educators with doctorates in education

2. A researcher interested in looking at resilience among patients with above-knee amputations recruited a sample from a population of patients in outpatient physical therapy facilities. The population in this study is
   1. targeted.
   2. accessible.
   3. clustered.
   4. stratified.

3. To select an appropriate study sample, researchers need to use _______________ during the recruitment process.

4. Which of the following statements are true regarding a sample? **Select all that apply.**
   1. They are "segments of a population based on a specific characteristic" (Polit & Beck, 2014, p. 178). **Select all that apply.**
   2. Most researchers work with samples rather than populations.
   3. A key criterion for samples is representativeness.
   4. Samples are selected the same way for every type of study.
   5. A sample refers to persons who participate in research.

5. Which of the following sample characteristics include an exclusion criterion?
   1. Subjects ages 20 to 30 years who are currently pursuing a BSN in nursing and are enrolled full time
   2. Patients 75 to 85 years of age with high-risk scores for pressure ulcers who are able to converse in English
   3. Academic educators in a 4-year college who are master's prepared, currently enrolled in a doctoral program, and have no other college degrees
   4. African American men, ages 50 to 60 years with a current diagnosis of benign prostatic hypertrophy and a history of three or more urinary tract infections

Probability Sampling Plans

6. Which of the following statements describes probability sampling?
   1. The researcher broadly defines the eligibility criteria to recruit a wide range of individuals to be recruited as the sample.
   2. "Every member (element) of the population has a probability higher than zero of being selected for the sample" (Burns & Grove, 2011, p. 545).
   3. Probability sampling is "sampling in which not every element of the population has an opportunity for selection" (p. 542).
   4. The procedure entails outlining the specific ways to obtain an appropriate sample for the study.

7. Which of the following research studies must use probability sampling?
   1. Descriptive studies
   2. Nonexperimental research
   3. Randomized clinical trials
   4. Quasi-experimental studies

8. How does a researcher do a stratified random sampling procedure? He or she
   1. establishes a sampling frame, assigns numbers to each element, and uses a table of random numbers to draw the sample (Polit & Beck, 2014).
   2. calculates a sampling interval and uses the interval to select each participant accordingly.
   3. divides the population into two or more layers and then selects randomly elements from each layer.
   4. assigns each element (from the sample) randomly to treatment groups.

9. The major advantage of a cluster sampling procedure compared with all the other probability procedures is that
   1. there are fewer errors and thus a lower probability of bias.
   2. data generated are easier to process.
   3. less time and money are spent.
   4. representativeness is maximized.

10. If the total accessible population of women with fibrocystic disease is 10,000 and the researcher needs 200 as a sample, what would be the sampling interval if systematic sampling is used?
    1. 100
    2. 1,000
    3. 500
    4. 50

11. Which of the following is true regarding probability sampling? Probability sampling
1. is the easiest method to obtain research participants.
2. obtains a representative sample from the population.
3. enables the researcher to handpick the participants.
4. is the most common method to use for all studies.

12. In which of the following situations would a probability sampling procedure not be considered appropriate? The researchers want to
1. explore the lived experience of children orphaned by HIV/AIDS.
2. determine the effectiveness of a new bed to reduce pressure ulcer development.
3. look at the effects of imagery on postoperative pain after a mastectomy.
4. study the relationship of music on sleep patterns of persons with arthritis.

13. In a study of "the effects of listening to non-commercial music on the quality of nocturnal sleep and relaxation indices in patients in medical surgical intensive care unit," Su et al. (2013) used random assignment of subjects. Random assignment means that
1. research participants were handpicked by the researchers.
2. the estimate of the number of subjects needed was calculated using power analysis.
3. participants were assigned to treatment conditions purely by chance.
4. a sampling interval was calculated as a guide to select the sample.

Nonprobability Sampling Plans

14. Which of the following statements is true regarding nonprobability sampling procedures? **Select all that apply.**
1. Findings of studies using nonprobability are less generalizable.
2. Risk of bias is greater than with other methods.
3. Nonprobability sampling procedures are costly to use.
4. Nonprobability samples are difficult to obtain.
5. More confidence could be achieved with careful selection of research participants.

15. Rydstrom et al. (2013) want to explore the experiences of adults growing up with innate or early-acquired HIV infection. Which sampling procedure would be appropriate for this study?
1. Probability, simple random
2. Nonprobability, purposive
3. Nonprobability, quota
4. Probability, systematic

16. Which of the following statements applies to snowball sampling?
1. Participants are selected through referrals from other participants.
2. Research participants are handpicked by the researcher.
3. The most accessible persons are recruited as participants.
4. A sampling interval of 10 deems every 10th person a participant.

17. "A quota sample of 913 working adults from nine occupational categories were recruited" (Lam, Lee, Wong, & Wong, 2012, p. 205). The quota sample means that the researchers
1. used the most readily available or accessible persons to participate in the study.
2. handpicked the sample considered to be typical and knowledgeable of the research issue.
3. subdivided the population into subgroups or strata based on some characteristics.
4. identified the population strata and calculated how many people are needed from each stratum.

18. A convenience sample of 200 adults provided informed consent to participate in a study to examine the influence of rheumatoid arthritis–related fatigue on symptoms of depression, health impairment perception, and satisfaction with ability (Ashley & Harrell, 2012). The use of the convenience sample means that the researchers
    1. identified the strata of the population and obtained participants from each stratum.
    2. handpicked each participant considered to be knowledgeable of the research topic.
    3. used the most accessible persons as subjects for the study.
    4. calculated a sampling interval to guide in picking the research participants.

Sample Adequacy

19. The procedure to determine sample adequacy in quantitative studies is called ______________.

20. When does data saturation in qualitative studies occur?
    1. The process occurs when data have been systematically organized and synthesized.
    2. No new data have emerged; redundancy has occurred.
    3. Data are reanalyzed in another investigation to answer new questions.
    4. The process occurs when themes or codes are identified in the data.

Critiquing the Sampling Procedure of a Quantitative Study

21. In critiquing the sampling procedures of a quantitative study, what questions would be appropriate to ask? **Select all that apply.**
    1. Was the sampling strategy appropriate to the study?
    2. What biases were evident in the sampling procedure used?
    3. Did the researcher use the best method of capturing the study phenomena?
    4. What steps did the researcher take to control extraneous variables?
    5. What factors affected representativeness?

ANSWERS AND RATIONALES

The correct answer number and rationale for why it is the correct answer are given in **boldface blue type**. Rationales for why the other possible answer options are incorrect also are given, but they are not in boldface type.

1. 1. The phrase might indicate a characteristic of a sample.
   2. **This could be the target population of a study. The key word in the option is "all."**
   3. The phrase might indicate a characteristic of a sample.
   4. The phrase might indicate a characteristic of a sample.

   TEST-TAKING TIP: A key word in the question stem is *population*, which means "the total group of persons or objects." *Total* means "all"; only option 2 has the word *all*.

   Content Area: *Basic Sampling Terminology;* ***Cognitive Level:*** *Analysis;* ***Question Type:*** *Multiple Choice*
   CRITICAL THINKING FACILITATOR: Think of when the word *population* is used. What is the population of a country? It is all the people living there. This notion is the same as the concept of population in research.

2. 1. The target population is "the entire population in which a researcher is interested and to which he or she would like to generalize the study results" (Polit & Beck, 2014, p. 393).
   2. **An accessible population is one that is "available for a study, often a nonrandom subset of the target population" (p. 374).**
   3. The term *cluster* refers to sampling wherein a researcher "develops a sampling frame that includes a list of all the states, cities, institutions, or organizations with which elements of the identified population can be linked" (Burns & Grove, 2011, p. 302).
   4. The term *stratified* refers to the stratified random sampling procedure that is "used in situations in which the researcher knows some of the variables in the population that are critical for achieving representativeness. Stratification ensures that all levels of the identified variables are adequately represented in the sample" (p. 301). For instance, basic nursing education might be used to stratify the sample of registered nurses in a study.

   TEST-TAKING TIP: A key phrase in the question stem is *patients in outpatient physical therapy facilities*. These facilities offer rehabilitation services for persons who have had an amputation. These facilities provide therapy for muscle strengthening and for learning how to use a prosthesis.

   Content Area: *Basic Sampling Terminology;* ***Cognitive Level:*** *Analysis;* ***Question Type:*** *Multiple Choice*
   CRITICAL THINKING FACILITATOR: Where do researchers recruit subjects for their studies? They need to find large numbers of persons who might be eligible to participate. Researchers could recruit successfully in a diabetic clinic if the intended sample consists of people with diabetes. Where would one find a population of persons with chronic illness? Most likely, these persons would be clients of home healthcare agencies. Think of other accessible populations.

3. **eligibility criteria.**

   TEST-TAKING TIP: To qualify, or be eligible, for something, one must possess certain characteristics. For instance, a job applicant must possess certain educational and experiential qualities to be eligible for a particular position.

   Content Area: *Basic Sampling Terminology;* ***Cognitive Level:*** *Knowledge;* ***Question Type:*** *Fill-in-the-Blank*
   CRITICAL THINKING FACILITATOR: What are the purposes of eligibility criteria? Don't they limit or restrict the number of possible subjects who are eligible? Eligibility criteria are used to screen or select applicants for a position so that those who apply have the characteristics desired. What were the eligibility criteria for any positions you have held?

4. 1. **The statement is correct. The key word in the option is *segments*. A segment of the population is the sample.**
   2. **The statement is a correct one. Working with populations rather than samples is extremely costly, time consuming, and labor intensive. Think of the U.S. Census, which looks at the entire U.S. population. A research study does not have the money and resources to study an entire population.**
   3. **Because only a sample and not the entire population is studied, it is essential that the sample is representative of the population from which it is drawn.**
   4. The statement is not accurate. Sample selection differs depending on the type of study design.
   5. The statement is not completely accurate. Samples are not just persons. They could be records, events, situations, and so on. For instance, a researcher studying falls might use the records of patients as the sample.

TEST-TAKING TIP: A key word in the question stem is *sample*. A sample means a segment of a whole, so it has to be representative of that whole. Studying a segment of the population is more feasible for many reasons including cost, time, and energy. If one samples a piece of a whole pie, then one could conclude that it is apple pie without eating the whole pie.

Content Area: *Basic Sampling Terminology;* ***Cognitive Level:*** *Knowledge;* ***Question Type:*** *Multiple Response*
CRITICAL THINKING FACILITATOR: Think of a population and the segment that is the sample. If one knows the population, what should the sample look like? What are the advantages of using a sample instead of the entire population? Think how much time and resources are needed to study the population.

5. 1. The phrase lists eligibility criteria.
2. The phrase identifies eligibility criteria.
3. The phrase includes eligibility criteria and adds an exclusion criterion. The term *no* is a clue in the option.
4. The phrase lists eligibility or inclusion criteria.

TEST-TAKING TIP: A key word in the question stem is *exclusion*. Exclusion indicates a restriction or a reason why one is ineligible to participate.

Content Area: *Basic Sampling Terminology;* ***Cognitive Level:*** *Comprehension;* ***Question Type:*** *Multiple Choice*
CRITICAL THINKING FACILITATOR: What is the purpose of exclusion criteria? Think of the eligibility criteria. If these are ways to make the sample more homogenous and to control extraneous variables, then what would you conclude about exclusion criteria?

6. 1. The statement relates to recruitment of interested persons; it does not define probability sampling.
2. The statement defines probability sampling. In this approach, every member of the population has an equal probability of being selected.
3. The statement is an incorrect definition of probability sampling. The statement is true for nonprobability sampling.
4. The statement is a correct one about recruitment of a sample, but it does not specifically indicate probability sampling.

TEST-TAKING TIP: The key word in the question stem is *probability*, which means "likelihood." The correct option includes the words "every member."

Content Area: *Probability Sampling;* ***Cognitive Level:*** *Knowledge;* ***Question Type:*** *Multiple Choice*
CRITICAL THINKING FACILITATOR: Sometimes thinking of opposite situations helps in arriving at a correct response. For example, if only the first 100 people who report are asked to participate in a study, then those who come after the first 100 have zero probability of being selected. Will all who participate in a raffle have equal probability of getting the winning number?

7. 1. Descriptive studies are nonexperimental in design and therefore do not use probability sampling procedures. Although practical and useful, descriptive studies do not test for cause and effect.
2. Nonexperimental designs include all designs that do not actively manipulate an independent variable. They do not test for cause and effect and do not require probability sampling procedures.
3. A randomized clinical trial requires probability sampling procedures because the independent variable is manipulated, and all types of controls are imposed on the research situation. These designs are the strongest for testing cause and effect.
4. Quasi-experimental designs are a step below the experimental designs. There is active manipulation of the independent variable, and some controls are imposed. However, the usual element missing is probability sampling.

TEST-TAKING TIP: The key word in the question stem is *probability*. Probability sampling uses some type of random process. Only a randomized clinical trial, as the name indicates, uses a random process.

Content Area: *Probability Sampling;* ***Cognitive Level:*** *Analysis;* ***Question Type:*** *Multiple Choice*
CRITICAL THINKING FACILITATOR: Review the levels of purposes of research studies. Those that aim to test the effectiveness of an intervention (independent variable) must have tight controls over all aspects of the research study. All known extraneous variables are addressed. One important control imposed is on the sampling procedure.

Because probability sampling procedures are more likely to produce a representative sample, there is a great deal of effort spent on this to strengthen the study's validity.

Look at a randomized clinical trial or an experimental study.. You will find that probability sampling is a critical part of the study.

8. 1. The process that is described is random sampling.
2. The process that is described is systematic sampling.
3. The process that is described is stratified random sampling. A key word in the option is *layers*, which mean strata.
4. The process describes random assignment to experimental or control groups.

TEST-TAKING TIP: The key word in the question stem is *stratified*. To stratify means to create layers. Therefore, layers of the population are created, and then the sample is randomly selected from each layer, or stratum.

Content Area: *Probability Sampling;* ***Cognitive Level:*** *Comprehension;* ***Question Type:*** *Multiple Choice*

CRITICAL THINKING FACILITATOR: If you wanted a representative sample, for instance, of nurses who work in critical care, how would you get one using a stratified random sampling? You might want to use educational background as a stratum, or age group. What would your final sample look like using this procedure?

9.
1. Compared with the other probability sampling procedures, cluster sampling has more errors (Haber, 2010). This is a disadvantage.
2. Data from cluster sampling are more difficult to process (Haber, 2010). This is a disadvantage.
3. **The statement indicates the advantage of cluster sampling (Haber, 2010).**
4. Representativeness is not maximized in cluster sampling because one of its major disadvantages is having more errors compared with the other random sampling procedures.

TEST-TAKING TIP: Each type of probability sampling procedure has advantages and disadvantages. Procedures used by the most stringent designs tend to be more costly and time consuming. However, sampling errors are fewer. Therefore, the others with possibility of more errors (a disadvantage) would have some other advantages.

Content Area: *Probability Sampling;* ***Cognitive Level:*** *Comprehension;* ***Question Type:*** *Multiple Choice*

CRITICAL THINKING FACILITATOR: Create a grid of the different types of probability sampling procedures. For each one, think of an advantage and a possible disadvantage. Look at a sample research study that used a probability sampling procedure. Provide a possible rationale for the researcher's choice. Then look at the discussion section and see whether the researcher discussed any limitations regarding this sampling procedure.

10.
1. The researcher would not use 100 as the sampling interval, known as the kth in systematic sampling. The sampling interval is calculated by dividing the total population by the required sample.
2. The sampling interval can be calculated by dividing the total population by the required number as the sample; 1,000 is an incorrect answer.
3. This is not the correct sampling interval.
4. **The sampling interval is 50. Therefore, each 50th person will serve as part of the sample; 10,000 divided by 200 is 50.**

TEST-TAKING TIP: The key words in the question stem are *sampling interval*, which means "standard distance between cases" (Polit & Beck, 2014, p. 181). Given the total number of the population, how does one calculate the distance between cases? It is done by dividing the larger number (population) by the smaller number (required sample). The quotient is the sampling interval.

Content Area: *Probability Sampling;* ***Cognitive Level:*** *Application;* ***Question Type:*** *Multiple Choice*

CRITICAL THINKING FACILITATOR: How do you arrive at an interval or an equal time or distance between cases? Say you have $1,000, and you have 10 people to share this equally. How much would each person get? Divide 1,000 by 10, and you get $100, which is the interval. Therefore, every $100 goes to a person. This is a nonresearch example, but it conveys the concept.

11.
1. The statement is not accurate. To use probability sampling, the population must be included before a representative sample could be extracted. The methods are also costly and time consuming.
2. **The probability sampling procedures have a greater likelihood of a sample that is representative of the population. Sampling biases and errors are minimized. Experimental designs, with purposes of prediction and explanation, use probability sampling procedures.**
3. The statement is not an accurate one regarding probability sampling procedures. Handpicking research participants is a process used in purposive sampling, a nonprobability sampling.
4. Probability sampling procedures are costly and time consuming. Therefore, not all types of studies use them. Only studies with purposes of prediction and control such as experimental designs and randomized clinical trials use these procedures. Studies that have purposes of identification, description, and exploration use nonprobability sampling procedures.

TEST-TAKING TIP: The key word is *probability*, which means that given a population, what is the likelihood that subjects will have an equal chance of being selected? If subjects are handpicked or selected because they are accessible or they meet a quota, then the process is

not an assurance that everyone has an equal likelihood of getting picked.

Content Area: *Probability Sampling;* ***Cognitive Level:*** *Comprehension;* ***Question Type:*** *Multiple Choice*
CRITICAL THINKING FACILITATOR: Representativeness is an essential element in quantitative studies. If researchers do not have representative samples, how will they address the generalizability (applicability) of their findings to the target population?

If you look at the different types of probability sampling, each attempts to obtain a representative sample because the rationale for the use of these is to minimize errors.

With minimal errors, research consumers (nurses and other healthcare providers) would have higher levels of confidence in using the findings in evidence-based practice.

12. 1. **A probability sampling procedure is not appropriate to use for the study. The study is a qualitative study, and a purposive sampling procedure, a nonprobability method, would be more appropriate. In this study, the researcher handpicks the participants who possess the lived experience.**
2. The information indicates that the study is a quantitative one with the purpose of explanation or prediction. The key word in the option is *effectiveness*. The researcher is looking to test the new bed's (independent variable) effectiveness in preventing pressure ulcers (dependent variable). A probability sampling procedure would be appropriate for this study.
3. The information indicates that the study is a quantitative one. The researcher is interested in looking at the effects. *Effect* is the key word in the option. The researcher would actively manipulate imagery, the independent variable, and watch for the change in the outcome or dependent variable, which is postoperative pain. This study would use probability sample if the purpose of the study is prediction or explanation.
4. The information indicates that the study is a quantitative one. A key word in the option is *relationship*. The term suggests a hypothesis that proposes a relationship between two or more variables. The independent variable to be manipulated is music, and the dependent variable is sleep patterns. One of the probability sampling procedures would be used. It is also possible to use a nonprobability procedure. However, in this instance, the level of confidence in the validity and generalizability of the findings is lessened.

TEST-TAKING TIP: Think of the basic concepts of probability sampling. Then look at the options. Option 1 contains the key term *lived experience*. Exploring the lived experience of persons is a qualitative study. Also recall the basic assumptions of the positivist paradigm for quantitative research. One assumption is control of sampling bias, which can be done with a probability sampling procedure.

Content Area: *Probability Sampling;* ***Cognitive Level:*** *Analysis;* ***Question Type:*** *Multiple Choice*
CRITICAL THINKING FACILITATOR: Look at a sample qualitative study and identify the sampling procedures that were used. How appropriate were the procedures? Compare and contrast them with probability sampling procedures.

13. 1. The statement is a process in purposive sampling.
2. The statement refers to the process of obtaining an adequate sample in quantitative studies.
3. **The statement is true of random assignment.**
4. The statement is a process in systematic sampling, one of the probability sampling procedures.

TEST-TAKING TIP: The key word in the question stem is *random*, which means "by chance."The random process eliminates or decreases errors. The fewer the errors, the more confidence in the validity of findings.

Content Area: *Probability Sampling;* ***Cognitive Level:*** *Comprehension;* ***Question Type:*** *Multiple Choice*
CRITICAL THINKING FACILITATOR: What is the goal of random assignment? Would this process eliminate bias in sampling? What are the other advantages and disadvantages of random assignment? When is it appropriate to use?

14. 1. **Nonprobability sampling procedures are less likely to produce representative samples; therefore, sampling bias and errors might occur. With these factors in mind, findings from studies that used nonprobability sampling procedures have less generalizability.**
2. **The statement is true of nonprobability sampling procedures in which not every member of the population has an equal probability of being selected.**
3. The statement is not an accurate one. Nonprobability sampling procedures are not as costly and time consuming as probability sampling procedures.

4. Nonprobability samples are not as difficult to obtain compared with probability samples. Convenience or accessible, quota, snowball, and purposive sampling require participants who possess the experience of the phenomena of interest.
5. **The statement is true for nonprobability sampling. For instance, a qualitative study on the lived experience of women after the loss of a breast from cancer would use purposive sampling. Careful identification and selection of these women would result in more confidence in the validity of the findings. Qualitative studies are gauged by different criteria. These include trustworthiness, transferability, and credibility.**

TEST-TAKING TIP: The key word in the question stem is *nonprobability*, which means "not by chance." Samples are obtained because they were accessible, they met the quota, they were referred by someone, or they were handpicked by the researcher. Keeping these definitions and what you already know about probability sampling in mind should help you choose the correct options.

Content Area: *Nonprobability Sampling;* ***Cognitive Level:*** *Comprehension;* ***Question Type:*** *Multiple Response*
CRITICAL THINKING FACILITATOR: Create a grid of all the different types of nonprobability sampling procedures. Think of hypothetical studies and the appropriate sampling procedure that should be used for each.

15. 1. The statement indicates that the study is qualitative. Therefore, none of the probability sampling procedures would be appropriate.
2. **The statement indicates the study is qualitative. A purposive sampling procedure would be appropriate. The researchers would handpick adults with innate or early-acquired HIV infection.**
3. A quota sample, a type of nonprobability sampling procedure, would not be appropriate. The size of the sample in qualitative studies is not specified at the beginning of the study. The researchers would stop collecting data when saturation is reached (no new data have emerged). In some qualitative studies, data saturation could be reached after as few as four participants.
4. A systematic sampling, a probability procedure, would not be appropriate for a qualitative study.

TEST-TAKING TIP: The key word in the question stem is *experiences*, which means that the researchers would conduct in-depth interviews with research participants who would describe their experiences. These descriptions are narrative data. Narrative data are not collected in quantitative studies.

Content Area: *Nonprobability Sampling;* ***Cognitive Level:*** *Analysis;* ***Question Type:*** *Multiple Choice*
CRITICAL THINKING FACILITATOR: Think of phenomena in nursing and healthcare that would be the foci of qualitative studies. Some examples to get you started are the lived experience of organ transplant donors, the experience of nurses transitioning from tertiary-care practice to restorative practice, or a study of the nursing clinical group in a community setting. How would researchers recruit participants for these studies?

16. 1. **Referrals are the means to get a snowball sample, also known as network sampling.**
2. Handpicking participants is characteristic of purposive sampling.
3. The statement describes convenience sampling.
4. The statement describes systematic sampling, a probability sampling procedure.

TEST-TAKING TIP: The key word in the question stem is *snowball*. Imagine a snowball rolling down a hill. As it rolls, it picks up more snow and becomes larger. This is the idea of snowball sampling, also known as network sampling.

Content Area: *Nonprobability Sampling;* ***Cognitive Level:*** *Comprehension;* ***Question Type:*** *Multiple Choice*
CRITICAL THINKING FACILITATOR: How do you disseminate information using a snowball technique? You depend on an initial core group to tell others. Over time, the network becomes bigger than when it started. The snowball technique is used in many situations in life and is an effective recruitment approach for obtaining a sample.

17. 1. The statement describes a convenience sampling procedure.
2. The statement describes purposive sampling.
3. The statement describes a part of stratified random sampling.
4. **The statement describes quota sampling.**

TEST-TAKING TIP: The key words in the question stem are *quota* and *occupational categories*. Categories can be treated as strata that delineate different occupations. *Quota* means that equal numbers from

each of the categories are extracted as research participants.

Content Area: *Nonprobability Sampling;* ***Cognitive Level:*** *Analysis;* ***Question Type:*** *Multiple Choice*
CRITICAL THINKING FACILITATOR: Suppose that a vice president of a tertiary health-care facility is interested in learning about the job satisfaction of all registered nurses employed by the facility. If the vice president uses a quota sampling procedure, what possible categories could be used to extract a sample?

18. 1. The statement describes quota sampling.
2. The statement describes purposive sampling.
3. The most accessible persons are the convenience sample.
4. The statement describes systematic sampling.

TEST-TAKING TIP: The key word in the question stem is *convenience*. The most accessible persons form a convenience sample. Time and effort tend to be minimal in this type of sample compared with other sampling procedures.

Content Area: *Nonprobability Sampling;* ***Cognitive Level:*** *Analysis;* ***Question Type:*** *Multiple Choice*
CRITICAL THINKING FACILITATOR: Using a grid comparing each of the nonprobability sampling procedures, look at some of the qualitative research in the Appendix of your core textbook. Did each of the studies use an appropriate sampling method? Why or why not?

19. power analysis

TEST-TAKING TIP: Recall from your statistics course that power has something to do with a large sample. Therefore, you could deduce that an adequate sample and a larger one would give the researcher power in the statistical process.

Content Area: *Sample Adequacy;* ***Cognitive Level:*** *Knowledge;* ***Question Type:*** *Fill-in-the-Blank*
CRITICAL THINKING FACILITATOR: What is an adequate sample? Are larger samples better? Recall some of these concepts from statistics and review how you interpreted results as statistically significant when you consulted your F table.

20. 1. The statement describes what needs to be done before data are interpreted.
2. The statements describe data saturation in qualitative studies.
3. The process described is relevant to secondary analysis.
4. The statement refers to data analysis in qualitative studies.

TEST-TAKING TIP: The key words in the question stem are *qualitative studies*. You know that data in qualitative studies are descriptive statements made by research participants. Because these statements cannot be statistically analyzed, some other process must be used. In a qualitative study in which the researcher is talking to research participants about a lived experience, would there be some indication that participants might share commonalities in their experiences? If the researcher labels these as themes (i.e., identifies each of these in every participant), would there be a point when there are no more new themes? When no new data emerge or a redundancy is evident, data saturation has been reached.

Content Area: *Data Saturation;* ***Cognitive Level:*** *Comprehension;* ***Question Type:*** *Multiple Choice*
CRITICAL THINKING FACILITATOR: Look at a sample phenomenological study. Note that in the body of the report, there are highlighted subheadings under the Results section. These are the themes identified by the researcher in the descriptive statements of the participants. Under each theme are examples of statements of participants that support the theme. Read on until the end of the section; there you would find a statement about data saturation. Now compare what you found with the analyses of data in a quantitative study. The difference between quantitative and qualitative approaches will become clearer.

21. **1. The question is a specific one to ask in critiquing the sampling procedure. Note the word *sampling* in the question.**
2. The question is a specific one to ask in critiquing the sampling procedure. Note the word *sampling* in the question.
3. The question is not an appropriate one to ask in critiquing the sampling procedure. The question is appropriate in critiquing data collection methods.
4. The question is appropriate to ask if one is critiquing the design of a study.
5. The question is a specific one to ask when critiquing the sampling procedure of a study. Note the word *representativeness*, which is a concept in sampling.

Content Area: *Critiquing Sampling Procedures;* ***Cognitive Level:*** *Analysis;* ***Question Type:*** *Multiple Response*
CRITICAL THINKING FACILITATOR: Review probability and nonprobability sampling procedures. When are they appropriate to use? What are the advantages and disadvantages of each? When would you consider the sampling strategy used as a strength of the study?

13 Examining Data Collection Methods

KEY WORDS

The following words include English vocabulary, nursing/medical terminology, concepts, principles, or information relevant to content specifically addressed in the chapter or associated with topics presented in it. English dictionaries, your nursing textbooks, and medical dictionaries such as *Taber's Cyclopedic Medical Dictionary* are resources that can be used to expand your knowledge and understanding of these words and related information.

Biophysiologic methods
Interval
In vitro
In vivo
Levels of measurement
Measurement
Measurement errors
Nominal
Observation
Obtained score
Ordinal
Ratio
Response set bias
Self-report
Semantic differential
True score
Visual analog

QUESTIONS

Measurement and Levels of Measurement

1. Which of the following statements describes measurement in research?
1. "The process of selecting a group of people, events, behaviors, situations, or other elements that are representative of the population being studied" (Burns & Grove, 2011, p. 548)
2. "The process of assigning numbers to objects, events, or situations, in accordance to some rule" (p. 541)
3. "The identification of subjects and the precise, systematic gathering of information (data) relevant to the research purpose or the specific objectives, questions, or hypotheses of a study" (p. 535)
4. "A structured or unstructured oral communication between the researcher and the subject during which information is obtained for a study" (p. 540)

2. Which of the following is/are true regarding the nominal level of measurement? **Select all that apply.**
1. Data can be "organized into categories of a defined property" (Burns & Grove, 2011, p. 329).
2. Categories of data cannot be put in rank order.
3. It is the lowest level of measurement.
4. Weight in pounds can be considered nominal data.
5. There is a ranking order of the data with specific distances in between.

3. Which of the following is/are true of the interval level of measurement? **Select all that apply.**
   1. It is the third level of measurement with ratio as the highest.
   2. Interval data provide information about the magnitude of the attribute.
   3. It ranks people, events, and situations on a relative standing on an attribute.
   4. Interval data cannot be mathematically computed.
   5. "Interval data can be averaged" (Polit & Beck, 2014, p. 201).

Errors in Measurement

4. An obtained score on a research instrument includes the true score and ______________.

5. Which statement best describes response set bias?
   1. "A measurement distortion arising from the study participant's awareness of being observed, or more generally, from the effect of the measurement procedure itself" (Polit & Beck, 2014, p. 390).
   2. "The measurement error resulting from the tendency of some participants to respond to items in characteristic ways (e.g., always agreeing) independently of the item content" (p. 391).
   3. "The fluctuation of the value of a statistic from one sample to another drawn from the same population" (p. 391).
   4. "The effect on the dependent variable resulting from subjects' awareness that they are participants in a study" (p. 381).

Types of Data

6. Which of the following studies would use existing data? **Select all that apply.**
   1. A survey of the "consumption of added sugars among US adults, 2005-2010" (Ervin & Ogden, 2013, p. 1)
   2. Del Pino-Casado, R., Frías-Osuna, A., Palomino-Moral, P. A., & Ramón Martínez-Riera, J. (2012). Gender differences regarding informal caregivers of older people: A secondary analysis
   3. A correlational cross-sectional study of "psychosocial health of infertile Ghanaian women and their infertility beliefs" (Naab, Brown, & Heidrich, 2013, p. 132)
   4. Rao, A. (2012). The contemporary construction of nurse empowerment: an integrative review
   5. Su, C. P., Lai, H. L., Chang, E. T., Yiin, L. M., Perng, S. J., & Chen, P. W. (2013). A randomized clinical trial of the effects of listening to non-commercial music on nocturnal sleep and relaxation indices in patients in medical intensive care

7. New data would be used for which of the following studies?
   1. Wang, P. (2013). The effectiveness of cranberry products to reduce urinary tract infections in females: A literature review
   2. Kao, H. F., & An, K. (2012). Effect of acculturation and mutuality on family loyalty among Mexican-American caregivers of elders
   3. Cahill, J., LoBiondo-Wood, G., Bergstrom, N., & Armstrong, T. (2012). Brain tumor symptoms as antecedents to uncertainty: An integrative review
   4. Hellström, A., & Willman, A.. (2011). Promoting sleep by nursing interventions in health care settings: A systematic review

Methods of Data Collection

8. Friese and Manojlovich (2012) explored nurses' perception of their relationships with physicians in ambulatory oncology settings. What type of data collection method was used in this study?
   1. Observation
   2. Biophysiologic methods
   3. Self-report
   4. Visual analog

9. Lam et al. (2012) assessed weight, height, and waist and hip circumferences of subjects who participated in a study on obesity. What type of data collection method was used?
   1. Observation
   2. Biophysiologic, in vivo
   3. Self-report
   4. Biophysiologic, in vitro

10. Which of the following statements is/are true regarding a semantic differential scale? **Select all that apply.** The semantic differential
    1. "is composed of a set of scales, using pairs of adjectives that reflect opposite feelings" (Fain, 2009, p. 136).
    2. "is different from Likert scales because only two extremes are labeled" (p. 137).
    3. "requires subjects to respond to series of statements to express a viewpoint" (p. 132).
    4. has "response choices [that] commonly address agreement, evaluation, or frequency" (p. 132).
    5. can be used to measure attitudes or beliefs.

11. What data collection tool is used when "subjects are asked to mark a point on the line indicating the amount of the phenomena experienced at that time?" (Fain, 2009, p. 138).
    1. Visual analog scale
    2. Observation tool
    3. Likert scale
    4. Semantic differential scale

12. Which of the following is/are classified as a self-report method? **Select all that apply.**
    1. Questionnaire
    2. Interview schedule
    3. Biophysiologic, in vitro
    4. Observation
    5. Likert scale

13. Which of the following is/are true of a self-report tool such as a questionnaire? **Select all that apply.**
    1. Can be costly to produce and distribute
    2. Can be distributed widely, especially via the Internet
    3. Provide minimal valid and reliable data
    4. Are less intimidating than interviews
    5. Could protect the anonymity of respondents

14. Which of the following are advantages of an interview as a self-report method? **Select all that apply.**
    1. It could provide the researcher with a higher percentage of willing respondents.
    2. It would be useful for those who have difficulty completing a questionnaire.
    3. It would guarantee confidentiality and anonymity.
    4. It would offer opportunities for interacting with and observing the respondents.
    5. The researcher might get superficial data.

15. A self-report method of data collection is evident in which of the following? **Select all that apply.**
    1. Yoon and Kim (2013) looked at "women's demographic and job characteristics, job-related stress, emotional labor, and depressive symptoms" (p. 169).
    2. "Three bilingual *promotoras* collected data from 193 Mexican-American adult caregivers of community-dwelling elders using three scales designed for Mexican-Americans" (Kao & An, 2012, p. 111).
    3. In a study by Ervin and Ogden (2013) on the consumption of added sugars, part of the data analyzed came from "blood and urine specimens provided by participants during the physical examination" (p. 7).
    4. Respondents in Davidson and Rourke's (2012) "study unanimously identified five essential learning needs for nursing clinical instructor" (p. 1).
    5. Fakhouri et al. (2012) looked at the "prevalence of obesity among older adults in the United States, 2007-2010" (p. 1). The heights and weights of the adults were measured.

16. Which of the following could be obtained by using a biophysiologic in-vivo measure?
    1. Blood pressure
    2. Potassium levels
    3. Hemoglobin
    4. T cell count

17. Which are the advantages of biophysiologic measures? **Select all that apply.**
    1. Easy to use
    2. Objective measurements of the variable
    3. Not easily distorted
    4. Readily available to anyone
    5. Usually accurate and precise

18. A researcher wanted to examine the levels of cortisol in persons who report disturbance in their sleep patterns. What type of data collection measurement would be appropriate to use?
    1. Self-report of stress
    2. Biophysiologic, in vitro
    3. Observation of behavior
    4. Biophysiologic, in vivo

19. When are observations as data collection measurements appropriate to use? **Select all that apply.** Observations are appropriate when researchers want to
    1. examine cultural practices of an ethnic group.
    2. study how first-time mothers bond with their newborns.
    3. explore the relationship between regular exercise and cardiac efficiency.
    4. describe the lived experience of individuals with above-knee amputations.
    5. ascertain the perceptions of self-concept in women who have lost a breast.

Critiquing Data Collection Methods

20. Which of the following questions would be appropriate in critiquing a study's data collection methods?
    1. "Were the study participants subjected to any physical harm, discomfort, or psychological distress?" (Polit & Beck, 2014, p. 93).
    2. "Did the researchers use the best method for capturing the study phenomena?" (p. 193).
    3. "Were adequate steps taken to safeguard participants' privacy?" (p. 93).
    4. "Are key characteristics of the sample described?" (p. 183).

ANSWERS AND RATIONALES

The correct answer number and rationale for why it is the correct answer are given in **boldface blue type.** Rationales for why the other possible answer options are incorrect also are given, but they are not in boldface type.

1. 1. Sampling is described in this statement. A clue in this incorrect option is the word *selecting*.
   2. Measurement is described in this statement. "Assigning numbers" indicates that something is quantitative and therefore can be measured.
   3. The process described is data collection even though some form of measurement is used in quantitative studies. Data in qualitative studies are descriptive and not numerical.
   4. The statement describes an interview, which is a type of self-report method of data collection.

   TEST-TAKING TIP: ***Measurement* implies numbers, and numbers can be subjected to operations such as addition, subtraction, multiplication, and division.**

   Content Area: *Measurement and Levels of Measurement;* ***Cognitive Level:*** *Comprehension;* ***Question Type:*** *Multiple Choice*
   CRITICAL THINKING FACILITATOR: When someone asks you to rate a feeling state, such as pain, on a scale from 1 to 5, that person is asking for a measurement. Your response would be one of the numbers from 1 to 5. In this situation, you have just "created" a measurement of pain. The process of measurement is related to numbers designating levels or degrees of feelings, attitudes, attributes, and other situations. Look at the instruments or the data collection methods used in quantitative studies and decide what was measured.

2. **1. A key word in the option is *categories*, which means some sort of classification. Classifications cannot be subjected to statistical analysis. Therefore, the data are nominal.**
   2. Key words in the option are *rank order*, which means "in succession" or "some type of organizational method." The statement refers to ordinal data. Ordinal pertains to succession.
   3. Because ordinal data only indicate rank order and cannot be subjected to statistical analysis, ordinal data are considered the lowest level of measurement.
   4. Weight is an attribute that could have an absolute zero. Therefore, it can be considered ratio scale and is the highest form of measurement.
   5. The statement describes interval scale measurement. The key words in the option are *specific distances in between*. So, if the data are 2, 4, 6, one can say that the distance of 6 is twice the distance of 4 from 2.

   TEST-TAKING TIP: **The word *nominal* means "pertaining to a name." Names cannot be subjected to statistical analyses.**

   Content Area: *Measurement and Levels of Measurement;* ***Cognitive Level:*** *Analysis;* ***Question Type:*** *Multiple Response*
   CRITICAL THINKING FACILITATOR: What are some examples of nominal data? Let us say you come up with numbers assigned to football players. Can you do any mathematical operations on these numbers? No, you cannot average the numbers or add or subtract them. The numbers provide another way to name the athletes they are assigned to.

3. **1. This statement describes interval scale measurement. It is the third highest level of measurement.**
   2. Interval scale measurements "have equal numerical distances between intervals. These scales follow the rules of mutually exclusive categories, exhaustive categories, and rank ordering and are assumed to represent a continuum of values. Thus, the magnitude of the attribute can be more precisely defined" (Burns & Grove, 2011, p. 330).
   3. A key word that makes this option incorrect is *rank*. Rank is related to ordinal measurement.
   4. This statement is incorrect. Interval data can be subjected to mathematical operations.
   5. This statement is correct because interval data can be subjected to mathematical operations such as the computation of an average.

   TEST-TAKING TIP: **The key word in the question stem is *interval* that means specified points with distances between points.**

   Content Area: *Measurement and Levels of Measurement;* ***Cognitive Level:*** *Analysis;* ***Question Type:*** *Multiple Response*
   CRITICAL THINKING FACILITATOR: What are some examples of interval data? Interval data provide the ranking of an attribute with specific distances between data points. Take the following scores on an examination: 100, 90, 80, and 70. These scores are ranked from high to low. There is a 10-point interval

between each score. The difference between 100 and 90 is 10, the difference between 90 and 80 is 10, and so on.

4. error

TEST-TAKING TIP: The obtained score is not perfect. The true score is the one "that would be obtained if a measure were infallible" (Polit & Beck, 2014, p. 394). Any flaws in the instrument could cause errors.

***Content Area:** Measurement and Levels of Measurement; **Cognitive Level:** Knowledge; **Question Type:** Fill-in-the-Blank*

CRITICAL THINKING FACILITATOR: No research situation, regardless of the controls imposed, is ever a perfect situation. Any number of factors, external or internal, could influence the obtained score. Think of examinations you have taken. Would your obtained score (grade) be pure (no influences)? How did you feel during the examination? Was there a disturbance in the room? Were there terms on the examination that you did not understand?

5. 1. The definition is applicable to reactivity. A clue in the option is the word *effect*, which means "a reaction."
   2. **This definition is correct. The key word in this option is *tendency*, which means "inclination" or "disposition."**
   3. This definition applies to sampling error. Measurement has to do with data. This statement includes the words *sample* and *population*. These terms are relevant to sampling, not measurement.
   4. This statement refers to the Hawthorne effect. The statement addresses the dependent variable not the overall measurement of variables.

TEST-TAKING TIP: A clue in the question stem is *bias*, which means "an inclination or tendency."

***Content Area:** Measurement and Levels of Measurement; **Cognitive Level:** Analysis; **Question Type:** Multiple Choice*

CRITICAL THINKING FACILITATOR: Think of situations when someone has an almost immediate response to something without considering all aspects of the situation. Perhaps the reaction or response is related to previous experiences or other factors. In any case, the reaction is almost always similar in other circumstances. The person has a "tendency" to react or respond in the same way each time.

6. 1. The title of this study suggests new, not existing data were used. A survey "obtains information about people's activities, beliefs, preferences, attitudes via direct questioning" (Polit & Beck, 2014, p. 393).
   2. **The title of this study suggests existing data, not new, were used. Secondary analysis is "a form of research in which the data collected in one study are reanalyzed in another investigation to answer new questions" (p. 391).**
   3. The title of this study contains the word *correlation*. Correlation research examines "the relationship between two or more variables to explain the nature of relationships in the world; does not examine cause and effect" (Burns & Grove, 2011, p. 535). Nothing in the title suggests using existing data. The study is an original investigation by the researchers.
   4. **This title contains the term *integrative review*. An integrative review is "conducted to identify, analyze, and synthesize the results of independent studies to determine the current knowledge (what is known and not known) in a particular area" (p. 540).**
   5. A randomized clinical trial (RCT) is a "full experimental test of an intervention, involving random assignment to treatment groups" (Polit & Beck, 2014, p. 390). There is nothing in the title to suggest that the researchers used existing data. This is an original study by the researchers.

TEST-TAKING TIP: The key words in the question stem are *existing data*. These mean data are already available or present. Studies that use existing data are those that take data collected by others and do additional analyses. Examples of these types of studies are integrative reviews, systematic reviews, and secondary analysis.

***Content Area:** Types of Data; **Cognitive Level:** Analysis; **Question Type:** Multiple Response*

CRITICAL THINKING FACILITATOR: Think of a paper you need to write on a topic. Unless you are the first person to write about it, you will use what has been written and published about the topic. You search for existing literature, read the articles, and then synthesize the information to answer the criteria for the assignment. Nursing and other disciplines rely on existing information and use these as foundation. Think of the expression "it makes no sense to reinvent the wheel." Also look at a sample article that is a systematic or integrative review. There are usually tables summarizing the studies used and showing how the relevant information is analyzed.

7. 1. The title of this study indicates that it is a literature review. A literature review "involves identification and analysis of relevant publications that contain information pertaining to the research problem" (Fain, 2009, p. 53).

2. **The title suggests a study in which the researchers ascertained the effects of independent variables, acculturation and mutuality, on a dependent variable, family loyalty. This is an original study by the researchers, and they collected new data from their participants, Mexican-American caregivers of elders.**
3. The title indicates that the study is an integrative review. An integrative review is "conducted to identify, analyze, and synthesize the results from independent studies to determine the current knowledge" (what is known and not known) in a particular area" (Burns & Grove, 2011, p. 540). An integrative review uses existing data from many studies. No new data are collected by the researcher(s).
4. The title indicates that the study is a systematic review. "A systematic review is a structured, comprehensive synthesis of quantitative and outcome studies in a particular healthcare area to determine the best research evidence available for expert clinicians to use to promote evidence-based practice" (p. 550). Existing data from many studies were used for this study.

TEST-TAKING TIP: The key words in the question stem are *new data*. These mean data that are the latest or additional. Studies that use new data are those wherein the researchers collected their own data as part of their research study. Surveys, all types of nonexperimental, experimental, and qualitative studies, all collect new data.

Content Area: *Types of Data;* ***Cognitive Level:*** *Analysis;* ***Question Type:*** *Multiple Choice*

CRITICAL THINKING FACILITATOR: Look at a sample study and determine what type of data were collected and used. There is a section in each article where data collection procedures are described. Data collection procedures would be under the methods section. Reading this section will help you determine your response.

8. 1. An observation has the aim of watching something such as behavior or conditions. Perceptions cannot be observed but are reported or described by the person.
2. Biophysiologic methods measure physiologic functions and processes. Machines or equipment are used to measure these functions. For example, temperature, as a biophysiologic factor, is measured using a thermometer.
3. **A self-report method obtains information from the research participant herself or himself. Depending on the type of study, the self-report method might obtain numerical data (quantitative study) or descriptive data (qualitative study). The study is exploring perceptions of nurses. The nurses themselves have to describe these to the researcher, making the method of data collection a self-report one.**
4. A visual analog scale is a type of scale that is "useful for measuring subjective phenomena (e.g., pain, fatigue, shortness of breath, anxiety). The scale is unidimensional, quantifying intensity only" (Fain, 2009, p. 138).

TEST-TAKING TIP: The key word in the title of the study is *perception*. A perception is subjective, so it can only be reported by the person experiencing it.

Content Area: *Methods of Data Collection;* ***Cognitive Level:*** *Analysis;* ***Question Type:*** *Multiple Choice*

CRITICAL THINKING FACILITATOR: Get familiar with what types of data could be collected using the different data collection methods. Look at a sample studies and determine which studies used self-report methods to obtain data.

9. 1. Although the variables in the study could be observed, one could only come up with estimates, and the variables could be described, not measured, such as describing the weight as under or over, tall or short for height, or wide or narrow for waist or hip circumference.
2. **Weight, height, and waist and hip circumferences are physiologic factors. Therefore, biophysiologic measures are appropriate to use. Rather than estimates, the researcher would use a scale and a tape measure to ascertain the actual measurements of these factors. In addition, in-vivo measures are "those performed directly within or on living organisms" (Polit & Beck, 2014, p. 192).**
3. Self-report measures might be appropriate but not accurate. People might report the weights they obtain from a home scale that might not provide reliable readings. People can also describe their weights as under or over. Accuracy is an essential requirement for research tools.
4. Biophysiologic in-vitro measures use biophysiologic materials from research participants, and these are then sent for analysis in a laboratory. Examples are blood, urine, sputum, cerebrospinal fluid, and so on.

TEST-TAKING TIP: The key words in the title of the study are *weight, height,* and *waist and hip circumferences*. These are anatomic and physiologic indicators. To measure these accurately, some type of apparatus or equipment is needed.

Content Area: *Methods of Data Collection;* ***Cognitive Level:*** *Analysis;* ***Question Type:*** *Multiple Choice*
CRITICAL THINKING FACILITATOR: Differentiate biophysiologic measures that are in vivo and in vitro. Remember that in-vitro ones require some type of specimen from the research subject. Identify some of these in-vitro measures, and think of how these are measured. You will encounter these in your clinical work. For example, a culture and sensitivity would be considered in vitro because a swab of fluids will be needed such as drainage from a wound, mucus from the throat, or urine, just to name a few.

10. 1. **The semantic differential uses bipolar adjectives.**
    2. **This statement identifies the difference between the semantic differential and a Likert scale, on which responses are ranked from strongly agree to strongly disagree.**
    3. This statement describes a Likert scale.
    4. This statement describes a Likert scale.
    5. **This statement is true about a semantic differential.**

TEST-TAKING TIP: The key word in the question stem is *differential*. Derived from the word *different*, it means "not the same." The scale would have opposite adjective pairs to express the respondent's feelings about a particular situation.

Content Area: *Methods of Data Collection;* ***Cognitive Level:*** *Analysis;* ***Question Type:*** *Multiple Choice*
CRITICAL THINKING FACILITATOR: Create semantic differentials using situations from your clinical experiences. Take, for example, your feelings about doing clinical in a community health setting. What are opposite adjective pairs you could use to describe your feelings, such as overwhelming versus manageable or growth facilitating versus growth inhibiting? Think of some more.

11. 1. **The statement describes a visual analog scale.**
    2. An observation is used for studying situations such as behaviors, verbal and nonverbal communication, activities, and environmental conditions (Polit & Beck, 2014).
    3. A Likert scale "consists of several declarative statements (items) that express a viewpoint on a topic" (p. 186).
    4. A semantic differential scale is "composed of a set of scales, using pairs of adjectives that reflect opposite feelings" (Fain, 2009, p. 136).

TEST-TAKING TIP: The key part of the statement is *subjects are asked to mark a point on the line*. To mark a point on a line, the subject will have to use her or his vision to answer a question posed by the researcher.

Content Area: *Methods of Data Collection;* ***Cognitive Level:*** *Analysis;* ***Question Type:*** *Multiple Choice*
CRITICAL THINKING FACILITATOR: Think of some clinical applications of visual analogs. A common example of a visual analog is the Wong-Baker FACES pain scale. When is this tool useful?

12. 1. **A questionnaire is a "printed self-report form designed to elicit information that can be obtained through written or verbal responses of the subject" (Burns & Grove, 2011, p. 545).**
    2. **An interview is an interaction between a research subject and the researcher wherein information is provided by a subject in response to questions posed by the researcher. This is a self-report method.**
    3. Biophysiologic in-vitro methods are performed on research subjects by extracting biophysiologic material that can be analyzed. These are not self-report methods.
    4. An observation is used for studying situations such as behaviors, verbal and nonverbal communication, activities, and environmental conditions (Polit & Beck, 2014). Observation is not considered a self-report method.
    5. **A Likert scale "consists of several declarative statements (items) that express a viewpoint on a topic" (p. 186). A scale ascertains a research subject's viewpoints and is considered a self-report method.**

TEST-TAKING TIP: The key word in the question stem is *self-report*. A self-report method would allow the research subject to express her or his own responses to the questions, oral or printed, posed by the researcher.

Content Area: *Methods of Data Collection;* ***Cognitive Level:*** *Comprehension;* ***Question Type:*** *Multiple Response*
CRITICAL THINKING FACILITATOR: Think of subjective and primary sources of data in relation to the assessment phase of the nursing

process. Data obtained are directly from the individual who reports the data herself or himself.

13. 1. This statement is incorrect. The cost of reproducing and distributing questionnaires is low with the availability of modern technology.
   2. Many questionnaires are posted on Web sites such as Survey Monkey, and the distribution is wide.
   3. This statement is incorrect. A well-developed questionnaire could elicit a large amount of valid and reliable data.
   4. A questionnaire can be completed without interacting with a researcher or a data collector. So, respondents could complete it in a relaxed atmosphere and at their own pace and possibly outside a formal research setting.
   5. Because a questionnaire could be completed outside a research setting and without interacting with a researcher, there is a higher probability that anonymity would be maintained.

TEST-TAKING TIP: Think of an online survey that you were asked to complete. Compare this experience with another way to get information from you such as a telephone interview. In the telephone interview, the interviewer would have to be paid, making the process more costly. Also, when subjects are asked a question by the interviewer, they feel a certain degree of pressure to give an answer in a short period of time. Making these comparisons will help you come up with the correct answer.

Content Area: *Methods of Data Collection;* ***Cognitive Level:*** *Analysis;* ***Question Type:*** *Multiple Response*
CRITICAL THINKING FACILITATOR:
Think of the other self-report methods of data collection. Evaluate their appropriateness to the research question as well as their advantages and disadvantages. Look at a research study that used interviews to collect data. Identify the advantages and disadvantages of using interviews for data collection.

14. **1. This statement can be considered an advantage. Potential research participants would be more willing and receptive if they had a personal connection with the researcher who could answer concerns or issues. A person, rather than a piece of paper (questionnaire), might make the research more real for the potential participant.**
   2. There are many reasons why people would rather be interviewed than complete a questionnaire. Some people might have a low literacy level; others could be intimidated by online questionnaires. Others might have visual issues. Some people prefer a connection with a person rather than a paper or online questionnaire.
   3. Interviewing does not guarantee anonymity and confidentiality. In fact, it raises the possibility that the interviewer might know the participant.
   4. This statement is an advantage of an interview. Some people enjoy the encounter with a researcher and see the interview as an opportunity to express their feelings and perceptions about a topic of interest. Research participants might appreciate participating when they know the significance of the study and the benefits to others.
   5. This statement is incorrect. An interview has the potential for obtaining rich data from research participants. Such is the case in qualitative studies in which participants are asked to describe their experiences relating to the phenomenon of interest.

TEST-TAKING TIP: Try this: Compare and contrast an interview and questionnaire. You can guess what the advantages are by analyzing why a researcher would use an interview versus a questionnaire.

Content Area: *Methods of Data Collection;* ***Cognitive Level:*** *Analysis;* ***Question Type:*** *Multiple Response*
CRITICAL THINKING FACILITATOR:
Evaluate a patient interview you conducted such as a nursing history. Think of the patient's attitude and demeanor. Was the patient receptive and attentive to you? Did the patient attempt to answer your questions? How willing was the patient to share her or his experiences? What was the overall nonverbal communication conveyed during the interview?

15. **1. The title suggests that the researchers used self-report methods to ascertain participants' perceptions.**
   2. The title suggests that the researchers used self-report methods.
   3. The information from the study report indicates the use of biophysiologic in-vitro measurements because blood and urine samples were used.
   4. The researchers indicate in the statement that respondents identified essential learning needs. Identifying learning needs is considered self-reporting.

5. The researchers use height and weight as data. These are considered biophysiologic in-vivo measurements.

TEST-TAKING TIP: The key word in the question stem is *self-report*. Self-report means that responses are provided by the research participants.

Content Area: *Methods of Data Collection;* ***Cognitive Level:*** *Analysis;* ***Question Type:*** *Multiple Response*
CRITICAL THINKING FACILITATOR:
Identify assessment tools that are self-reports. How do you find out what types of foods your patients eat? What are the cultural practices that influence health habits? What illnesses have the patients experienced in the past 10 years? Data obtained would be considered self-reports.

16. **1. Blood pressure is a biophysiologic in-vivo measurement. In-vivo measurements are performed directly on the person. There is no material extracted from the person.**
2. Potassium levels are biophysiologic in-vitro measurements. Blood needs to be extracted to measure potassium levels. The blood is then analyzed in the laboratory.
3. To determine hemoglobin levels, someone has to obtain a blood sample and have this sample analyzed. Therefore, hemoglobin levels are considered biophysiologic in-vitro measures.
4. A laboratory needs a blood specimen to do a T-cell count. Therefore, this is a biophysiologic in-vitro measure.

TEST-TAKING TIP: The key words in the question stem are in vivo. This means measures performed directly on the person and that do not require any kind of specimen such as blood, urine, feces, sputum, and so on.

Content Area: *Methods of Data Collection;* ***Cognitive Level:*** *Analysis;* ***Question Type:*** *Multiple Choice*
CRITICAL THINKING FACILITATOR:
Identify other in-vivo measures. List different kinds of biophysiologic tests you have encountered in the clinical setting. What types of specimens were used for in-vitro measures?

17. 1. Although some biophysiologic measures are easy to use, some, especially the in-vitro ones, require specialized training.
2. Data collected from biophysiologic measures yield objective data. The data are readings from instruments or machinery and are not reports by the person.
3. Biophysiologic measures cannot be distorted intentionally. Unintentional and random errors might occur if the equipment malfunctions or procedures to obtain the data have flaws.
4. Some biophysiologic measures can be easily obtained by anyone. However, those that are used to analyze in-vitro data can be costly and require trained personnel.
5. A biophysiologic measure that is valid and reliable will provide accurate and precise data.

TEST-TAKING TIP: Think of two biophysiologic instruments such as a thermometer and a blood component analyzer machine. Using a set of criteria to compare them, what are your resulting judgments about each instrument? Some examples of criteria to use include ease of obtaining data, amount of time needed to complete measurement, skills, or knowledge required to perform the measurement, and so on. After you have completed this process, you should be able to answer the question.

Content Area: *Methods of Data Collection;* ***Cognitive Level:*** *Analysis;* ***Question Type:*** *Multiple Response*
CRITICAL THINKING FACILITATOR:
Compare several biophysiologic instruments that you have used or encountered in the clinical setting. What are their advantages and disadvantages?

18. 1. Self-report of stress is not an appropriate method to determine cortisol levels.
2. A blood specimen would be needed to determine cortisol levels. Therefore, this is considered a biophysiologic in-vitro measure.
3. Behaviors indicative of stress can be observed, but checking cortisol levels is considered a biophysiologic in-vitro measure.
4. Biophysiologic in-vivo measures are performed directly on the person, and no materials from the person are required.

TEST-TAKING TIP: A key word in the question stem is *cortisol*. This is a hormone. Therefore, its level is determined by using a blood sample.

Content Area: *Methods of Data Collection;* ***Cognitive Level:*** *Analysis;* ***Question Type:*** *Multiple Choice*
CRITICAL THINKING FACILITATOR:
What are some body materials (liquids and solids) that can be used as measures of physiologic variables? One example is blood urea nitrogen levels to determine ability of the kidney to clear nitrogenous wastes. Can you think of other examples?

19. 1. **Cultural practices can be studied more appropriately by observation.**
2. **How first-time mothers bond with their infants can be studied by observation.**
3. Cardiac efficiency can be measured using biophysiologic measures.
4. Self-reporting through an interview would be appropriate when individuals with above-knee amputations describe their lived experiences.
5. Perceptions would be considered self-report. Observations would not be appropriate.

TEST-TAKING TIP: A key word in the question stem is *observation*. Behaviors and practices can be observed. Biophysiologic data must be measured using some type of equipment. Self-reports include tools such as interviews and questionnaires that can ascertain feelings, attitudes, and other variables from the research participant.

Content Area: *Methods of Data Collection;* ***Cognitive Level:*** *Application;* ***Question Type:*** *Multiple Choice*

CRITICAL THINKING FACILITATOR:
Identify situations that can be appropriately studied using observation. In your clinical experiences, how do your clinical instructors determine your psychomotor skills? How do caregivers interact with care recipients who are clients of a home care agency? Comment on how you know that a nurse uses space effectively as a way to communicate.

20. 1. This question is appropriate in critiquing the ethical aspects of research.
2. **This question is appropriate in critiquing the data collection methods of a study.**
3. This question is appropriate in critiquing the ethical aspects of research.
4. This question is appropriate in critiquing the sampling procedures.

TEST-TAKING TIP: The key words in the question stem are *data collection methods*. This term means how information could be obtained on the variables or phenomena of interest.

Content Area: *Critique of Data Collection Methods;* ***Cognitive Level:*** *Evaluation;* ***Question Type:*** *Multiple Choice*

CRITICAL THINKING FACILITATOR:
Look at two or more sample studies and determine the phenomena of interest or the variables. For each variable or phenomenon, was the data collection method appropriate to use? Why?

14 Analyzing the Properties of Research Instruments

KEY WORDS

The following words include English vocabulary, nursing/medical terminology, concepts, principles, or information relevant to content specifically addressed in the chapter or associated with topics presented in it. English dictionaries, your nursing textbooks, and medical dictionaries such as *Taber's Cyclopedic Medical Dictionary* are resources that can be used to expand your knowledge and understanding of these words and related information.

Concurrent validity
Construct validity
Contrasted groups approach
Convergent validity
Criterion-related validity
Cronbach's alpha
Equivalence
Factor analysis
Homogeneity
Interrater reliability
Kuder-Richardson coefficient
Reliability
Sensitivity
Specificity
Test–retest procedure
Validity

QUESTIONS

Reliability of a Measurement Instrument

1. Which of the following statements is correct regarding reliability? Reliability is
   1. "the extent to which an instrument measures the attributes of a concept accurately" (LoBiondo-Wood & Haber, 2010, p. 288).
   2. "the inference that the data are representative of similar phenomena in a population beyond the studied sample" (p. 578).
   3. "the degree to which it can be inferred that the experimental treatment, rather than an uncontrolled condition, resulted in the observed effects" (p. 579).
   4. "the extent to which the instrument yields the same results on repeated measures" (p. 295).

Types of Reliability and Tests

2. Which of the following statements is/are true regarding instrument stability? **Select all that apply.** Stability
1. "indicates to what degree the subject's performance on the measurement instrument and the subject's actual behavior are related" (LoBiondo-Wood & Haber, 2010, p. 290).
2. "is the degree that the measurement instrument and the items it contains are representative of the content domain that the researchers intend to measure" (p. 288).
3. is a concern when the instrument is "expected to measure a concept consistently over a period of time" (p. 296).
4. is estimated by using test–retest procedure and alternate or parallel form approaches.
5. is exhibited "when the same results are obtained on repeated administration of the instrument" (p. 296).

3. An admissions officer wants to establish the reliability of an entrance examination into the nursing program. The examination was administered to 30 high school seniors. After 1 week, the same examination was administered to the same seniors. This test of the examination's reliability is called
1. parallel form.
2. alternate form.
3. test–retest procedure.
4. split-half procedure.

4. A researcher wants to establish the stability of an instrument. In the morning, she administers Form A of the instrument to a group of volunteers. In the afternoon, she administers Form B to the same volunteers. What test of reliability did the researcher use?
1. Split-half procedure
2. Test–retest procedure
3. Parallel form
4. Odd–even form

5. Which of the following statements are true regarding internal consistency? **Select all that apply**. Internal consistency
1. is synonymous with homogeneity.
2. can be established by doing factor analysis.
3. can be established by doing a Cronbach's alpha.
4. means the items are complementary to each other.
5. is concerned with consistency of the instrument over time.

6. Which of the following statements is true? Cronbach's alpha
1. "simultaneously compares each item on the scale with the others" (LoBiondo-Wood & Haber, 2010, p. 299).
2. "provides a measure of consistency in terms of sampling of the content" (p. 300).
3. "[is] an estimate of homogeneity used for instruments that have a dichotomous response format" (p. 301).
4. expresses "the consistency or agreement among observers using the same measurement instrument" (p. 301).

7. An instrument is considered reliable after doing the split-half method when there is
1. a strong relationship between each of the items and the total scale.
2. consistency among observers using the same instrument.
3. consistency between the odd and even numbered items of the instrument.
4. very little variation of the scores on two administrations of the instrument.

8. Which test is used to measure the internal consistency of an instrument that has a dichotomous format?
   1. Kuder-Richardson coefficient
   2. Cronbach's alpha
   3. Item-to-item consistency
   4. Interrater reliability

9. Which of the following statements is correct regarding equivalence as a test of reliability? Equivalence means that
   1. "the same results are obtained on repeated administration of the instrument" (LoBiondo-Wood & Haber, 2010, p. 296).
   2. there is "agreement among observers using the same measurement instrument, (p. 301).
   3. there is a strong correlation between each of the items and the total scale.
   4. each item on the instrument is compared simultaneously with other items.

10. The Physical Performance Test (PPT) evaluates a participant's ability to perform physical demands with different levels of difficulty in an appropriate and timely manner. Tests of reliability indicate that the interrater reliability of the PPT is 0.93 to 0.99 (Turner, Hochschild, Burnett, Zulfiqar, & Dyer, 2012). Which of the following statements describes interrater reliability? Interrater reliability
    1. "involves having two or more observers or coders who make independent observations. An index of agreement is then calculated with these data to evaluate the strength of the relationship" (Polit & Beck, 2014, p. 204).
    2. "focuses on the instrument's susceptibility to time-related influences such as participant fatigue. The researchers administer the measure to a sample twice and then compare the scores" (p. 202).
    3. "examines the relationship between scores on an instrument and an external criterion. A coefficient is computed by using a mathematical formula that correlates the two scores" (p. 206).
    4. "concerns the degree to which an instrument has an appropriate sample of items for the construct being measured. Conceptualization of the construct comes from a thorough literature review, a concept analysis, or findings from a qualitative inquiry," (p. 205).

11. Which of the following statements is/are true regarding the reliability coefficient? **Select all that apply**. The reliability coefficient
    1. expresses the relationship among the error, true score, and observed score.
    2. ranges from + or – 0 to 1.
    3. is closer to 1 when the error is high.
    4. is closer to 1 in a reliable instrument.
    5. reported to be 0.50 is considered acceptable.

12. Which of the following statements can be used to critique the reliability of a research instrument?
    1. Were measures taken to ensure that established protocols were carried out when using the instrument to measure the variable? (Burns & Grove, 2011).
    2. "What measurement methods were used to measure each study variable?" (p. 336).
    3. "Did the researchers provide adequate description of the measurement methods to judge the extent of the measurement errors?" (p. 336).
    4. "Did the sample produce saturation and verification of the information in the area of the study?" (p. 319).

Validity of Measurement Instruments

13. Which of the following statements describe validity? Validity is the
    1. "extent to which an instrument consistently measures a concept" (Burns & Grove, 2011, p. 546).
    2. "accuracy with which the population parameters have been estimated within a study" (p. 544).
    3. "difference between what exists in reality and what is measured by a research instrument" (p. 541).
    4. "extent to which an instrument accurately reflects the abstract construct (concept) being examined" (p. 552).

Types of Validity and Tests

14. Which question addresses the main concern in establishing content validity of a research instrument?
    1. Would the "same results be obtained on repeated administration of the instrument"? (LoBiondo-Wood & Haber, 2010, p. 296).
    2. Would the items within the instrument measure the same concept?
    3. Do the items of the instrument reflect what the researcher wants to measure?
    4. Does the instrument give "the appearance of measuring the content"? (p. 289).
15. The General Self-Efficacy Scale (GSES) has criterion-related validity. "Positive coefficients were found with favorable emotions, dispositional optimism and work satisfaction" (Rew et al. 2001; as cited in Taylor & Reyes, 2012, p. 4). Criterion-related validity means that the GSES as a research instrument
    1. consists of items that are "representative of the content domain that the researcher intends to measure" (LoBiondo-Wood & Haber, 2010, p. 288).
    2. "indicates to what degree the subject's performance on the measurement instrument and the subject's actual behavior are related" (p. 290).
    3. "represents the universe of content or the domain of a given construct" (p. 288).
    4. "assesses the degree to which the individual items on a scale truly cluster together around one or more dimensions" (p. 293).
16. The Resilience Scale (RS) has five underlying characteristics, including "self-reliance, meaning, equanimity, perseverance, and existential aloneness. The instrument has demonstrated content and construct validity" (Taylor & Reyes, 2012, p. 3). Construct validity means that the instrument
    1. "indicates to what degree the subject's performance on the measurement instrument and the subject's actual behavior are related" (LoBiondo-Wood & Haber, 2010, p. 290).
    2. has validated "a body or theory underlying the measurement by testing of the hypothesized relationship" (p. 290).
    3. "represents the universe of content or domain of a given construct" (p. 288).
    4. "yields the same results on repeated measures" (p. 295).
17. A factor analysis of the Expectations of Family Loyalty of Children Toward Elderly Relatives Scale revealed a two-factor structure, respect and priority (Kao & An, 2012). What type of validity testing is factor analysis?
    1. Content
    2. Criterion related
    3. Construct
    4. Equivalence

18. The Diabetes Knowledge Test (DKT) is an instrument used to measure participants' knowledge about diabetes. The validity of this instrument was established by studying two different groups (Hawkins, 2010). The test of validity for the DKT is known as
    1. split-half procedure.
    2. contrasted group validity approach.
    3. factor analysis.procedure.
    4. concurrent.validity approach.

19. Which of the following statements is true regarding convergent validity? Convergent validity
    1. "is a procedure that gives the researcher information about the extent to which a set of items measures the same underlying construct or dimension of a construct" (LoBiondo-Wood & Haber, 2010, p. 293).
    2. "also known as discriminant validity, uses measurement approaches that differentiate one construct from others that may be similar" (p. 292).
    3. "refers to a search for other measures of the construct" (p. 292). A test of relationship between the scores on theoretically similar measures would yield a correlation.
    4. "indicates to what degree the subject's performance on the measurement instrument and the subject's actual behavior are related" (p. 290).

20. Of the following statements, which one would a consumer of research find most acceptable regarding the requirements in research instruments?
    1. The Resilience Scale has demonstrated reliability with alpha coefficients ranging from 0.85 to 0.94. It has demonstrated content and construct validity (Taylor & Reyes, 2102).
    2. The Quality of Work Life has a Cronbach's alpha of 0.93 for the total scale and 0.73 to 0.89 for the subscales (Lee et al., 2013).
    3. The modified Breast Cancer Knowledge Scale with scores of 0 to 22 had a Cronbach's alpha of 0.68. Its constructs had internal consistency coefficients ranging from 0.49 to 0.87 (Othman et al., 2012).
    4. The Short Portable Mental Status Questionnaire has a "test-retest reliability of 0.45 for 8 of the 10 items. Criterion-related validity has been established" (Hawkins, 2010, p. 223).

Evidence-Based Practice and Diagnostic and Screening Tests

21. Evidence-based practice includes the use of reliable and valid diagnostic and screening tests. What dimensions of a test are inherent in this statement? **Select all that apply.**
    1. Sensitivity of the test
    2. Low cost
    3. A gold standard for comparison
    4. Specificity of the test
    5. Ease of administration

22. Yoon and Kim (2013) reported that the Korean version of the Center for Epidemiologic Studies Rating Scale for Depression with a "cut-off point of 21 indicated a 95% specificity and sensitivity for the relationship with the diagnosis of major depression in a community study" (p. 171). Which of the following statements describes sensitivity of the instrument? Sensitivity is
    1. "the proportion of those with disease who test positive" (Kirton, 2010, p. 451). An instrument with a high degree of this quality will show few false negatives.
    2. "the proportion of those without disease who test negative" (p. 451). "An instrument with a high degree of this quality will show few false positives" (p. 451).
    3. "the most accurate means of currently diagnosing a particular disease and serves as a basis for comparison for newly-developed diagnosing or screening tests" (Burns & Grove, 2011, p. 341).
    4. "the measure of the amount of random error in the measurement technique and includes dependability, precision, stability, consistency, and reproducibility" (p. 333).

23. What are the most important concerns regarding the use of biophysiologic measures in relation to instrument quality? **Select all that apply.**
    1. Error
    2. Accuracy
    3. Ease of administration
    4. Costs
    5. Precision

24. The quality of biophysiologic measures can be affected by errors. What are the different types of possible errors? **Select all that apply.**
    1. Environmental factors
    2. Users of the test
    3. Subject sampling
    4. Interpretation of the data
    5. Volume of data processed

ANSWERS AND RATIONALES

The correct answer number and rationale for why it is the correct answer are given in **boldface blue type**. Rationales for why the other possible answer options are incorrect also are given, but they are not in boldface type.

1. 1. This statement is a description of validity, another characteristic of research measurements.
2. This statement describes the concept of generalizability.
3. This statement describes the concept of internal validity.
4. This statement is a definition of reliability.

TEST-TAKING TIP: The key word in the question stem is "reliability." It is synonymous with dependability and consistency. Something that is reliable could be expected to perform or work in a consistent manner over time. Option 4 has the word "repeated," which gives a clue to the correct option.

Content Area: *Reliability of Measurement Instruments;* ***Cognitive Level:*** *Comprehension;* ***Question Type:*** *Multiple Choice*

CRITICAL THINKING FACILITATOR: When do you use the word "reliable"? Perhaps you use it to describe your car because it starts every time. Maybe it relates to a friend who borrows money from you and pays you back as promised.

2. 1. This statement describes criterion-related validity.
2. This statement describes content validity.
3. This statement describes stability, a test of reliability. A key word in the option is "consistently."
4. This statement describes the procedures to establish stability. Note that the test–retest procedure and the alternate or parallel form require more than one administration. Therefore, consistency is inherent.
5. This statement describes stability. The key words are "same" and "repeated." Consistency is inherent in these procedures.

TEST-TAKING TIP: The key word in the question stem is "stability," which means constancy. In relation to reliability, stability or constancy indicates no change or very little change.

Content Area: *Types of Reliability and Tests;* ***Cognitive Level:*** *Analysis;* ***Question Type:*** *Multiple Response*

CRITICAL THINKING FACILITATOR: The word "stable" is a common term in healthcare, so you should be familiar with it. Clinicians speak of vital signs as stable or of a condition as stable. In either situation, there is constancy, so no change or very little change is seen. This example should help you in understanding stability as an aspect of reliability.

3. 1. Although administering a parallel form is a test of reliability, this is not the one described in the situation. A parallel form is a comparable form of the same test.
2. Administering an alternate form is a test of reliability, but this is not the one described in the situation. An alternate form, as the name implies, is a different version of the test.
3. The test–retest procedure is described in the situation.
4. The split-half procedure is a test of internal consistency or homogeneity, not stability. This involves "dividing a scale into two halves and making a comparison" (LoBiondo-Wood & Haber, 2010, p. 300).

TEST-TAKING TIP: The key words in the question stem are "same examination" and "same seniors." In other words, the same test was administered twice.

Content Area: *Types of Reliability and Tests;* ***Cognitive Level:*** *Comprehension;* ***Question Type:*** *Multiple Choice*

CRITICAL THINKING FACILITATOR: How do you determine the reliability of the equipment you use to take blood pressure? One way is to take two consecutive readings. If the instrument is reliable and conditions are unchanged, you should get identical or very similar readings. Think of other situations when you would do something twice to confirm your assessments.

4. 1. The split-half procedure involves administration of the two halves of the instrument and then comparing the scores on each half. A higher correlation between the two halves indicates a higher reliability coefficient.
2. The test–retest procedure involves administering the same test to the same group twice. A comparison of the two sets of scores is then done to determine the reliability.
3. A parallel form of the test is administered. "Parallel forms or tests contain the same items that are based on the same concept, but the wording of the items is different" (LoBiondo-Wood & Haber, 2010, p. 296). Scores on the forms of the test, A and B, are then compared to determine reliability.

4. The odd–even procedure entails administering the even-numbered items to a group and then the odd-numbered items. The scores on the odd and even items are then compared to determine reliability.

TEST-TAKING TIP: The key words in the question stem are "Form A" and "Form B." Two forms of the test are parallel forms. A meaning of "parallel" is the same or similar.

Content Area: *Types of Reliability and Tests;* ***Cognitive Level:*** *Application;* ***Question Type:*** *Multiple Choice*

CRITICAL THINKING FACILITATOR: What happens when a student has to miss a scheduled examination? Generally, the instructor administers a parallel form of the examination, one that tests the same content but words the items differently. Most academic educators have parallel forms of their examinations to use as make-up examinations. To ensure a just evaluation of the student, the faculty member would have to establish the reliability of the make-up test.

5. 1. Homogeneity is synonymous with internal consistency.

2. Factor analysis is a test for construct validity.

3. A Cronbach's alpha is the most common way to establish internal consistency, an aspect of reliability.

4. The statement describes internal consistency, an aspect of reliability.

5. The statement describes stability, an aspect of reliability.

TEST-TAKING TIP: The key words in the question stem are "internal consistency." *Consistency* means agreement or harmony. In option 1, *homogeneity* means of the same or similar make or composition. In option 4, the term *complementary* means together to make a whole. If you know the definition of Cronbach's alpha, you can choose option 3.

Content Area: *Types of Reliability and Tests;* ***Cognitive Level:*** *Comprehension;* ***Question Type:*** *Multiple Response*

CRITICAL THINKING FACILITATOR: Why is it important to establish reliability by doing a test of internal consistency? Let's say you are taking an examination on the cardiovascular system, but some of the questions are about musculoskeletal problems. How does the examination's lack of internal consistency affect you? The test is not homogenous. Therefore, it is not a reliable measure of your knowledge of cardiovascular nursing.

6. 1. The statement describes Cronbach's alpha.

2. The statement describes split-half reliability.

3. The statement describes the Kuder-Richardson coefficient.

4. The statement describes interrater reliability.

TEST-TAKING TIP: Look at all the answer options and eliminate as many incorrect statements as you can. Option 2 has the phrase "sampling of the content." This does not relate to the Cronbach's alpha. Option 3 has the phrase "dichotomous response." The Cronbach's alpha is used for instruments with a Likert format, not dichotomous responses. Option 4 has the phrase "among observers," and this relates to interrater reliability.

Content Area: *Types of Reliability and Tests;* ***Cognitive Level:*** *Comprehension;* ***Question Type:*** *Multiple Choice*

CRITICAL THINKING FACILITATOR: Get familiar with the different ways of establishing reliability. Then look at the instrument section of a sample quantitative study. (The section might be labeled "measures" instead of "instruments.") Read about the reliability of the instrument(s) used in the study. See whether you understand the information that describes the instrument's reliability.

7. 1. The statement is descriptive of internal consistency.

2. The statement is descriptive of interrater reliability.

3. The statement describes the split-half method, wherein odd-numbered items are administered and then even-numbered items are administered. The score on the odd items is compared with the score on the even items, and a correlation is calculated.

4. The statement is indicative of the test–retest procedure to establish stability.

TEST-TAKING TIP: The key words in the question stem are "split half." Some type of process to divide the instrument was done. One way is comparing the upper half with the lower half. Another way is to separate the even-numbered items from the odd-numbered items.

Content Area: *Types of Reliability and Tests;* ***Cognitive Level:*** *Comprehension;* ***Question Type:*** *Multiple Choice*

CRITICAL THINKING FACILITATOR: If you took an examination consisting of 30 items on a specific topic, how would your score on the first 15 items compare with your score on the last 15 items? If the examination is reliable, your scores should be ____________. If the test has a low reliability, your scores would be ______________.

8. 1. The Kuder-Richardson coefficient estimates reliability on instruments that have a dichotomous response format (yes/no, true/false, agree/disagree).

2. Cronbach's alpha is used for instruments with a Likert scale response format.

3. Item-to-item consistency measures the relationship between each of the items and the total scale.
4. Interrater reliability involves at least two raters or observers, and reliability is estimated based on the percentage of agreement between the scores.

TEST-TAKING TIP: The key words in the question stem are "dichotomous format." *Dichotomous* means two. Options 2 and 3 involve Likert scale–type responses (giving a range of 3, 5, or 7 from most to least/always to never/etc.). Option 4 focuses on observations of behaviors by observers or coders.

Content Area: *Types of Reliability and Tests;* ***Cognitive Level:*** *Knowledge;* ***Question Type:*** *Multiple Choice*
CRITICAL THINKING FACILITATOR: What are some instruments you know that have a two-response format? The more common ones are attitude scales or inventories. You might encounter a dichotomous questionnaire in your doctor's office. The questionnaire is part of your history and physical examination and asks you to check Yes or No to record your history or experience of health problems. Most research studies reported in journals do not include a copy of the instruments used. If you have an interest in instruments, consult with your school's reference librarian, who should be able to direct you to a research measurement manual.

9. 1. The statement describes the test–retest procedure as a procedure for establishing stability.
2. The statement describes interrater reliability, a procedure to establish equivalence.
3. The statement describes item-to-item consistency, a procedure to establish internal consistency or homogeneity.
4. The statement describes Cronbach's alpha, a procedure to establish internal consistency or homogeneity.

TEST-TAKING TIP: The key word in the question stem is "equivalence," which implies equality. The only option that has this meaning is option 2 with the word "agreement."

Content Area: *Types of Reliability and Tests;* ***Cognitive Level:*** *Knowledge;* ***Question Type:*** *Multiple Choice*
CRITICAL THINKING FACILITATOR: Establishing reliability by interrater reliability testing is quite common. Check out a couple of the research studies in your core textbook and locate the section in each report that describes reliability. What aspects of reliability were done by the researchers or others? Could you identify all those that were done?

10. 1. The statement describes interrater reliability, a test of equivalence. A clue in the statement is the phrase "two or more observers or coders."
2. The statement describes test–retest reliability to test stability.
3. The statement describes criterion-related validity.
4. The statement describes content validity.

TEST-TAKING TIP: The key word in the question stem is "rater," which indicates a person using the measurement instrument to make sure that the items are consistently measuring what they are supposed to be measuring.

Content Area: *Types of Reliability and Tests;* ***Cognitive Level:*** *Comprehension;* ***Question Type:*** *Multiple Choice*
CRITICAL THINKING FACILITATOR: Imagine that a student is appealing a grade on a written assignment. One or more faculty members might be asked to evaluate the same paper. If all three faculty members evaluated the paper using the same criteria and arrived at grades with little variation, then the original grade would be considered consistent via multiple raters.

11. 1. The statement is a definition of the reliability coefficient.
2. The range of + or –0 to 1 is the correlation coefficient. The reliability coefficient is from 0 to 1, with no plus or minus.
3. The statement is not accurate. If the error is high, then the reliability coefficient is far from 1.
4. The statement is true. A research instrument with a reliability coefficient close to 1 is considered highly reliable.
5. Most experts would agree that an acceptable reliability coefficient is 0.70 (minimum) or above.

TEST-TAKING TIP: Researchers want their measurements to have a high degree of reliability. If 1 is perfect, then the closer the number is to 1, the more reliable it is (option 4). What do you know about a score on an instrument? There is the score that is obtained, but there is also the true score, devoid of errors. So the reliability coefficient has all three components (option 1).

Content Area: *Types of Reliability and Tests;* ***Cognitive Level:*** *Comprehension;* ***Question Type:*** *Multiple Response*
CRITICAL THINKING FACILITATOR: Look at a sample quantitative study and read over the description of an instrument's reliability. What

was the coefficient reported? Was there more than one test of reliability done? In some cases, the researchers might also do their own reliability studies on the instrument when the reliability coefficient is not deemed high enough. What are the implications of using instruments that lack acceptable reliability?

12. 1. The question is not appropriate to critique reliability. The question is appropriate in critiquing the intervention (independent variable).
2. The question is appropriate to critique the data collection methods of the study, not reliability.
3. **The question is appropriate to critique the reliability of measurement instruments.**
4. The question is an appropriate one to use in critiquing sample adequacy in qualitative studies.

TEST-TAKING TIP: Read each answer option carefully. Option 1 has the words "protocols" and "treatment," which imply an intervention. Option 2 asks for a measurement method, referring to data collection. Option 3 has the words "measurement errors," which relate to the quality of the research instruments. Option 4 has the words "saturation and verification of information," which imply data in the study.

***Content Area:** Critique of Reliability; **Cognitive Level:** Application; **Question Type:** Multiple Choice*

CRITICAL THINKING FACILITATOR: By now you should be familiar with the guidelines for critiquing a research study. The guidelines are found just before the end of each chapter in most nursing research textbooks. Take a part of a study and read it. As a research consumer, what kinds of questions would you ask to determine the validity of the study?

13. 1. Reliability of a measurement instrument is described.
2. Precision is described.
3. Measurement error is described.
4. **The statement describes validity.**

TEST-TAKING TIP: The key word in the question stem is "validity." It is synonymous with accuracy and appropriateness. Option 2 contains the word "accuracy," but it refers to the population. Research instrument validity is the focus of the question. Option 4 has the relevant terms "accuracy" and "instrument."

***Content Area:** Validity of Measurement Instruments; **Cognitive Level:** Comprehension; **Question Type:** Multiple Choice*

CRITICAL THINKING FACILITATOR: Consider the validity of an examination. How can you tell if the scores on an examination are a valid indication of the students' knowledge? Is an examination for advanced practice nurses a valid one to use for practitioners who have only baccalaureate degrees?

14. 1. The question focuses on the test–retest procedure as a way to establish stability, an aspect of reliability.
2. The question is relevant to item-to-item correlation as a way to establish internal consistency, an aspect of reliability.
3. **The question is relevant to establishing the content validity of a measurement instrument.**
4. The question is asking about face validity. The word "appearance" relates to face.

TEST-TAKING TIP: The key word in the question stem is "content," which means that which is contained. In a research instrument, the content includes the items (statements or questions) used to measure the concept or variable. Option 1 contains the words "same results," which imply consistency or reliability. Option 2 has the words "same concept." These imply consistency among items, an aspect of reliability. Option 4 has the word "appearance." Only option 3 has the key words that are relevant to content validity, "reflect" and "what the researcher wants to measure."

***Content Area:** Types of Validity and Tests; **Cognitive Level:** Analysis; **Question Type:** Multiple Choice*

CRITICAL THINKING FACILITATOR: After items for an instrument are created, how do researchers decide whether the items are representative of the content domain being tested? Who decides whether the instrument has content validity?

15. 1. The descriptive information is consistent with content validity.
2. **The information is reflective of criterion-related validity. The tool, General Self-Efficacy Scale, is valid (accurate) in relating it to other criteria, including favorable emotions, dispositional optimism, and work satisfaction.**
3. The information is consistent with content validity.
4. The information is consistent with the factor analytical approach for establishing construct validity.

TEST-TAKING TIP: The key words in the question stem are "criterion-related

validity." *Criterion* means some type of standard. In criterion-related validity, the instrument is used to measure a person's performance in relation to another measure, which is the criterion. For example, Scholastic Aptitude Test (SAT) scores are correlated with success in college (criterion). If the SAT as an instrument has criterion-related validity, it can be said that SAT scores are accurate and appropriate to measure success in college.

Content Area: *Types of Validity and Tests;* ***Cognitive Level:*** *Analysis;* ***Question Type:*** *Multiple Choice*
CRITICAL THINKING FACILITATOR: What are some applications of criterion-related validity? Does the Graduate Record Exam (GRE) have criterion-related validity to success in a graduate program?

16. 1. The information is consistent with criterion-related validity.
2. **The information is consistent with construct validity, which is "based on the extent to which a test measures a theoretical construct, attribute, or trait" (LoBiondo-Wood & Haber, 2010, p. 290).**
3. The information is consistent with content validity.
4. The information indicates a test of reliability, test–retest, a procedure to establish stability.

TEST-TAKING TIP: The key words in the question stem are "construct validity." A *construct* is an "abstraction or concept that is deliberately invented (constructed) by researchers for a scientific purpose" (Polit & Beck, 2014, p. 377). Option 2 contains the relevant words "theory underlying the measurement." Concepts are the building blocks of theories.

Content Area: *Types of Validity and Tests;* ***Cognitive Level:*** *Comprehension;* ***Question Type:*** *Multiple Choice*
CRITICAL THINKING FACILITATOR: What are some constructs you have encountered in the clinical setting? Quality of life, medication adherence, and cultural competence are a few examples. How would you go about developing a tool on these constructs? When the tool is developed, what type of validity would be established, and what procedures are used to do this?

17. 1. Content validity is established by using a panel of experts.
2. Criterion-related validity can be established by predictive or concurrent validity. In both, a validity coefficient is calculated by "using a mathematical formula that correlates the two scores" (Polit & Beck, 2014, p. 206). One score comes from the measurement instrument, and the other score comes from the second measurement, which is the criterion.
3. **Factor analysis is a procedure to establish construct validity. It is a "procedure that gives the researcher information about the extent to which a set of items measures the same underlying construct or dimensions of a construct" (LoBiondo-Wood & Haber, 2010, p. 293).**
4. Equivalence is an aspect of reliability, not validity.

TEST-TAKING TIP: The key words in the question stem are "two-factor structures," "respect," and "priority." The key word in the title of the instrument is "loyalty." This is the construct or concept. The two factors that were underlying loyalty were respect and priority. Therefore, factor analysis is concerned with construct validity.

Content Area: *Types of Validity and Tests;* ***Cognitive Level:*** *Comprehension;* ***Question Type:*** *Multiple Choice*
CRITICAL THINKING FACILITATOR: Examine a study's description of its validity. If there is a description of validity and factor analysis was used to establish validity, what factors underlie the construct that is the focus of the instrument?

18. 1. Split-half is a test to establish stability of an instrument and is concerned with reliability.
2. **The contrasted group approach is used to test construct validity. Two groups that are expected to score either high or low in the characteristic being measured are administered the instrument. If the instrument is sensitive, the scores from the groups should differ significantly. The difference between the groups attests to the construct validity of the instrument (LoBiondo-Wood & Haber, 2010).**
3. Factor analysis is a procedure to establish construct validity. It "uses a statistical procedure for determining the underlying dimensions or components of a variable" (p. 578). The procedure does not entail comparing the scores of two different groups.
4. Concurrent approach to validity "refers to the degree of correlation of one test with the scores of another, more established instrument of the same concept when both are administered at the same time" (p. 290).

TEST-TAKING TIP: The key words in the question stem are "two different groups." Only option 2 is concerned with groups.

Content Area: *Types of Validity and Tests;* ***Cognitive Level:*** *Application;* ***Question Type:*** *Multiple Choice*

CRITICAL THINKING FACILITATOR: The contrasted group approach is a test of construct validity. By now you should be familiar with the different approaches for establishing validity. Create a grid of the different types of validity and identify specific procedures used to establish each type.

19. 1. The statement describes the factor analytical approach for establishing construct validity.
2. The statement is incorrect. Divergent, not convergent, validity is also known as discriminant validity.
3. The statement describes convergent validity.
4. The statement refers to criterion-related validity.

TEST-TAKING TIP: The key word in the question stem is "convergent" from the verb *converge*, which means to come together. In convergent validity, the researcher attempts to search for other measures of the construct. Upon finding another measure, the correlation of the measures is calculated. A positive correlation means that there is convergent validity.

Content Area: *Types of Validity and Tests;* ***Cognitive Level:*** *Comprehension;* ***Question Type:*** *Multiple Choice*

CRITICAL THINKING FACILITATOR: Differentiate convergent validity from discriminant validity. Look at any of the quantitative study you have and locate the discussion on validity. Can you identify the difference between convergent validity and divergent validity? Be sure to ask your instructor if you are not clear on these.

20. **1. The information indicates acceptable reliability and validity. Both characteristics must be present in a research instrument.**
2. Although the reliability coefficients are high, the statement mentions nothing about validity.
3. The reliability for the total scale is below the acceptable 0.70. Also some of the constructs have reliability coefficients below 0.70.
4. The reliability coefficient is below the acceptable level but the instrument has validity. (One would wonder why a valid instrument has a low reliability coefficient.)

TEST-TAKING TIP: The key words in the question stem are "most acceptable."

Content Area: *Reliability and Validity;* ***Cognitive Level:*** *Comprehension;* ***Question Type:*** *Multiple Choice*

CRITICAL THINKING FACILITATOR: Think of the relationship between reliability and validity. Which of these two is the more important?

21. **1. "Sensitivity is the proportion of those with disease who test positive; that is, sensitivity is a measure of how well the test detects disease when it is really there, a highly sensitive test has few false negatives" (Kirton, 2010, p. 451).**
2. The low cost of an instrument is not relevant to its diagnostic and screening qualities.
3. "The gold standard is the most accurate means of currently diagnosing a particular disease and serves as a basis for comparison for newly-developed diagnostic or screening tests" (Burns & Grove, 2011, p. 341). This is a relevant concern in the use of biophysiologic instruments.
4. "Specificity is the proportion of those without disease who test negative. It measures how well the test rules out disease when it is really absent; a specific test has few false positives" (Kirton, 2010, p. 451).
5. A test that is easily administered is not a concern in reliability and validity of diagnostic and screening tests.

TEST-TAKING TIP: The key words in the question stem are "reliable" and "valid." Because diagnostic and screening tests guide practitioners in designing care approaches, it is imperative that they are accurate in terms of specificity and sensitivity.

Content Area: *Evidence-Based Practice and Diagnostic and Screening Tests;* ***Cognitive Level:*** *Analysis;* ***Question Type:*** *Multiple Response*

CRITICAL THINKING FACILITATOR: Think of the many diagnostic and screening tests performed in the clinical setting. Are these tests sensitive and specific enough? What happens if these qualities are lacking in a screening and diagnostic test? Think of the implications for the individual, the family, and the healthcare provider.

22. **1. The statement defines the sensitivity of a diagnostic or screening test.**
2. The statement defines the specificity of a diagnostic or screening test.

3. The statement describes the gold standard for diagnostic or screening tests.
4. The definition relates to reliability testing.

TEST-TAKING TIP: The key word in the question stem is "sensitivity," which pertains to acuteness in detecting something. A sensitive instrument can detect minor fluctuations or changes. Therefore, a highly sensitive test has high accuracy.

Content Area: *Evidence-Based Practice and Diagnostic and Screening Tests;* ***Cognitive Level:*** *Comprehension;* ***Question Type:*** *Multiple Choice*

CRITICAL THINKING FACILITATOR:
What are the advantages and disadvantages of using biophysiologic measures as diagnostic and screening tools? Check out a quantitative study and locate a description of a biophysiologic tool. How are the reliability and validity of the tool established?

23.
1. **Biophysiologic measures should have no to few errors, particularly if these are used as diagnostic and screening tools. Clinicians depend on them and use the data from these tools to create appropriate treatment protocols for patients.**
2. **Accuracy is also a major concern. Accuracy is synonymous with validity. Therefore, a tool should be accurate or valid when it is used for making decisions about people's lives.**
3. Ease of administration is a concern but not a major one. There are biophysiologic measures that require sophisticated skills and knowledge. This is one reason why clinicians undergo rigorous training to be become experts.
4. Cost is a concern also, but when one is dealing with people's lives and health, other concerns are more important.
5. **Precision is a major concern. A biophysiologic measure must be precise in doing what it is intended to do. If it is not precise, errors that can cause death, injury, suffering, and other serious effects could occur.**

TEST-TAKING TIP: The key words in the question stem are "most important." Most important concerns are major concerns. When biophysiologic tools are used for diagnostic and screening purposes, they must be error free, accurate, and precise. Clinicians such as physicians depend on these measures to guide them in prescribing appropriate therapies for patients' diseases. If a test is not accurate in determining the level of glucose in the blood, how would a physician know the amount of insulin that a patient requires?

Content Area: *Evidence-Based Practice and Diagnostic and Screening Tests;* ***Cognitive Level:*** *Analysis;* ***Question Type:*** *Multiple Response*

CRITICAL THINKING FACILITATOR:
Think of situations when errors in diagnosis were made. Were errors made by the instrument? What were the implications of these errors?

24.
1. **Environmental factors such as "temperature, barometric pressure and static electricity" (Burns & Grove, 2010, p. 339) could contribute to errors.**
2. **Variations in the user might also produce errors.**
3. Subject sampling is not related to errors in biophysiologic instruments.
4. **Misinterpretation of data could also lead to errors.**
5. The volume of data is not related to errors.

TEST-TAKING TIP: The key word in the question stem is "errors." An error is an inaccuracy or mistake. If you have biophysiologic instrument such as a piece of machinery, what could possibly produce errors? Errors might be produced by conditions that influence the running of the machine, by those who run it, or by those who read the data produced by the machine.

Content Area: *Evidence-Based Practice and Diagnostic and Screening Tests;* ***Cognitive Level:*** *Analysis;* ***Question Type:*** *Multiple Response*

CRITICAL THINKING FACILITATOR:
What are measures to prevent errors in biophysiologic instruments? Some machines are housed in temperature-controlled environments. In addition, users are trained in the operation of the machine, and experts periodically calibrate delicate machines. Finally, manuals and protocols are in place to guide interpretation of the data. If you have the opportunity, meet with personnel in the laboratory in one of your clinical settings to learn more about measures to prevent errors in biophysiologic instruments.

15 Understanding the Concepts and Processes in Analyzing Quantitative Data

KEY WORDS

The following words include English vocabulary, nursing/medical terminology, concepts, principles, or information relevant to content specifically addressed in the chapter or associated with topics presented in it. English dictionaries, your nursing textbooks, and medical dictionaries such as *Taber's Cyclopedic Medical Dictionary* are resources that can be used to expand your knowledge and understanding of these words and related information.

ANCOVA
ANOVA
Chi square
Correlation
Descriptive statistics
Frequency distribution
Inferential statistics
Level of significance
Mean
Median
Mode
Multiple regression
Nonparametric tests
Normal distribution or curve
Probability (*p*)
Post hoc analysis
Range
Repeated measures ANOVA
Statistical significance
t test
Type I and II errors

QUESTIONS

Quantitative Data Analysis

1. What does a researcher do to prepare quantitative data for analysis? **Select all that apply.** The researcher
   1. checks for missing data.
   2. selects a computer program to process the data.
   3. eliminates analysis of some subjects if data cannot be collected.
   4. checks data for accuracy.
   5. tests the reliability and validity of the instrument(s) used.
2. Whereas a(n) ____________ is a characteristic of a population, an ____________ is a characteristic of a sample.
3. ____________ are subjects or data points with extreme values (values that are far from other plotted points on a graph) that seem unlike the rest of the sample.

Descriptive Statistics

4. Which is true regarding descriptive statistics? **Select all that apply.** Descriptive statistics

1. include measures of central tendency.
2. are used primarily to "describe the characteristics of the sample."
3. allow the researcher to predict whether findings can be applied to other populations.
4. identify whether the control or experimental groups are different.
5. are used to analyze data in some descriptive studies.

5. A way to organize numerical data is to create a(n) ____________, "a systematic arrangement of values from lowest to highest, together with a count or percentage of how many times each value occurred" (Polit & Beck, 2014, p. 215).

6. The registered nurses sampled in a study had 30 to 45 years of work experience. What is true about the range in this statement? **Select all that apply.** The range

1. is a measure of variability.
2. can be calculated by subtracting the lower number of years from the higher number of years.
3. is a stable measure of variability from one sample to another.
4. can be used to show variability when the means are the same.
5. can be considered in judging the "typicalness" of a sample (Polit & Beck, 2014).

7. **Research Study Information:** In their study, Stanley and Pollard (2013) described their sample as having a mean age of 36.64 years. What correct statement can be made about this mean?

1. The mean age can be identified by looking at the most occurring age of the participants.
2. The mean age would not be influenced by the extremes in the ages.
3. The mean is identified as the midpoint of all ages from youngest to oldest.
4. The mean was calculated by dividing the sum of the ages by the number of participants.

8. The following are the scores on an examination in a nursing course: **Set of scores on an exam: 100, 94, 94, 94, 88, 88, 86, 86, 84, 84, 82, 78, 76, 74, 60**. Which is the mode in the above scores?

1. 94
2. 86
3. 40
4. 84.53

9. What is the median of this set of ages? **Set of ages: 90, 88, 88, 86, 84, 82.**

1. 88
2. 8
3. 87
4. 86.33

10. The normal curve is a "theoretical frequency distribution of all possible values in a population" (Burns & Grove, 2011, p. 379). What aspect of quantitative analysis uses the logic of the normal curve?

1. Level of significance
2. Relationship of two variables
3. Calculation of the mean
4. Power analysis

11. Using the normal distribution, if the scores on an examination fell within +1 and -1 standard deviation (SD) from the mean, the percentage of those who earned these scores will be ____________% of the total number of scores.

12. Using the normal distribution, if the weights of a sample of older adults fall within +2 SD from the mean, the percentage of those who have these weights would be ___________% of the total.

Level of Significance

13. Which of the following statements is true regarding level of significance or alpha? **Select all that apply.** Level of significance
   1. is usually set at 0.05 for most nursing studies.
   2. means that the research hypothesis was proven to be true.
   3. asks whether "the samples being tested are from the same population or of different populations" (Burns & Grove, 2011, p. 532).
   4. can be expressed by saying that findings approached significance.
   5. is a concept relevant to decision theory in analyzing quantitative data.

14. When does a type II error occur? It occurs when
   1. the level of significance is 0.05.
   2. the null hypothesis is rejected when it is true.
   3. there are flaws in the methodology.
   4. the level of significance becomes more extreme.

15. **Research Study Information:** Zhuang, An, and Zhao (2013) indicated that they used < 0.05 as a p in analyzing their data. What does this value represent?
   1. The probability of a type I error
   2. The intensity of the relationship between variables
   3. The probability of a type II error
   4. The probability of a relationship between variables

16. A correlation is a type of bivariate descriptive statistic. What statements are true about a correlation? **Select all that apply.** In a correlation,
   1. the question asked is, "To what extent are two variables related to each other?" (Polit & Beck, 2014, p. 222).
   2. the coefficient calculated could be 1.00.
   3. the product-moment coefficient is the most common one calculated.
   4. the variables could be negatively or positively correlated.
   5. the correlation coefficient is low when variables are unrelated.

17. **Research Study Information:** Stanley and Pollard (2013) studied the "relationship between knowledge, attitudes, and self-efficacy of nurses in the management of pediatric pain" (p. 165). Data analysis indicated that there is a positive relationship between the level of knowledge and pediatric nursing experience. The second statement means that
   1. level of knowledge and pediatric experience have an effect on the attitudes of nurses on their patients.
   2. nurses who had more years in pediatric nursing scored higher on the Pediatric Nurses' Knowledge and Attitudes Survey Regarding Pain.
   3. nurses who had more years in pediatric nursing scored lower on the Pediatric Nurses' Knowledge and Attitudes Survey Regarding Pain.
   4. there was no relationship between years of experience of pediatric nurses and their scores on the Pediatric Nurses' Knowledge and Attitudes Survey Regarding Pain.

18. If the correlation coefficient (r squared) between critical thinking and performance on a standardized exam is 64%, ___________ is the percentage of the unexplained variance between the two variables.

Post-Hoc Analysis

19. When study results show a significant difference among groups, the researcher must do a(n) ____________ to determine which groups are different.

20. A(n) ____________ is appropriate to use "to test for significant differences between two samples" (Burns & Grove, 2011, p. 404).

21. "In a one-tailed test of significance, the ____________ is directional, and extreme statistical values that occur in a single tail of the curve are of interest" (Burns & Grove, 2011, p. 380).

Inferential Statistics

22. What are the requirements for a study in order that the data can be analyzed using inferential statistics? **Select all that apply.**
    1. The study sample must be representative of the population.
    2. A probability sampling procedure must have been used.
    3. There must be an active manipulation of the independent variable.
    4. Data must be at the ratio level of measurement.
    5. The size of the sample depends upon the size of the population.

23. ____________ is used to test mean group differences of three or more groups.

24. **Research Study Information:** Hasson and Gustasson (2010) did a study on declining sleep quality among nurses. They used a repeated-measures ANOVA to analyze their data. The procedure indicated "a general significant decrease in sleep quality over time" (p. 3). What statement is true about a repeated-measures ANOVA? This procedure
    1. "tests the mean group differences of three or more groups" (Polit & Beck, 2014, p. 233).
    2. "tests the effect of two independent variables on an outcome variable" (p. 234).
    3. "summarizes the relationship magnitude and direction of a relationship between variables" (p. 236).
    4. "determines whether the means being compared are means at different points in time" (p. 234).

25. When a study has more than one independent variable, what statistic should be used?
    1. t test
    2. Analysis of variance
    3. Multiple regression
    4. Correlation

26. **Research Study Information:** Choi and Reed (2013) looked at the contributors to depressive symptoms among Korean immigrants with type 2 diabetes. What type of statistical procedure would be appropriate to analyze their data? **Select all that apply.**
    1. Descriptive
    2. Correlation
    3. Analysis of variance (ANOVA)
    4. Multiple regression
    5. Multiple analysis of variance (MANOVA)

27. **Research Study Information:** Yang et al. (2112) compared "two recovery room warming methods for hypothermia patients who had undergone spinal surgery" (p. 2). The data analyses "showed that the main effects of two rewarming methods were significantly different after controlling for the 'temperature, upon arrival at the post anesthesia care unit [PACU]" (p. 8). What inferential statistical procedure did the researchers use?
    1. Pearson's r
    2. Multiple regression
    3. ANOVA
    4. ANCOVA

28. When are nonparametric statistics used to analyze quantitative data?
    1. The sample is too small.
    2. The data are at the nominal or ordinal levels.
    3. There is one group of research participants.
    4. The sample was obtained using probability procedures.

29. **Research Study Information**: Powell-Young and Sprull (2013) looked at the views of Black nurses toward genetic research and testing. They used the chi-squared test "to test for group differences by education level" (p. 155). What is true about this test?
    1. To use the test, researchers must have interval or ratio data.
    2. The statistic is used to test whether the means of two groups are different.
    3. The statistic is considered a parametric procedure.
    4. The test is used to compare observed from expected frequencies of variables.

Statistical Significance

30. ____________ means that "the results from an analysis of sample data are unlikely to have been caused by chance, at a specified level of probability" (Polit & Beck, 2014, p. 392).

31. **Research Study Information:** A study looked at acupressure and the sleep quality of psychogeriatric patients. Selected data are as follows:

	Pretest M (SD)	Posttest M (SD)	t	*p*
Sleep latency (min)	34.93 (4.46)	30.07 (4.80)	3.61**	0.001

(Lu, Lin, Chen, Tsang, & Su, 2013, p. 134). What do the data mean? **Select all that apply.**
    1. There is a difference in the means and SDs between the pre- and posttests.
    2. The difference between the means is not statistically significant.
    3. The *p* value indicates the probability of a type II error.
    4. The difference between the means is statistically significant.
    5. The *p* value indicates the probability of a type I error.

Study Results

32. What type of study results are seen when "the theory used by the researcher to develop the hypothesis is in error"? (Burns & Grove, 2011, p. 409).
    1. Unpredicted
    2. Mixed
    3. Nonsignificant
    4. Unexpected

ANSWERS AND RATIONALES

The correct answer number and rationale for why it is the correct answer are given in **boldface blue type**. Rationales for why the other possible answer options are incorrect also are given, but they are not in boldface type.

1. 1. **This is a correct action of the researcher. "If enough data are missing for certain variables, the researcher may have to determine whether the data are sufficient to perform analyses using those variables" (Burns & Grove, 2011, p. 373).**
   2. This is not a process done in preparing the data. The computer program selected is related to the type of analysis the researcher wants to do.
   3. **This is a correct action by the researcher. The researcher makes a decision to exclude missing data and changes the total number of subjects. This is considered attrition.**
   4. **This is a correct action of the researcher. Ensuring accuracy of data is a responsibility of the researcher before he or she does the analysis.**
   5. This process is not part of data preparation. This process is essential before data collection when instruments are going to be used.

   TEST-TAKING TIP: The key phrase in the question stem is "to prepare quantitative data for analysis." This implies reviewing the raw data for completeness and accuracy so that the process of analysis will be done smoothly and the program to analyze the data can do its work.

   Content Area: *Processes in Quantitative Data Analysis;* ***Cognitive Level:*** *Knowledge;* ***Question Type:*** *Multiple Response*

   CRITICAL THINKING FACILITATOR: Every phase in a study has many substeps to accomplish the work of that phase. What issues could be avoided when all the steps in quantitative data analysis are carried out?

2. **parameter; statistic**

   TEST-TAKING TIP: The key words in the statement are "population" and "sample." Recall that the sample is derived from the population. Think of the population as the whole with boundaries (parameters). Then take a part of the whole (sample) to estimate the parameter (statistic).

   Content Area: *Concepts in Quantitative Data Analysis;* ***Cognitive Level:*** *Knowledge;* ***Question Type:*** *Fill-in-the-Blanks*

   CRITICAL THINKING FACILITATOR: Why do researchers report statistics instead of parameters?

3. **Outliers**

   TEST-TAKING TIP: The key words in the question stem are "extreme values," meaning data that are not within the defined boundaries.

   Content Area: *Concepts in Quantitative Data Analysis;* ***Cognitive Level:*** *Knowledge;* ***Question Type:*** *Fill-in-the-Blank*

   CRITICAL THINKING FACILITATOR: What does the researcher do with data that do not seem to "cluster" around the other obtained values? How do these types of data affect the rest of the data for analysis?

4. 1. **Measures of central tendency, frequency distributions, measures of dispersion, and standardized scores are all descriptive statistics.**
   2. **One of the purposes of descriptive statistics is to make known, in summary form, who the sample is and its characteristics.**
   3. This is not a correct statement about descriptive statistics. The statement is true of inferential statistics.
   4. Descriptive statistics do not differentiate the control from the experimental group. Both groups come from the sample and then are randomly assigned to either control or experimental group.
   5. **The statement is true. Descriptive statistics are used to analyze data in a descriptive study.**

   TEST-TAKING TIP: The key word in the question stem is "descriptive." It is derived from the verb "describe," which means to present information.

   Content Area: *Descriptive Statistics;* ***Cognitive Level:*** *Knowledge;* ***Question Type:*** *Multiple Response*

   CRITICAL THINKING FACILITATOR: Think of the data in a quantitative study and how these could be presented so that readers would have an organized summary of the data. Familiarize yourself with the different ways to summarize large amounts of quantitative data.

5. **frequency distribution**

   TEST-TAKING TIP: The key phrases in the question stem are "count or percentage of how many times" and "lowest to highest." The first phrase indicates frequency of occurrence, and the second phrase indicates how data are sequenced.

Content Area: Descriptive Statistics; ***Cognitive Level:*** *Knowledge;* ***Question Type:*** *Fill-in-the-Blank*
CRITICAL THINKING FACILITATOR: As a nursing student, how could you summarize your performance on examinations for the duration of your academic program? One way is by organizing your grades from lowest to highest and noting how many times you earned each grade.

6. 1. **The range and the SD are measures of variability. Variability is the "degree to which values in a set of scores are dispersed" (Polit & Beck, 2014, p. 394).**
2. **In the information, 15 is the range. To find the range, subtract 30 from 45.**
3. The statement is not correct. "Because the range is based on only two scores, however, the range is unstable: from sample to sample drawn from a population" (p. 219).
4. **The statement is accurate. Even when the means of two samples are the same, the range, a measure of variability, can be different.**
5. The statement is not correct. Descriptive statistics (mean, mode, and median) reflect typicalness.

TEST-TAKING TIP: The key words in the question stem are "range" and "30 to 45." One meaning of range is extent. The numbers 30 to 45 represents the extent of something between these two numbers.

Content Area: Descriptive Statistics; ***Cognitive Level:*** *Application;* ***Question Type:*** *Multiple Response*
CRITICAL THINKING FACILITATOR: What are instances when you had to describe numerical data? How did you present characteristics such as years of education, income levels, years of residence, and so on?

7. 1. The statement identifies a way to obtain the mode.
2. The statement is erroneous. Extreme values influence the mean.
3. The statement describes the median.
4. **The statement is correct. This describes how one calculates the mean.**

TEST-TAKING TIP: The key word in the question stem is "mean." In mathematics, the other name for the mean is average.

Content Area: Descriptive Statistics; ***Cognitive Level:*** *Application;* ***Question Type:*** *Multiple Choice*
CRITICAL THINKING FACILITATOR: When is the mean the most appropriate way to describe data? What must be taken into consideration when using the mean as a descriptive statistic?

8. 1. **The score of 94 is identified as the mode because it occurred three times. The mode is the "numerical value or score that occurs with the greatest frequency in a distribution but does not necessarily indicate the center of the data set" (p. 542).**
2. The score of 86 is the median. The median is "the exact center of the ungrouped frequency distribution" (p. 541).
3. Forty (40) is the range. The range is the simplest measure of dispersion. It is obtained by subtracting the lowest score from the highest score.
4. This number is the mean of the set of scores. It is calculated by adding all the scores and dividing the sum by the total number of scores.

TEST-TAKING TIP: The key word in the question stem is "mode," which means norm or prevailing.

Content Area: Descriptive Statistics; ***Cognitive Level:*** *Application;* ***Question Type:*** *Multiple Choice*
CRITICAL THINKING FACILITATOR: What are some situations in which the mode is an appropriate statistic to use?

9. 1. This number is the mode, the age that occurs most frequently.
2. This number is the range: 90 – 82 = 8.
3. **This number is the median. The median is the "exact center of the ungrouped frequency distribution" (Burns & Grove, 2011, p. 541). In an odd number of ages, the median might not show up as one of ages.**
4. This number is the mean of the ages (sum of all ages divided by the total number of ages).

TEST-TAKING TIP: The key word in the question stem is "median," which means middle.

Content Area: Descriptive Statistics; ***Cognitive Level:*** *Application;* ***Question Type:*** *Multiple Choice*
CRITICAL THINKING FACILITATOR: When is the median an appropriate descriptive statistic to use?

10. 1. **A level of significance is established before the analysis of the data. Level of significance is defined as "the probability level at which the results of statistical analysis are judged to indicate statistically significant difference between groups" (Burns & Grove, 2011, p. 541).**

2. The relationship between variables is calculated by a correlation.
3. A normal curve is not used to calculate the mean.
4. Power analysis is a "technique used to determine the risk of a type II error" (Burns & Grove, 2011, p. 544).

TEST-TAKING TIP: The key phrase in the question stem is "normal curve." The normal curve is a "theoretical frequency distribution of all possible values in a population" (Burns & Grove, 2011, p. 379).

Content Area: *Normal Distribution;* ***Cognitive Level:*** *Knowledge;* ***Question Type:*** *Multiple Choice*
CRITICAL THINKING FACILITATOR: Using the logic of the normal curve, what does an alpha, or level of significance, mean?

11. 68

TEST-TAKING TIP: The key phrase in the question stem is "+1 and –1 SD from the mean." The normal distribution has a mean of 50 and an SD of 10, a fixed percentage of cases falls within 1 SD above and below the mean. Ninety-five percent (95%) of cases fall within an SD +2 and –2. Only 2% of cases fall more than +3 and –3 SDs from the mean.

Content Area: *Normal Distribution;* ***Cognitive Level:*** *Knowledge;* ***Question Type:*** *Fill-in-the-Blank*
CRITICAL THINKING FACILITATOR: Knowing the mean and SD of a normal distribution, can you determine where a student's score of 75 on an exam would fall in relation to the class as a whole?

12. 47.5

TEST-TAKING TIP: The key phrase in the question stem is "+2 SDs from the mean." The normal distribution has a mean of 50 and an SD of 10, a fixed percentage of cases fall within 1 SD above and below the mean. Ninety-five percent (95%) of cases fall between +2 and –2 SDs from the mean. Divide 95% by 2 to get 47.5%.

Content Area: *Normal Distribution;* ***Cognitive Level:*** *Knowledge;* ***Question Type:*** *Fill-in-the-Blank*
CRITICAL THINKING FACILITATOR: Familiarize yourself with the probability levels of the normal distribution. Knowing at least two of the probability levels will facilitate calculation of the rest.

13. **1. The level of significance selected for most nursing studies is 0.05. This means that "if the level found in the statistical analyses is 0.05 or less, the experimental and comparison groups are considered to be significantly different (members of different populations)" (Burns & Grove, 2011, p. 377).**
2. The statement is not related to level of significance. Furthermore, researchers do not express this type of statement. The researcher might say that the data provide evidence of a strong relationship between or among variables.
3. The statement is correct. This is the definition of level of significance.
4. The statement is erroneous. "The level of significance is dichotomous, which means that the difference is either significant or not significant; there are no 'degrees' of significance" (p. 377).
5. Level of significance is a concept in decision theory. "Decision theory is inductive and assumes that all groups in a study (e.g., experimental and comparison groups) used to test a particular hypothesis are components of the same population relative to the variables under study." It is up to the researcher to provide evidence for a genuine difference between the groups, (p. 377).

TEST-TAKING TIP: The key phrase in the question stem is "level of significance." Values are based on the normal distribution.

Content Area: *Level of Significance;* ***Cognitive Level:*** *Comprehension;* ***Question Type:*** *Multiple Response*
CRITICAL THINKING FACILITATOR: If a researcher sets the alpha at 0.01, what does this mean in relation to the analysis of the data?

14. 1. When the level of significance is 0.05, the risk for a type I error increases.
2. The statement indicates a type 1 error.
3. Issues in methodology, such as having a small sample, lead to a type II error. A type II error occurs when "the researcher concludes that no significant difference exists between the samples examined, when in fact a difference exists; the null hypothesis is regarded as true when it is false" (Burns & Grove, 2011, p. 552).
4. When the level of significance becomes more extreme, a type I error occurs.

TEST-TAKING TIP: The key phrase in the question stem is "type II error." A clue indicating this type of error is a small sample.

Content Area: *Type I and II Errors;* ***Cognitive Level:*** *Comprehension;* ***Question Type:*** *Multiple Choice*

CRITICAL THINKING FACILITATOR: What measures could be implemented to avoid a type II error?

15. **1. The *p* value is the probability of a type I error. A type I error is "created by rejecting the null hypothesis that is true" (Polit & Beck, 2014, p. 394). The researcher concludes that there is a relationship between the variables when in fact there is none.**

2. The correlation coefficient describes the "intensity and direction of a relationship" (p. 222) of the variables in the study.
3. The probability of a type II error is called beta. It can be "estimated through power analysis" (p. 231).
4. The relationship between two variables can be calculated by a correlation.

TEST-TAKING TIP: The key phrase in the question stem is "< 0.05 as a *p* value." Recall that most nursing research studies use 0.05. "With a 0.05 significance level, we accept the risk that out of 100 samples from a population, a true null hypothesis would be wrongly rejected 5 times" (Polit & Beck, 2014, p. 231).

Content Area: *Probability;* ***Cognitive Level:*** *Comprehension;* ***Question Type:*** *Multiple Choice*

CRITICAL THINKING FACILITATOR: Why do most nursing studies use 0.05 as the p value?

16. **1. This is an appropriate question to ask. A correlation analyzes the relationship between two variables.**

2. Correlation coefficients range from –1.00 to +1.00.
3. **This is a true statement. The product-moment correlation coefficient is also known as Pearson's r.**
4. **The relationship between correlated variables could be either negative or positive.**
5. The statement incorrect. There is a relationship between variables even when the coefficient is low. The correct interpretation of a low correlation is that the relationship is weak.

TEST-TAKING TIP: The key word in the question stem is "correlational," which means the relationship of two variables is the focus. Recall the characteristics of a correlation study under the chapter on design.

Content Area: *Correlation: Test of Relationship;* ***Cognitive Level:*** *Comprehension;* ***Question Type:*** *Multiple Response*

CRITICAL THINKING FACILITATOR: Look at the results of a sample correlation study. What do the numbers mean in relation to the research question and hypothesis?

17. 1. The statement does not indicate the direction of the relationship.

2. **The statement indicates a positive correlation because the increase in one variable resulted in an increase in the second variable.**
3. The statement indicates a negative correlation. The increase in one variable resulted in a decrease in the second variable.
4. The statement is a null hypothesis that proposes the absence of a relationship between two variables.

TEST-TAKING TIP: The key phrase in the second statement is "positive relationship." Think of a positive correlation as a relationship between two people, in which both benefit equally.

Content Area: *Correlation: Test of relationship;* ***Cognitive Level:*** *Analysis;* ***Question Type:*** *Multiple Choice*

CRITICAL THINKING FACILITATOR: Think of pairs of clinically relevant variables that have a positive correlation. How would you use this knowledge to facilitate nursing care? For instance, the higher the level of circulating fluids in the body, the higher the blood pressure.

18. 36

TEST-TAKING TIP: The key phrase in the question stem is "correlation coefficient (r squared)." The r squared indicates the percentage of variance explained by the relationship" (Burns & Grove, 2011, p. 395) between two variables. Subtract the explained variance from 100%, which is the total, and you get the percentage of unexplained variance.

Content Area: *Correlation: Test of Relationship;* ***Cognitive Level:*** *Application;* ***Question Type:*** *Fill-in-the-Blank*

CRITICAL THINKING FACILITATOR: Recall that a perfect correlation is either +1 or –1. Convert these into percentages when computing the correlation coefficient. Consider hypothetical correlation coefficients between familiar variables in the clinical setting (e.g., nutrition and pressure ulcer development; unsteady gait and risk for falls) What would the percentages indicate?

19. post hoc analysis

TEST-TAKING TIP: The key phrase in the question stem is "study results showed." This phrase indicates something that is done after the initial analysis.

***Content Area:** Concepts in Quantitative Data Analysis; **Cognitive Level:** Knowledge; **Question Type:** Fill-in-the-Blank*

CRITICAL THINKING FACILITATOR: Why do researchers want to determine whether there was a difference between or among the groups in a study? Furthermore, why do they also want to know in which group the difference occurred? In answering these questions, think of a study that had an intervention.

20. t test

TEST-TAKING TIP: The key phrase in the question stem is "difference between two means." A t test is a post hoc analysis measure to determine whether the difference between two groups is significant.

***Content Area:** Test for Significance; **Cognitive Level:** Comprehension; **Question Type:** Fill-in-the-Blank*

CRITICAL THINKING FACILITATOR: What information does a researcher need in order to do a t test to analyze quantitative data?

21. Hypothesis

TEST-TAKING TIP: The key word in the statement is "directional." Recall that a hypothesis is a "statement of predicted relationship between variables or predicted outcomes" (Polit & Beck, 2014, p. 382). A directional hypothesis proposes a specific direction for the relationship (either tail of the normal curve).

***Content Area:** Level of Significance; **Cognitive Level:** Analysis; **Question Type:** Fill-in-the-Blank*

CRITICAL THINKING FACILITATOR: How would the normal curve be used in analyzing data of a study that has a nondirectional hypothesis?

22. 1. **A representative sample is a requirement for use of inferential statistics. A representative sample is one "whose characteristics are comparable to those of the population from which it is drawn" (Polit & Beck, 2014, p. 390).**
    2. **Probability sampling uses random procedures to select a representative sample. Probability sampling reduces bias and error.**
    3. This is not a requirement in using inferential statistics. This is a requirement of an experimental design.
    4. **Data for inferential statistics must be at the ratio level of measurement. This fourth level of measurement "has equal distances between scores and a true meaningful zero point" (p. 390).**
    5. This is not a correct statement. A large sample would add power. Power "is the ability of a design or analysis strategy to detect true relationships that exist among variables" (p. 388).

TEST-TAKING TIP: The key words in the question statement are "inferential statistics." Inferential statistics "permit inferences about whether results observed in a sample are likely to occur in the larger population" (Polit & Beck, 2014, p. 382).

***Content Area:** Inferential Statistics; **Cognitive Level:** Analysis; **Question Type:** Multiple Response*

CRITICAL THINKING FACILITATOR: List some examples of inferential statistical techniques and identify their specific uses.

23. Analysis of variance (ANOVA).

TEST-TAKING TIP: The key phrase in the question stem is "three or more groups." Recall that to determine the difference between two groups, a researcher would use a t test.

***Content Area:** Inferential Statistics; **Cognitive Level:** Knowledge; **Question Type:** Fill-in-the-Blank*

CRITICAL THINKING FACILITATOR: Think of a study on a variable when three or more comparison groups are used.

24. 1. The statement describes a basic ANOVA.
    2. The statement describes a basic ANOVA.
    3. The statement describes a correlation.
    4. **The statement describes a repeated-measures ANOVA.**

TEST-TAKING TIP: The key phrase in the third statement is "over time," which indicates more than one data collection after the initial one.

***Content Area:** Inferential Statistics; **Cognitive Level:** Application; **Question Type:** Multiple Choice*

CRITICAL THINKING FACILITATOR: What is the significance of using a repeated-measures ANOVA as a statistical procedure in intervention studies?

25. 1. A t test is a "parametric statistical test for analyzing the difference between two groups" (Polit & Beck, 2014, p. 394).
    2. An analysis of variance (ANOVA) is a "statistical procedure for testing mean differences among three or more groups by comparing variability between groups to variability within groups, yielding an F-ratio statistic" (p. 374).

3. Multiple regression is a "statistical procedure for understanding the effects of two or more independent (predictor) variables on a dependent variable" (p. 385).
4. A correlation looks at the "bond or association between variables, with variation in one variable systematically related to the variation in another" (p. 378).

TEST-TAKING TIP: The key phrase in the question stem is "more than one independent variable," which alludes to the term "multiple." ***To regress*** **means "to go back." Recall the "cause and effect" in experimental research. One could consider going back to see what caused (independent variable) the effect (dependent variable).**

Content Area: *Statistical Significance; Concepts in Quantitative Data Analysis;* ***Cognitive Level:*** *Comprehension;* ***Question Type:*** *Multiple Choice*
CRITICAL THINKING FACILITATOR:
Think of a clinical situation that has multiple causes such as pressure ulcers or falls. If you were to do a study to determine which of these causes is most likely to have the strongest effect, how would you process your data?

26. **1. Descriptive statistics would be appropriate to provide information on the demographic characteristics of the sample.**
2. A correlation can be done on selected variables and the relationship with the dependent variable, depression.
3. An ANOVA is not appropriate because there is only one group of research participants.
4. Multiple regression is appropriate because there could be more than one independent variable.
5. A MANOVA is not appropriate because this statistical test is used "to test the significance of differences between the means of two or more groups on two or more dependent variables, considered simultaneously" (Polit & Beck, 2014, p. 385).

TEST-TAKING TIP: The key phrase in the first statement is "contributors to depression." ***Contributors*** **indicate multiple "causes." In addition, there is no indication that there are comparison groups (experimental and control).**

Content Area: *Inferential Statistics;* ***Cognitive Level:*** *Comprehension;* ***Question Type:*** *Multiple Response*
CRITICAL THINKING FACILITATOR:
Create a grid of the different statistical techniques. Include types of data needed, the use of groups, and the number of independent and dependent variables.

27. 1. The statistic is used to analyze data in a correlational study that seeks to "determine relationships among variables" (Burns & Grove, 2011, p. 543). The information provided indicates that the study could be either a quasi-experimental or experimental design. There is an independent variable, rewarming methods, and a dependent variable, hypothermia.
2. Multiple regression is not an appropriate statistical procedure because there is only one independent variable.
3. An ANOVA is not appropriate because there were only two groups of research participants as implied in the two rewarming methods.
4. An analysis of covariance (ANCOVA) is the appropriate statistical test. This test would "reduce the variance within groups by partialing out the variance due to a confounding variable."

TEST-TAKING TIP: The key phrase in the third statement of the research information is "after controlling for." This is the distinct feature of an ANCOVA. Look for the confounding variable stated after the phrase "after controlling for."

Content Area: *Inferential Statistics;* ***Cognitive Level:*** *Analysis;* ***Question Type:*** *Multiple Choice*
CRITICAL THINKING FACILITATOR:
What are some variables (covariates) that can confound a study? Take one and describe how this variable can confound the results.

28. 1. For any study, a large sample is desirable. However, the size of the sample is more critical in a parametric test.
2. This is a correct statement about nonparametric tests. They are the choice of tests for nominal or ordinal data.
3. This is not a correct statement. Nonparametric tests can be used in studies with more than one group.
4. Nonparametric procedures are not based on probability sampling.

TEST-TAKING TIP: The key word in the question stem is "nonparametric." "Nonparametric statistics are not based on the estimation of population parameters, so they involve less restrictive assumptions about the underlying distribution" (Sullivan-Bolyai & Bova, 2010, p. 323). They are used when data are at the nominal and ordinal levels of measurement.

Content Area: *Nonparametric Statistics;* ***Cognitive Level:*** *Comprehension;* ***Question Type:*** *Multiple Choice*

CRITICAL THINKING FACILITATOR: How do nonparametric procedures compare with parametric procedures?

29. 1. The statement is incorrect. A chi-square test is nonparametric, and it uses nominal or ordinal level data.

2. The statement is incorrect. The statement refers to a t test.
3. The statement is not accurate because the chi-square test is nonparametric.
4. **The statement is an accurate one. The observed and expected frequencies are compared, and the level of significance of the difference is analyzed.**

TEST-TAKING TIP: The key word in the question stem is "nonparametric." "Nonparametric statistics are not based on the estimation of population parameters, so they involve less restrictive assumptions about the underlying distribution" (Sullivan-Bolyai & Bova, 2010, p. 323). They are used when data are at the nominal and ordinal levels of measurement.

Content Area: *Nonparametric Statistics;* ***Cognitive Level:*** *Comprehension;* ***Question Type:*** *Multiple Choice*

CRITICAL THINKING FACILITATOR: Look at a sample study where a chi-square statistic was used. Can you make sense of the data as analyzed by this statistic?

30. **Statistical significance**

TEST-TAKING TIP: The key phrase in the statement "unlikely to have been caused by chance." Statistical significance is guided by probability theory, which is "used to explain the extent of a relationship, the probability that an event will occur in a given situation, or the probability that an event can be accurately predicted" (Burns & Grove, 2011, p. 376).

Content Area: *Statistical Significance;* ***Cognitive Level:*** *Comprehension;* ***Question Type:*** *Fill-in-the-Blank*

CRITICAL THINKING FACILITATOR: Review the normal distribution and how it is used in establishing statistical significance.

31. 1. **The statement is a correct one. The mean at pretest was 34.93, and the mean at posttest was 30.07.**

2. This is not an accurate statement. Look at the *p* value. The ** sign under the t indicates statistical significance.
3. The *p* is the probability of a type I error.
4. **This is a correct statement. The ** sign after the t indicates statistical significance.**
5. **This is a correct statement.**

TEST-TAKING TIP: Review the concepts in descriptive statistics and probability. A researcher has to note the difference in the scores and decide whether the difference is significant. So, in reading tables, relate each number to these concepts.

Content Area: *Results;* ***Cognitive Level:*** *Analysis;* ***Question Type:*** *Multiple Response*

CRITICAL THINKING FACILITATOR: Take a table that reports results from quantitative data analysis and try to make sense of the numbers.

32. 1. Unpredicted results are those that are "opposite of those predicted by the researcher" (Burns & Grove, 2011, p. 409).

2. Mixed results occur when "one variable upholds predicted characteristics whereas another does not" (p. 409).
3. **Nonsignificant results are also called inconclusive results. These results might occur when the "theory used by the researcher to develop the hypothesis is in error" (p. 409).**
4. Unexpected results are "relationships found between variables that were not hypothesized and not predicted from the framework being used" (p. 410).

TEST-TAKING TIP: The key phrase in the question stem is "in error." When something has flaws, it will not produce anything that is useful.

Content Area: *Study Results;* ***Cognitive Level:*** *Knowledge;* ***Question Type:*** *Multiple Choice*

CRITICAL THINKING FACILITATOR: Look at the different types of results in research and identify potential gains for evidence-based practice.

16 Analyzing the Findings in Quantitative Studies

KEY WORDS

The following words include English vocabulary, nursing/medical terminology, concepts, principles, or information relevant to content specifically addressed in the chapter or associated with topics presented in it. English dictionaries, your nursing textbooks, and medical dictionaries such as *Taber's Cyclopedic Medical Dictionary* are resources that can be used to expand your knowledge and understanding of these words and related information.

Confidence interval
Generalizability
Implication
Limitation
Power analysis
Precision
p value
Recommendation
Response bias
Sampling bias

QUESTIONS

Concepts and Processes in Analyzing Findings

1. The appropriateness of a particular statistical procedure for analyzing research data is dependent on several factors. **Select all that apply.**
1. The level of purpose of the study (description, exploration, prediction, explanation)
2. The type of data collected (nominal, ordinal, interval, ratio)
3. The hypothesis to be tested
4. The sample size
5. The study design

2. The summary of analyzed data is often presented in tables in a research report. What should the reader ask when reading a table? **Select all that apply.**
1. Is the title of the table consistent with the purpose of the study?
2. Do the table headings support the title?
3. Does the table explain the data as they are given in the text of the report?
4. Are the statistical procedures appropriate for the level of data collected?
5. Are explanations given for the meaning of the data?

3. **Research Study Information:** Yoon and Kim (2013) looked at "job-related stress, emotional labor, and depressive symptoms among Korean nurses" (p. 169). They found that there was a "significant difference in age ($p = .001$)" among nurses who were depressed and nondepressed. What does the *p* value indicate?
1. "The probability that the obtained results are due to chance alone" (Polit & Beck, 2014, p. 387).
2. There is a correlation between depressive symptoms and age.
3. The possibility of an "error created by accepting a null hypothesis that is false" (p. 394).
4. The probability that older nurses are more likely to be depressed.

4. Decision theory guides the researcher in determining whether study findings are significant. What statements are true regarding decision theory when used in analyzing study data? **Select all that apply.**
   1. Decision theory can help explain the extent of a relationship between two variables.
   2. There is an assumption that all of the groups in a study come from different populations in relation to the study variables.
   3. The researcher selects a level of significance before the data analysis.
   4. The researcher is able to reject or accept the null hypothesis based on the level of significance.
   5. The level of significance can only be decided as significant or not significant ("no degrees of significance"), [Burns & Grove, 2011, p. 377].

5. ____________________ is the "degree to which an estimated population value (statistic) clusters around the estimate, usually expressed in terms of the width of the confidence intervals" (Polit & Beck, 2014, p. 389).

Analyzing the Use of Statistics

6. **Research Study Information:** Jacobsson, Friedrichsen, Goransson, and Hallett (2011) looked at the "psychological well-being in women suffering from coeliac [celiac] disease and living on a gluten free diet" (p. 766). The mean difference in depression between the two groups was 1.7. They used a 95% confidence interval (CI). The lower limit was 1.60, and the upper limit was 1.80. Which statement about CI is true?
   1. CI means that there is only a 5% possibility of committing a type II error.
   2. CI indicates that the researchers have made a decision to reject the null hypothesis.
   3. CI represents the "range of values within which a population parameter is estimated to lie at a specified probability" (Polit & Beck, 2014, p. 371).
   4. CI is also called alpha and is the "risk the researcher is willing to accept of making a Type I error" (p. 374).

7. **Research Study Information:** Romeo (2013) did a study on the "predictive ability of critical thinking, nursing GPA, and SAT scores on first-time NCLEX-RN performance" (p. 248). Under the design section of the research report, the following information was presented: **Power level: 0.80; alpha level: 0.05; estimated effect size: 0.40; and sample size: 100 subjects.** ____________________ is the process in evidence from the set of data in the above statement. It is also used to determine the risk of a type II error (Burns & Grove, 2011).

8. **Research Study Information:** "There were 98 (89%) women and 120 (11%) men in the study. Their ages ranged from 21-52 years with a mean age of 30.4 plus or minus 7.4 years. The median age was 28 years, and the interquartile range was 24-36 years" (Hasson & Gustavsson, 2010, p. 3). What does the information indicate?
   1. The use of statistics to identify a relationship between groups
   2. The use of statistics to describe the research sample
   3. The information identifies the target population for generalizability purposes.
   4. The statistics would help in making inferences about the other pieces of data.

9. **Research Study Information:** Lee, Dai, Park, and McCreary (2013) studied the effect of quality of work life (QWL) on nurses' intention to leave. They found "the seven dimensions of QWL were all significantly correlated (r = 0.15 - 0.66, $p < 0.05$)" (p. 163). The r is the ____________________ and indicates the degree of relationship between two variables.

10. **Research Data Information:** Yoon and Kim (2103) looked at "job-related stress, emotional labor, and depressive symptoms among Korean nurses" (p. 169). "A multivariate logistic regression analysis was used to explore and determine which factors are more strongly associated with depressive symptoms" (p. 171). These statements indicate the use of statistics to ____________________ the dependent variable, depressive symptoms.

11. **Research Study Information:** Jacobsson et al. (2011) studied the ":effects of an active method of patient education on the psychological well-being of patients with coeliac disease living on a gluten-free diet" (p. 766). They "used an independent t test to analyze the difference between groups at baseline and also to analyze the difference between groups in improvement from 0-10 weeks" (p. 769) after the intervention. What is true about the statistical procedure they used?
    1. The t test is used "to examine causality by testing for significant differences between two samples" (Burns & Grove, 2011, p. 404).
    2. The test can be used for nominal or ordinal data.
    3. A comparison was made between expected and observed values.
    4. As a parametric test it can "test for the relationship between two variables" (Burns & Grove, 2011, p. 394).

Analyzing the Study Results and Discussion

12. **Research Study Information:** Cho, Lee, Mark, and Yun (2012) did a study of the "turnover of new graduate nurses in their first job using survival analysis" (p. 63). "Seventeen percent reported overall job satisfaction. Job aspects with large proportions of nurses dissatisfied were working hours (37%) and pay (33%)" (p. 66). This research information is included in what section of a research report?
    1. Analysis of the data
    2. Study results
    3. Interpretation of findings
    4. Collection of data

13. **Research Study Information:** Taylor and Reyes (2012) did a study on self-efficacy and resilience in baccalaureate nursing students. The researchers indicated that "The study was conducted over a short period of time and may not be reflective of the changes in self-efficacy and resilience over an entire program of nursing study" (p. 9). What does the statement above indicate in the research report?
    1. Conclusion
    2. Interpretation
    3. Limitation
    4. Recommendation

14. **Research Study Information:** Powell-Young and Spruill (2013) looked at the "views of Black nurses toward genetic research and testing" (p. 151). Statements in their conclusion were as follows: "Sample representativeness may not be ideally characteristic of Black American nurses in the United States. Individuals who participated in this research project were self-selected. Future studies would likely benefit from a larger, more representative sample of Black nurses" (p. 156). What do these statements indicate?
    1. Sampling bias
    2. Lack of power
    3. Nonsignificant findings
    4. Mixed findings

15. In the discussion section, the researchers expressed their concern because "outcome measures were based on subjective self-report" (Yoon & Kim, 2013, p. 174). What type of bias is this?
    1. Experimental or control group
    2. Sampling
    3. Design
    4. Response

16. Which of the following statements is a conclusion of a study?
1. "The results presented in this report showed that the radiant warmer device required significantly less time for rewarming and was more efficient in raising body temperature than warm cotton blankest in post-spinal surgery hyperthermia patients" (Yang et al., 2012, p. 11).
2. "More longitudinal studies using various analytic methods are needed to advance turnover research and ultimately reduce turnover rates in the nursing workforce" (Cho et al., 2012, p. 69).
3. "However, a potential bias is the educational environment as for instance different organizational climates and locations may have an impact on stress and sleep" (Hasson & Gustavsson, 2010, p. 5).
4. "Further efforts should focus on studying underlying reasons for non-adherence in larger samples of older adults who are self-neglecting" (Turner et al., 2012, p. 748).

17. Research Study Information: Li et al. (2010) studied the "effects of music on physiological stress response and anxiety level of mechanically ventilated patients" (p. 978). They stated that "for music to elicit the expected therapeutic effect, nurses must include items on musical preferences when they conduct patient assessment if attempting to use music intervention" (p. 986). What does this research information represent?
1. Limitation
2. Interpretation
3. Conclusion
4. Implication

18. Research Study Information: Othman et al. (2012) studied the "influence of demographic factors, knowledge, and beliefs on Jordanian women's intention to undergo mammography screening" (p. 19). The researchers stated that "the significant contribution of perceived self-efficacy to the women's intention to engage in mammography is consistent with earlier studies [authors of studies were cited]" (p. 24). Where would these statements made by the researchers belong in a research report?
1. Results
2. Analysis of data
3. Implications
4. Discussion

19. Research Study Information: Yang et al. (2012) compared "two recovery room methods for treating hypothermia patients who had undergone spinal surgery" (p. 2). Under the discussion section, the researchers had this to say: "Only individuals who had undergone spinal surgery were selected. It is not clear whether these findings would be clinically relevant to patients undergoing different types of surgery, such as open thoracic or open abdominal surgery" (pp. 8-9). What does this research information indicate?
1. Lack of eligible subjects
2. Issue with generalizability
3. Study recommendation
4. Validity of findings

20. Mindful of evidence-based practice (EBP), what is the most important question to ask about the findings of a study?
1. Are the study findings statistically significant?
2. What is the degree of applicability of the findings to practice?
3. How can the study findings improve future research?
4. Why did findings fail to show statistical significance?

Critiquing a Study's Findings and Dicussion

21. What are appropriate questions to ask in critiquing the statistical procedures used in a research study? **Select all that apply.**
1. Were appropriate techniques used to analyze the data in relation to the study's purpose?
2. Was the level of data measurement appropriate for the procedures used?
3. Did the researcher provide a rationale for the use of specific procedures?
4. Did the researcher explain the use of the procedure in relation to previous studies?
5. Did the researcher include a description of the reliability of the method for data collection?

22. What are some appropriate questions to ask in critiquing the discussion section of a quantitative study? **Select all that apply.**
1. Was the intervention for the experimental group described and differentiated from what was given the control group?
2. Were the composition of the experimental and control group consistent?
3. Were recommendations for future research identified?
4. Did the researcher discuss data in relation to each hypothesis?
5. Did the researcher discuss the clinical significance of the findings?

ANSWERS AND RATIONALES

The correct answer number and rationale for why it is the correct answer are given in **boldface blue type**. Rationales for why the other possible answer options are incorrect also are given, but they are not in boldface type.

1. 1. **This is a factor to consider in determining appropriateness of a statistical procedure. If the purpose of a study is description, then descriptive statistics would be appropriate. For prediction, parametric inferential statistics would be appropriate.**
   2. **Whereas parametric statistical procedures require interval or ratio data, nonparametric tests only need nominal or ordinal data.**
   3. **The variables and their relationships are expressed in the hypotheses. The type of hypothesis and the number of variables help determine the appropriate tests.**
   4. **Sample size must also be considered particularly in selecting an inferential statistical procedure.**
   5. **The study design is a determining factor in the selection of statistical procedures. Whereas a correlational study would use a correlation such as the Pearson r, a randomized clinical trial would use t tests or analysis of variance (ANOVA) if investigating differences in groups.**

   TEST-TAKING TIP: The key phrase in the question stem is "in analyzing research data." Recall that lower level studies have simpler designs and lack the requirements that are essential in more complex designs that have higher levels of purposes.

   Content Area: *Quantitative Data Analysis;* ***Cognitive Level:*** *Analysis;* ***Question Type:*** *Multiple Response*
   CRITICAL THINKING FACILITATOR: Compare the statistical procedures for a descriptive or exploratory study with those used for quasi-experimental or experimental study. Look at the study's purpose, hypothesis, design, sample size, and type of data collected to facilitate understanding of these statistical procedures.

2. 1. **This is an appropriate question to ask. If the purpose of the study is description, then the table should be about descriptive data.**
   2. **This is a correct question to ask. If the table is about descriptive data, then the table should have information on the means, standard deviations, and percentages.**
   3. The table might repeat some data in the text; however, the table summarizes the data and presents it in an organized, visually concise way. The table does not provide explanation of the data in a narrative format.
   4. **The level of the data collected might not appear in the table. Only the statistical procedure would appear (e.g., correlation, t test, ANOVA) One can note whether the procedure was appropriate by reading about the level of data collected. This information would be under the methods section.**
   5. No explanations are given for the meaning of the data. However, the table might indicate which data are significant. This information is noted at the bottom portion of the table.

   TEST-TAKING TIP: The key word in the question stem is "table." A table in a report would have columns and rows of information. A table summarizes information to facilitate processing and understanding.

   Content Area: *Quantitative Data Analysis;* ***Cognitive Level:*** *Comprehension;* ***Question Type:*** *Multiple Response*
   CRITICAL THINKING FACILITATOR: Look at a table in a quantitative study. Other than numerical values, what other information is conveyed by the table?

3. 1. **This is the correct statement about a *p* value.**
   2. The statement is in error. The statement expresses a relationship, and this is not represented by the *p* value.
   3. The statement defines a type II error.
   4. The statement does not reflect the *p* value.

   TEST-TAKING TIP: The key words in the question stem are "*p* value." Researchers use probability theory to "explain the extent of a relationship, the probability that an event will occur in a given situation, or the probability that an event can be predicted" (Burns & Grove, 2011, p. 376).

   Content Area: *Quantitative Data Analysis;* ***Cognitive Level:*** *Analysis;* ***Question Type:*** *Multiple Choice*
   CRITICAL THINKING FACILITATOR: Look at a study table that reports data about the study and determine what *p* values were used.

4. 1. The statement does not define decision theory. The statement refers to probability and is expressed as a *p* value.
   2. The statement is erroneous. The correct assumption is that groups come from the

same population in relation to the study variables. It is the role of the researcher "to provide evidence for a genuine difference between the groups" (Burns & Grove, 2011, p. 377).
3. **This is a true statement. The level of significance guides the researcher in making a decision about the data.**
4. **The level of significance determines whether the difference seen in groups in relation to study variables would lead to rejection or acceptance of the null hypothesis (no difference between the groups).**
5. **This is a true statement. Level of significance is "dichotomous" (Burns & Grove, 2011, p. 377), significant or not significant.**

TEST-TAKING TIP: The key phrase in the question stem is "determining whether study findings are significant." The term "determining" relates to making a decision. Recall the concepts of the normal distribution to help you in selecting the correct options.

Content Area: *Decision Theory in Quantitative Analysis;* ***Cognitive Level:*** *Comprehension;* ***Question Type:*** *Multiple Response*
CRITICAL THINKING FACILITATOR: Many decisions have to be made by the researcher about the design and conduct of the study. Finally, when data have been collected and processed, what decisions must be made by the researcher?

5. **Precision**

TEST-TAKING TIP: The key phrase in the question stem is "clusters around the estimate." Recall that a researcher can provide only an estimate of population parameters. Therefore, the closer the statistic to the parameter, the more precise it is.

Content Area: *Concepts in Quantitative Data Analysis;* ***Cognitive Level:*** *Knowledge;* ***Question Type:*** *Fill-in-the-Blank*
CRITICAL THINKING FACILITATOR: What are measures to ensure precision of findings in quantitative studies? Why are precise findings critical for EBP?

6. 1. The statement is not accurate about CI.
   2. The statement indicates an action in using decision theory.
   3. **The statement describes the CI. In the research information, lower and upper limits include the estimated population parameter.**
   4. This is not an accurate statement. The alpha is not the same as the CI.

TEST-TAKING TIP: The key phrase in the question stem is "confidence interval." If someone asks you to estimate a distance, you might give that person a range, a lower and an upper limit of your estimate. Your CI is the "extent" of how close you think your estimate is to the real thing. For instance, you might say, "I am 50% sure."

Content Area: *Concepts in Quantitative Data Analysis;* ***Cognitive Level:*** *Comprehension;* ***Question Type:*** *Multiple Choice*
CRITICAL THINKING FACILITATOR: Look at the results of a quantitative study and see whether a CI is reported. Are you able to discern what it means in relation to the hypothesis that was tested?

7. **power analysis**

TEST-TAKING TIP: The key words in the research information are "power" and "sample size."

Content Area: *Concepts in Quantitative Analysis;* ***Cognitive Level:*** *Application;* ***Question Type:*** *Fill-in-the-Blank*
CRITICAL THINKING FACILITATOR: Recall that a type II error occurs "when the null hypothesis is regarded as true when it is false" (Burns & Grove, 2011, p. 352). One of the causes of this error is a small sample. Locate information under study design that describes sample size and makes sense why a certain number of participants is essential.

8. 1. The statement is incorrect because the statistics provided are descriptive. They summarize information about the sample; they do not identify a relationship.
   2. **This statement is correct because it presents descriptive information about the sample.**
   3. The target population is not identified in the information.
   4. The statistics are descriptive and are not used for making inferences.

TEST-TAKING TIP: The key words in the question stem are "mean, median, and interquartile range." Recall that these are descriptive statistics and are measures of central tendency.

Content Area: *Analyzing the Use of Statistics;* ***Cognitive Level:*** *Application;* ***Question Type:*** *Multiple Choice*
CRITICAL THINKING FACILITATOR: Look at the results section of a sample quantitative study. What is the first set of data presented by the researcher? What is the purpose of this set of data?

9. Pearson product–moment correlation

TEST-TAKING TIP: The key word in the question stem is "correlated." Correlation is a test of relationship between variables. The r (for relationship) tests for correlation.

Content Area: *Analyzing the Use of Statistics;* ***Cognitive Level:*** *Knowledge;* ***Question Type:*** *Fill-in-the-Blank*

CRITICAL THINKING FACILITATOR: Look at a sample correlational study. Are you able to understand the meanings of the symbols and numbers after them?

10. predict

TEST-TAKING TIP: The key word in the research information is "determine." One meaning of *determine* is "to ascertain." After something is ascertained, a prediction can be made. For instance, a number of factors might cause one to arrive late for class. Heavy traffic during a certain time of the day might be the strongest factor to cause lateness. Knowing this factor, lateness can then be predicted.

Content Area: *Analyzing the Use of Statistics;* ***Cognitive Level:*** *Application;* ***Question Type:*** *Fill-in-the-Blank*

CRITICAL THINKING FACILITATOR:
What clinical situations can be examined using multiple regression? Think of situations that have multiple influencing factors.

11. 1. **The statement is correct about a t test.**
2. Interval or ratio level data are required to do a t test.
3. The statement describes the statistic called chi square.
4. The statement is erroneous. A correlation is a test for a relationship between variables.

TEST-TAKING TIP: The key phrase in the research information is "analyze the difference." The difference referred here is the "effect" of the intervention on the groups of research participants. Recall that a study with an intervention must have at least two groups, an experimental group and a control group. The research information does not imply more than two groups; therefore, a t test is appropriate.

Note that at times there might only be one group in a study, that is, when this one group is tested before the intervention and then after the intervention. This one group acts as its own control.

Content Area: *Analyzing the Use of Statistics;* ***Cognitive Level:*** *Application;* ***Question Type:*** *Multiple Choice*

CRITICAL THINKING FACILITATOR:
Compare the different statistical procedures that test for causality, including ANOVA, analysis of covariance (ANCOVA), and chi square.

12. 1. The information is not the analysis. Analysis is the "phase that involves a critical appraisal of the logical links connecting one study element with another" (Burns & Grove, 2011, p. 532).
2. **The research information indicates study results. The researchers are presenting data as collected with no analysis or interpretation.**
3. The research information is not interpretation. Interpretation "involves making sense of the study results and examining their implications" (Polit & Beck, 2014, p. 52).
4. The collection of data includes all the procedures for getting information from research participants, including training the data collectors.

TEST-TAKING TIP: The key terms in the research information are the percentages "17%, 37%, and 33%." Percentages are descriptive statistics. These are part of the results of a study.

Content Area: *Study Results;* ***Cognitive Level:*** *Knowledge;* ***Question Type:*** *Multiple Choice*

CRITICAL THINKING FACILITATOR:
What types of information are generally included in the results section of a study? Consult one of the studies in a sample study.

13. 1. Conclusions are "syntheses and clarifications of the meanings of study findings" (Burns & Grove, 2011, p. 534).
2. Interpretations "involve making sense of the study results and examining their implications" (Polit & Beck, 2014, p. 52).
3. **The statement indicates a limitation. Limitations are "theoretical and methodological restrictions in a study that may decrease the generalizability of the findings" (Burns & Grove, 2011, p. 541).**
4. Recommendations are "suggestions provided by a study's researcher for ways to design a better study next time" (p. 546).

TEST-TAKING TIP: The key words in the research information are "over a short period of time" and "may not be reflective." These are situations that could restrict or limit the study in some manner.

Content Area: *Study Results;* ***Cognitive Level:*** *Application;* ***Question Type:*** *Multiple Choice*

CRITICAL THINKING FACILITATOR: Read over the discussion section of a sample quantitative study and identify some of the constraints acknowledged by the researcher. Is this information useful to others? Why or why not?

14. **1. Sampling bias is indicated in the statements. "Sampling bias is seen when a sample is not representative of the population from which it was drawn" (Polit & Beck, 2014, p. 391).**
2. Lack of power is not indicated in the research information. Power is "the ability of a design or strategy to detect true relationships that exist among variables" (p. 388).
3. Findings are not expressed in the research statements.
4. Mixed findings are not indicated in the research statements. Mixed results "include both significant and nonsignificant findings" (Burns & Grove, 2011, p. 542).

TEST-TAKING TIP: The key words in the research information are "representativeness" and "self-selected." Both of these concepts relate to bias in the sampling procedure.

Content Area: *Concepts in Quantitative Data Analysis;* ***Cognitive Level:*** *Analysis;* ***Question Type:*** *Multiple Choice*
CRITICAL THINKING FACILITATOR: An effective research report includes a description of any bias in the study. Knowledge of these biases facilitates revisions in design and methodology. These revisions are critical in the conduct of valid research studies that contribute to EBP.

15. 1. The bias described does not relate to the comparison groups in the study.
2. Sampling bias is not reflected in the statement.
3. There is nothing in the statement that the bias relates to design.
4. The bias is in the response of the research participants.

TEST-TAKING TIP: The key phrase in the research information is "subjective self-report," which expresses a response by the research participants.

Content Area: *Concepts in Quantitative Data Analysis;* ***Cognitive Level:*** *Analysis;* ***Question Type:*** *Multiple Choice*
CRITICAL THINKING FACILITATOR:
Compare outcomes from a standardized objective instrument with those from a subjective self-report tool. Recall the requirements for research instruments to avoid bias.

16. **1. The statement is a conclusion of the researchers. Conclusions are "syntheses and clarifications of the meanings of study findings" (Burns & Grove, 2011, p. 534).**
2. The statement is a recommendation. Recommendations are "suggestions provided by a study's researcher for ways to design a better study next time" (p. 546).
3. The statement expresses a limitation of the study.
4. The statement is a recommendation for future studies.

TEST-TAKING TIP: The key phrases in the research information is "required significantly less time" and "was more efficient." These phrases indicate a judgment on the part of the researchers after their analysis and interpretation of the data.

Content Area: *Discussion of Findings;* ***Cognitive Level:*** *Application;* ***Question Type:*** *Multiple Choice*
CRITICAL THINKING FACILITATOR: Read the discussion section of a sample study and identify the different statements included. What is the value of this section to EBP?

17. 1. The statement is not a limitation. Limitations are "theoretical and methodological restrictions in a study that may decrease the generalizability of the findings" (Burns & Grove, 2011, p. 541).
2. The statement is not an interpretation. An interpretation "involves making sense of the study results and examining their implications" (Polit & Beck, 2014, p. 52).
3. The statement is not a conclusion. Conclusions are "syntheses and clarifications of the meanings of study findings" (Burns & Grove, 2011, p. 534).
4. The statement is an implication. An implication is the meaning of research conclusions for the body of knowledge, theory, and practice (p. 539).

TEST-TAKING TIP: The key phrase in the research information is "nurses must." This phrase implies specified guidelines for practice.

Content Area: *Discussion of Findings;* ***Cognitive Level:*** *Application;* ***Question Type:*** *Multiple Choice*
CRITICAL THINKING FACILITATOR: How should nurses, as consumers of research, process recommendations for practice? What guidelines do they need to use to determine the applicability of findings to EBP?

18. 1. The research information does not present results. Results in quantitative studies are numerical values calculated using the appropriate statistical procedures.
2. The research information is not the analysis of the data but rather is the meaning attached to the data by the researcher. In so doing, the researcher relates the data to the research question, purpose, and hypothesis.
3. The research information is not an implication of the study. Implications are the "meaning of the research conclusions for the body of knowledge, theory, and practice" (Burns & Grove, 2011, p. 539).
4. **The research information is part of the discussion section of the report. This section "ties together the other sections of the research report and gives them meaning" (p. 59).**

TEST-TAKING TIP: The second statement in the research information provides a clue to the answer. In the discussion section of a research report, researchers present their data in light of previous related studies. They cite the works of other researchers.

Content Area: *Discussion of Findings;* ***Cognitive Level:*** *Application;* ***Question Type:*** *Multiple Choice*
CRITICAL THINKING FACILITATOR: Read the discussion section of a sample study.. What statements were made by the researcher in relation to the findings of others on the same topic? Note in particular how the researcher discusses the findings in relation to the study's hypothesis and how these findings help add to the body of knowledge on the topic.

19. 1. The research information does not indicate a lack of subject availability.
2. **It is evident from the research information that there is an issue with generalizability. *Generalizability* means the "inference that the data are representative of similar phenomena in a population beyond the studied sample" (LoBiondo-Wood & Haber, 2010, p. 578).**
3. The research statements are not recommendations. A recommendation is an "application of a study to practice, theory, and future research" (Polit & Beck, 2014, p. 584).
4. The research information does not address the study's validity.

TEST-TAKING TIP: Read over the last statement in the research information, "It is not clear whether these findings would be clinically relevant to patients undergoing different types of surgery, such as open thoracic or open abdominal surgery," which provides a clue to the answer. What might future studies examine based on this statement?

Content Area: *Discussion of Findings;* ***Cognitive Level:*** *Analysis;* ***Question Type:*** *Multiple Choice*
CRITICAL THINKING FACILITATOR: Review the concept of external validity in relation to this question. Look for the researcher's acknowledgment of this under the discussion section of a study.

20. 1. Although this is a question that needs to be asked, it is not the most important one.
2. **The overall purpose of research is improvement of patient outcomes. Therefore, the applicability of findings that have the potential for improving outcomes is the most important question to ask.**
3. Although this is another important question to ask, it is not the most important.
4. This is not the most important question to ask. The researchers might be concerned about nonsignificant findings. This question would guide future research on the topic and potential changes in design and methodology.

TEST-TAKING TIP: The key words in the question stem are "evidence-based practice." Therefore, a question that asks about clinical application is the most important.

Content Area: *Critiquing Findings;* ***Cognitive Level:*** *Analysis;* ***Question Type:*** *Multiple Choice*
CRITICAL THINKING FACILITATOR: What are the expectations of healthcare providers who read the findings of a study? Compare these with the expectations of others such as researchers or educators.

21. 1. **The question is appropriate to ask. The purpose of the study guides the selection of appropriate procedures. For example, a study with a purpose of description would use descriptive statistics.**
2. **The level of data determines the type of procedure to be used. For instance, nominal-level data cannot be analyzed using an ANOVA.**
3. **This is an appropriate question to ask. Every researcher provides a rationale for the use of specific procedures to facilitate understanding by the reader/consumer.**

4. The question would be appropriate to ask when critiquing the review of the literature or the methods section of the report.
5. The question is appropriate to ask in critiquing the methods section of a report.

TEST-TAKING TIP: The key phrase in the question stem is "statistical procedures." The phrase implies the use of some measure to process numbers.

Content Area: *Critiquing Findings;* ***Cognitive Level:*** *Application;* ***Question Type:*** *Multiple Response*
CRITICAL THINKING FACILITATOR: Take one specific statistical procedure that you understand well. Describe the requirements and the outcomes in using this procedure.

22. 1. The question is not asked in critiquing the discussion section. This question is appropriate to ask in critiquing the methods section.
2. This question is not asked in critiquing the discussion but is asked in critiquing the methods section.
3. **The question is appropriate to ask because in the discussion section the researcher summarizes the findings and reviews what needs to be done in building the knowledge base of the topic.**
4. **The question is appropriate to ask because part of the discussion includes the findings and conclusions in relation to the study hypothesis(es). It is also important to find out which hypothesis was not supported and the reasons given by the researcher.**
5. **This question needs to be asked to ascertain the significance of the study's contribution to EBP.**

TEST-TAKING TIP: The key phrase in the question stem is "discussion section." This section would be the overall summary of the study report. Before you get to the discussion section (after having read and understood the other sections), what are your expectations of what should be included?

Content Area: *Critiquing Findings;* ***Cognitive Level:*** *Application;* ***Question Type:*** *Multiple Response*
CRITICAL THINKING FACILITATOR: Every journal presents the last section of a research report differently. Overall, what are the commonalities in their presentation? How did these commonalities facilitate your overall holistic perspective about the topic of this study?

17 Exploring the Paradigm for Qualitative Studies

KEY WORDS

The following words include English vocabulary, nursing/medical terminology, concepts, principles, or information relevant to content specifically addressed in the chapter or associated with topics presented in it. English dictionaries, your nursing textbooks, and medical dictionaries such as *Taber's Cyclopedic Medical Dictionary* are resources that can be used to expand your knowledge and understanding of these words and related information.

Confirmability
Credibility
Data saturation
Dependability
Emergent design
Informants
Mixed methods
Themes
Transferability

QUESTIONS

The Naturalistic Paradigm for Qualitative Research

1. Which of the following beliefs underlies the paradigm for qualitative studies?
1. "There is a reality out here that can be studied and known" (Polit & Beck, 2014, p. 7).
2. "Phenomena are not haphazard, but rather have antecedent causes" (p. 7).
3. "Reality is not a fixed entity but rather a construction of the people participating in the study" (p. 8).
4. "Nature is ordered and regular, and reality exists outside of human observations" (p. 7).

2. The naturalistic paradigm for qualitative research is also known as the constructivist paradigm. Which of the following statements helps explain what *constructivist* means?
1. Reality is not fixed; there are multiple interpretations by humans.
2. The research process generates numerical information about the world.
3. Findings are used to build the scientific base of the discipline.
4. Reality already exists, and its causes can be studied.

3. Which of the following research activities is done by a qualitative researcher? A qualitative researcher
1. "selects a representative sample and determines [sample] size before collecting data" (Barroso, 2010, p. 87).
2. generates a narrative summary of the participant information describing the human experience.
3. generates a numerical summary of data collected using measurement tools.
4. imposes controls over extraneous variables and the research context.

4. In a qualitative study, the researcher is considered a(n) ______________________ because he or she is involved in the entire process and is an active participant.

5. **Research Study Information:** Beck and Watson's (2010) qualitative study found that subsequent childbirth after a previous birth trauma has the potential to either heal or retraumatize women. Based on their study of these women, the researchers recommended that "during pregnancy women need permission and encouragement to grieve their prior traumatic birth to help remove the burden of their invisible pain" (p. 241). From the information given, how did the researchers come to their recommendation?
   1. The researchers are experts in dealing with women who have experienced traumatic birth.
   2. The conclusion is based on an inductive mode of reasoning.
   3. The deductive mode of reasoning is evident in the recommendation.
   4. The logical reasoning of the scientific method is evident in the recommendation.

6. Which of the following situations could be studied through a qualitative approach?
   1. Home care visiting and diabetic adherence to a therapeutic regimen
   2. The lived experience of loss of a parent through HIV/AIDS
   3. Nurse executive leadership style and job satisfaction among registered nurses
   4. Use of reflexology and the control of mild hypertension

7. Which of the following research conclusions suggests a qualitative study?
   1. "Overall, and for both men and women, the percentage of adults screened for cholesterol was lower for Hispanic adults than for non-Hispanic white, non-Hispanic black, and non-Hispanic Asian adults" (Carroll, Kit, Lachner, & Yoon, 2013, p. 5).
   2. "The relationship between depression and diabetes impact on QOL [quality of life] was stronger for men than women (b=.67, p=.020)" (Choi & Reed, 2013, p. 115) in this study of 164 adults with type 2 diabetes.
   3. "Participants with high and low metabolic control levels reported similar themes related to reaction of others, knowledge about type 1 diabetes, and believed healthcare providers used authoritarian interactions" (Scholes et al., 2013, p. 1235).
   4. The researchers reported that "workplace spirituality explained 16% of the variation in organizational citizenship behavior, while it explained 35% of the variation in commitment among nurses" (Kazemipour, Salmiah, & Poursedi, 2012, p. 302).

8. Where is a single qualitative study placed in the hierarchy of evidence for evidence-based practice (EBP)?
   1. Level 1
   2. Level 2
   3. Level 6
   4. Level 7

Activities, Concepts, and Processes in Qualitative Approaches

9. What is the first activity necessary to do a qualitative study?
   1. Do a review of the literature.
   2. Decide on the type of qualitative approach.
   3. Determine whether a sample is accessible.
   4. Focus on a topic of which little is known.

10. What is the concern about doing a review of the literature in a qualitative study?
    1. The literature must be current within the past 5 years.
    2. The literature could "influence the conceptualization of the phenomenon under study" (Polit & Beck, 2014, p. 54).
    3. The literature might not elucidate what is known about the phenomenon of interest (Polit & Beck, 2014).
    4. The literature might present many inconsistencies and gaps that are not going to be helpful.

11. What essential activity must be done by the qualitative researcher before going into the field to collect data?
    1. Search for reliable and valid research instruments, including checklists and scales.
    2. Recruit an adequate and representative sample from the accessible population.
    3. Ensure that all data collectors have been oriented and trained.
    4. Collaborate with gatekeepers to gain entrée into the "world" of research participants.

12. Sampling, data collection, data analysis, and data interpretation typically occur (how) ________________ in a qualitative study.

13. Qualitative studies have flexible designs that can be changed during the course of the study. Therefore, qualitative research designs are often said to be ________________ designs.

14. The persons providing the data for a qualitative study are appropriately identified as
    1. respondents.
    2. subjects.
    3. informants.
    4. the sample.

15. How are data from qualitative studies primarily organized and presented in a written report? Data are presented as
    1. tables.
    2. themes.
    3. graphs.
    4. boxes.

16. Which of the following examples shows data from a qualitative study?
    1. "Among the 27 hospitals excluded from the analysis, 23 hospitals had less than 100 admissions in total, and four hospitals were excluded because of missing data" (He, Almenoff, Keighley, & Li, 2013, p. 226).
    2. "As shown in Table 3, the total mean on the SET (Nurses' Self-Efficacy in Managing Children's Pain) was 26.28 (maximum score = 30), indicating that overall, the participants had a high level of self-efficacy in regard to pediatric pain management" (Stanley & Pollard, 2013, p. 168).
    3. "Three main categories emerged from the analysis: the dependent body reflects changes in the women's bodily strength and performance, as they moved from being care providers into those who need care; this was associated with experiences of a sense of paralysis, shame, and burden" (Zellani & Seymour, 2012, p. 99).
    4. "Independent t test revealed that the quantity of sleeping in the experimental group was significantly higher than control group ($t = 3.18$, $p < 0.05$) (Table 2). Therefore, hypothesis 1 was supported" (Ryu, Park, & Park, 2011, p. 732).

17. ______________________ is "the collection of qualitative data to the point where a sense of closure is attained because new data yield redundant information" (Polit & Beck, 2014, p. 391).

18. What is true regarding the number of research participants in a qualitative study?
    1. The number of participants is usually small for most of the qualitative approaches.
    2. The number of research participants is determined by power analysis.
    3. A large number of participants is required, usually a minimum of 30 per variable.
    4. The number of research participants depends on the size of the accessible population.

19. Which of the following statements explains the concept of credibility in qualitative research?
    1. It is a "criterion for evaluating integrity and quality in qualitative studies, referring to confidence in the truth of the data" (Polit & Beck, 2014, p. 378).
    2. It is a "criterion for integrity and quality in a qualitative inquiry, referring to the objectivity or neutrality of the data and the interpretations" (p. 377).
    3. It is a "criterion for evaluating integrity in qualitative studies, referring to the stability of data over time and over conditions" (p. 379).
    4. It is the "extent to which qualitative findings can be transferred to other settings and groups" (p. 393).

Mixed Methods

20. Which of the following indicates use of a qualitative method mixed with a quantitative method?
    1. "The students' experiences are characterized by emotional strains of various sorts—stress, ambivalence, disgust, frustration, and conflict—that arise in three different types of relationships: relationships with parents, with the clinical instructors, and with other students who are in their teams" (Arieli, 2013, p. 192).
    2. "Korean women in the study reported 'resentment regarding previous role strain.' This psychosocial burden was heightened by a noted pattern of 'self-sacrificing in favor of others,' which complicated both their lives and their ability to take care of themselves physically" (Park & Wenzel, 2013, p. 1400).
    3. The study "examined the effects of a 6-month program of self-regulated, home-based exercise in addition to the standard care provided by the CF Center" (Happ, Hoffman, DiVirgilio, Higgins, & Orenstein, 2013, p. 306). Parent–child dyads were interviewed at 2 months and again at 6 months to explore the experience of the program.
    4. The researchers "explored how an educational intervention related to organ donation affected the knowledge and attitudes of a randomized two group sample of baccalaureate nursing students. The introduction of specific educational strategies improved the attitudes and knowledge base of the experimental group" (Whisenant & Woodring, 2012, p. 1).

ANSWERS AND RATIONALES

The correct answer number and rationale for why it is the correct answer are given in **boldface blue type**. Rationales for why the other possible answer options are incorrect also are given, but they are not in boldface type.

1. 1. This belief underlies the paradigm for quantitative studies.
2. This belief underlies the paradigm for quantitative studies.
3. This belief underlies the paradigm for qualitative studies.
4. This belief underlies the paradigm for quantitative studies.

TEST-TAKING TIP: Recall the assumptions of the positivist paradigm for quantitative research. These are opposite to the beliefs that underlie the naturalistic paradigm.

Content Area: *Paradigm for Qualitative Research;* ***Cognitive Level:*** *Knowledge;* ***Question Type:*** *Multiple Choice*

CRITICAL THINKING FACILITATOR: Review the beliefs and assumptions of the naturalistic paradigm to facilitate understanding of the activities essential in doing a qualitative study.

2. 1. This statement helps explain why the naturalistic paradigm is also known as the constructivist paradigm. Multiple realities exist and are "constructed" from the participants' experience.
2. This statement is applicable to the quantitative paradigm. Note the word "numerical," which means numbers. Also, data are subjected to statistical analysis in quantitative studies.
3. This is a true statement about research findings, but it does not help explain the constructivist paradigm.
4. This is an assumption of the positivist paradigm, the paradigm for quantitative studies.

TEST-TAKING TIP: The key word in the question stem is "constructivist." The term means to put together or build. Note that a belief of the paradigm is that an objective reality does not exist. Therefore, reality is "constructed" by research participants through their descriptions of their experiences.

Content Area: *Paradigm for Qualitative Research;* ***Cognitive Level:*** *Comprehension;* ***Question Type:*** *Multiple Choice*

CRITICAL THINKING FACILITATOR: What takes place between research participants and the researcher in "constructing reality"? Compare this process with the data collection process in quantitative research.

3. 1. The statement is not true of qualitative researchers. Quantitative researchers select a representative sample of adequate size to meet the criterion of validity.
2. The statement is true regarding qualitative researchers. A summary of each participant's narrative is constructed that is a synthesis of that participant's experience.
3. The statement is not true of qualitative researchers. Numerical summaries are compiled by quantitative researchers, who then subject the data to statistical analyses and interpretation.
4. The statement is not true about qualitative researchers. For a quantitative study to be valid, controls must be imposed over extraneous variables and the entire research context.

TEST-TAKING TIP: The key words in the question stem are "qualitative researcher." Review the activities quantitative researchers perform to carry out a valid study. Also note that option 2 contains the clue words "narrative summary" and "human experience." These terms are consistent with qualitative research.

Content Area: *Paradigm for Qualitative Research;* ***Cognitive Level:*** *Comprehension;* ***Question Type:*** *Multiple Choice*

CRITICAL THINKING FACILITATOR: Think of the type of data collected by qualitative researchers. How do researchers analyze and interpret these data?

4. instrument

TEST-TAKING TIP: The key phrase in the question stem is "involved in the entire process." Recall that the qualitative researcher interacts actively in the data collection, analysis, and interpretation of the study findings to facilitate understanding of the phenomena. You may have heard the statement "He or she was *instrumental* in getting the work done."

Content Area: *Paradigm for Qualitative Research;* ***Cognitive Level:*** *Comprehension;* ***Question Type:*** *Fill-in-the-Blank*

CRITICAL THINKING FACILITATOR: Compare the activities of qualitative and quantitative researchers. Familiarity with the activities of quantitative researchers should facilitate the work of identifying some of the activities of the qualitative researcher.

5. 1. Experts are included in tradition and authority as sources of knowledge. Tradition and authority are not considered logical reasoning.
2. **The statement is correct. Inductive reasoning proceeds from specific observations to general conclusions. The researchers' observations of specific women are the basis for their recommendations to women in general. The assumptions and beliefs of the paradigm that underlie qualitative studies are consistent with the inductive mode of reasoning.**
3. The deductive mode of reasoning proceeds from general statements or rules to specific cases. The assumptions and beliefs that underlie the paradigm for quantitative studies are consistent with this mode.
4. This is an incorrect statement. The scientific method "is a set of orderly, systematic, controlled procedures for acquiring dependable, empirical—and typically quantitative—information; the methodologic approach associated with the positivist paradigm" (Polit & Beck, 2014, p. 391).

TEST-TAKING TIP: The key phrases in the question stem are "qualitative study" and "based on the study of these women." Recall that quantitative studies use deductive reasoning. If you recall that the assumptions, beliefs, and activities of qualitative research are opposite those of quantitative research, then you should be able to come up with inductive reasoning as the answer.

Content Area: *Paradigm for Qualitative Research;* ***Cognitive Level:*** *Analysis;* ***Question Type:*** *Multiple Choice*

CRITICAL THINKING FACILITATOR: Review inductive reasoning and look at a sample qualitative study and see whether you could apply inductive reasoning to the study's conclusions.

6. 1. The situation suggests an intervention, home care visiting, that could have an influence on diabetics' adherence to a therapeutic regimen, the dependent variable. The situation could be studied more appropriately using a quantitative approach.
2. **The situation could be studied by using a qualitative approach. The researcher would interview research participants about their experience. Data would consist of descriptions of the experience by the participants.**
3. The situation suggests an independent variable, nurse executive leadership style, and its effects on job satisfaction, the dependent variable. The situation indicates that a quantitative approach is appropriate.
4. The situation suggests an independent variable, reflexology, and its effects on mild hypertension, the dependent variable. A quantitative approach is appropriate to use.

TEST-TAKING TIP: The key words in the question stem are "qualitative approach." Look at option 2 carefully, and note the words "lived experience." To study this, the researcher would have to collect descriptive narrative data from research participants. The collection of these types of data is a research activity in qualitative studies.

Content Area: *Paradigm for Qualitative Research;* ***Cognitive Level:*** *Analysis;* ***Question Type:*** *Multiple Choice*

CRITICAL THINKING FACILITATOR: Can you think of clinical situations that can be studied by using a qualitative approach?

7. 1. The research information indicates the study is quantitative. The data are numerical, and the term "lower" expresses a comparison of percentages in cholesterol levels among the groups studied.
2. The research information indicates the study is quantitative. The study information also indicates a proposed relationship between variables.
3. **The research information indicates that the study is qualitative. No numerical data are mentioned, but "themes" are reported. A theme is "a recurring regularity emerging from an analysis of qualitative data" (Polit & Beck, 2014, p. 393).**
4. The research information indicates the study is quantitative because of numerical data that were subjected to statistical analysis.

TEST-TAKING TIP: Look at each option carefully. Note that option 3 has the term "theme." Options 1, 2, and 4 have information consistent with quantitative studies.

Content Area: *Paradigm for Qualitative Research;* ***Cognitive Level:*** *Analysis;* ***Question Type:*** *Multiple Choice*

CRITICAL THINKING FACILITATOR: Identify different key words that are commonly used in qualitative studies. Can you identify some of these in a sample qualitative study?

8. 1. In the EBP hierarchy, level 1 includes systematic reviews of randomized clinical trials.
2. In the hierarchy, a well-designed randomized clinical trial is placed at level 2.
3. A single descriptive or qualitative study is at level 6 of the hierarchy.
4. Opinions of experts or reports of expert committees are the lowest level, level 7.

TEST-TAKING TIP: Because EBP depends on outcomes for effective and safe practice, where would randomized clinical trials be placed? Contrast this information when you recall the purpose of qualitative studies. Understanding phenomena that are important to nursing is a major goal of qualitative studies and not interventions or predictions of outcomes.

Content Area: *Qualitative Studies and EBP;* ***Cognitive Level:*** *Comprehension;* ***Question Type:*** *Multiple Choice*

CRITICAL THINKING FACILITATOR:
Think of the hierarchy of research evidence and match these with levels of purposes of research. Studies that have the purposes of prediction and control are higher in the hierarchy. Where would studies that have a goal of description (of phenomenon) be placed?

9. 1. A review of the literature is part of the planning phase, but it is not the first activity.
2. The type of qualitative approach is not selected as the first activity.
3. Although this is part of the planning phase, it is not the first activity.
4. "Qualitative researchers usually begin with a broad topic, often focusing on an aspect about which little is known" (Polit & Beck, 2014, p. 53).

TEST-TAKING TIP: Recall the sequential steps that must be followed in doing a quantitative study. Also recall that the positivist paradigm guides quantitative approaches and that one of the assumptions is that "reality already exists." The paradigm for qualitative studies has assumptions and beliefs that are the opposite.

In qualitative research, "reality does not exist." Therefore, identifying and focusing on something about which little is known seems a logical place to start for a qualitative study.

Content Area: *Activities and Processes in Qualitative Studies;* ***Cognitive Level:*** *Application;* ***Question Type:*** *Multiple Choice*

CRITICAL THINKING FACILITATOR:
What are some phenomena that can be studied using a qualitative approach? What is the purpose of these studies?

10. 1. The statement is not a concern of a qualitative study but rather is a concern of a quantitative study.
2. Qualitative researchers are interested in constructing reality from the viewpoints of those being studied. Therefore, a review of the literature might interfere with this process because of preconceived ideas about the phenomenon being studied.
3. The statement does not indicate a concern of a qualitative study. The phenomenon of interest is elucidated by the data provided by the research participants, not by what is available in the literature.
4. Inconsistencies and gaps in the literature are identified by the quantitative researcher who places the proposed study within the context of other studies.

TEST-TAKING TIP: A key word in the question stem is "concern." A concern could be something that could pose a difficulty or barrier. Look at the options and eliminate those that are common concerns in quantitative studies.

Content Area: *Activities and Processes in Qualitative Studies;* ***Cognitive Level:*** *Comprehension;* ***Question Type:*** *Multiple Choice*

CRITICAL THINKING FACILITATOR:
What makes the role of the qualitative researcher different from that of the quantitative researcher? What are the concerns of a qualitative researcher that are different from those of the quantitative researcher?

11. 1. This activity is not done by a qualitative researcher. This is an essential activity of a quantitative researcher that he or she uses as a control measure.
2. This activity is a requirement for quantitative researchers. An adequate and representative sample eliminates bias and controls for some extraneous variables.
3. This is an activity done by quantitative researchers, who must ensure that research protocols for the collection of data or the intervention (the independent variable) are consistent and accurate.
4. This is the first activity of qualitative researchers before collecting data in a naturalistic setting. A naturalistic setting is one used "for the collection of research data that is natural to those

being studied (e.g., homes, places of work, and so on)" (Polit & Beck, 2014, 385). These naturalistic settings are the "worlds" of research participants.

TEST-TAKING TIP: The key phrase in the question stem is "before going into the field to collect data." The research sites for qualitative studies are naturalistic settings, or the real world. These include homes, places of employment, and other places where research participants spend time. Therefore, entering those sites, which may be unfamiliar to the researcher, requires facilitation by someone who knows the population and area before the researcher collects data.

Content Area: *Activities and Processes in Qualitative Studies;* ***Cognitive Level:*** *Application;* ***Question Type:*** *Multiple Choice*

CRITICAL THINKING FACILITATOR: Differentiate the research sites for qualitative studies from those in quantitative studies. What should be considered when research sites are selected for qualitative studies?

12. iteratively

TEST-TAKING TIP: Think of the qualitative study process as a one-on-one process with each research participant. The processes of recruiting a participant, interviewing her or him, and analyzing and interpreting the data occur repeatedly and as many times as it takes until no new data emerge.

Content Area: *Activities and Processes in Qualitative Studies;* ***Cognitive Level:*** *Comprehension;* ***Question Type:*** *Fill-in-the-Blank*

CRITICAL THINKING FACILITATOR: After each research participant's data are collected, what are the steps that the qualitative researcher must do before repeating the processes of sampling, collecting, analyzing, and interpreting the data?

13. emergent

TEST-TAKING TIP: The key phrase in the question stem is "can be changed during the course of the study." The specific design for a qualitative study is not "fixed" at the beginning like a quantitative study. As data are collected, analyzed, and interpreted, the design of the study could change to enable the researcher to "build a rich description of a phenomena" (Polit & Beck, 2014, p. 55). The term "emerge" means to come into full view.

Content Area: *Activities and Processes in Qualitative Studies;* ***Cognitive Level:*** *Comprehension;* ***Question Type:*** *Fill-in-the-Blank*

CRITICAL THINKING FACILITATOR: Think of a qualitative study as a process of building something. The materials for the structure come from the research participants. With the data from the first participant, you begin to build. As the structure begins to take a shape, you sort out the data to see what could be added. As you acquire more data, you might need to change the structure so that all pieces could come together as a coherent whole.

14. 1. *Respondents* usually refers to the persons who complete a questionnaire or a telephone or face-to-face interview (Polit & Beck, 2014).
    2. In a quantitative study, the persons being studied are called *subjects*.
    3. **In qualitative studies, persons providing the data are commonly identified as *informants*.**
    4. A *sample* is the "subset of the population selected to participate in a study" (Polit & Beck, 2014, p. 391). *Sample* is the collective identity for all research participants and is not specific to the type of study.

TEST-TAKING TIP: The key word in the stem question is "providing." From the verb *provide*, it means "to give or supply." Because research participants provide descriptive information about their experiences, they are appropriately called *informants*.

Content Area: *Activities and Processes in Qualitative Studies;* ***Cognitive Level:*** *Knowledge;* ***Question Type:*** *Multiple Choice*

CRITICAL THINKING FACILITATOR: The roles persons assume in an activity or process determine how they are identified. For instance, think of older people and their roles. In a senior center where social activities are the main foci, they are called *participants*. In a nursing home or extended care facility, they are referred to as *residents*. If they are in a hospital, they are *patients* or *clients*.

15. 1. Tables consist of columns showing numbers that are data in a quantitative study.
    2. **Themes are identified in the descriptive statements of research participants in a qualitative study. A *theme* is a "recurring regularity emerging from an analysis of qualitative data" (Polit & Beck, 2014, p. 393). Data are organized into themes, and the themes collectively describe the phenomenon of interest.**
    3. Graphs are used to indicate relationships among pieces of information. Arrows, lines, points, or other symbols might be

used to indicate the suggested relationships. Graphs are used for quantitative data.
4. Boxes are spaces for selected information that a writer might use to highlight or emphasize, or summarize. These are not always used for qualitative data.

TEST-TAKING TIP: The key phrase in the question stem are "organized and presented." Recall that data in qualitative studies are narrative descriptions of research participants about their experiences. Organizing and presenting data in tables or graphs would not be appropriate for narrative data. Although boxes might be used, these would only highlight or summarize narrative information.

Content Area: *Activities and Processes in Qualitative Studies;* ***Cognitive Level:*** *Knowledge;* ***Question Type:*** *Multiple Choice*

CRITICAL THINKING FACILITATOR: Locate the data from a sample qualitative study and determine whether there are other ways of organizing or presenting the data.

16. 1. The data are from a quantitative study. The data are numerical and are not narrative descriptions of research participants about their experience of the phenomena under study.
2. The data are from a quantitative study. Note the mention of a table that highlights some of the data in the study.
3. The data are from a qualitative study. The data reflect descriptions of the women regarding the phenomenon under study. The data also indicate that experiences of the women were analyzed and synthesized.
4. The data are from a quantitative study. A statistical test is mentioned as well as a comparison between an experimental group and a control group.

TEST-TAKING TIP: Recall the type of data collected from a quantitative study. Look at options 1, 2, and 4. How do those data look compared with those reported in option 3?

Content Area: *Activities and Processes in Qualitative Studies;* ***Cognitive Level:*** *Analysis;* ***Question Type:*** *Multiple Choice*

CRITICAL THINKING FACILITATOR: Review data reporting and presentation in quantitative studies and compare these with qualitative studies. Look at a qualitative study and note the physical appearance of the data.

17. Data saturation

TEST-TAKING TIP: The key phrase in the statement is "redundant information." ***Redundant*** **means "excess."** ***Saturation*** **means that the capacity of something has been reached.**

Content Area: *Activities and Processes in Qualitative Studies;* ***Cognitive Level:*** *Knowledge;* ***Question Type:*** *Fill-in-the-Blank*

CRITICAL THINKING FACILITATOR: Data saturation is an aspect in qualitative research that is different from quantitative research. Can you think of some of the other differences?

18. 1. This statement is applicable in qualitative studies. Large samples are not needed because data are not subjected to statistical analysis. The point when data collected no longer contributes anything new about the phenomenon of interest is reached after only several participants.
2. The statement is applicable in quantitative studies. Power analysis "is the mathematical procedure to determine the number for each arm (group) of a study" (LoBiondo-Wood & Haber, 2010, p. 583).
3. This statement is a general guideline for determining the size of the sample in quantitative studies.
4. This statement is not an accurate one even when applied to quantitative studies.

TEST-TAKING TIP: Recall the activities in quantitative studies. To achieve power, larger samples are needed. The concept of power is not applicable in qualitative research, so it makes sense that smaller samples are common. In addition, because data from qualitative studies are analyzed differently, larger samples do not necessarily contribute to the depth and richness of the data.

Content Area: *Activities and Processes in Qualitative Studies;* ***Cognitive Level:*** *Knowledge;* ***Question Type:*** *Multiple Choice*

CRITICAL THINKING FACILITATOR: What justifies the small sample in qualitative studies? Compare this element with the sample requirement in quantitative studies.

19. 1. The statement is a definition of ***credibility*** **of findings in qualitative studies.** ***Credibility*** **is "analogous to internal validity in quantitative research" (Polit & Beck, 2014, p. 278).**
2. The statement is a definition of *confirmability* in qualitative study findings.

3. The statement is a definition of *dependability* of findings in qualitative studies. It is "analogous to reliability in quantitative research" (Polit & Beck, 2014, p. 379).
4. The statement is a definition of *transferability* of findings of qualitative studies.

TEST-TAKING TIP: The key word in the question stem is "credibility," derived from *credible* or *believable*. Note the clue in option 1, "truth of the data."

Content Area: *Activities and Processes in Qualitative Studies;* ***Cognitive Level:*** *Knowledge;* ***Question Type:*** *Multiple Choice*
CRITICAL THINKING FACILITATOR: Determine how qualitative study findings would fulfill the criteria of credibility, confirmability, dependability, and transferability.

20. 1. The study used only a qualitative approach. Note the word "experience," which is often the focus in a qualitative study.
2. The study used only a qualitative approach. Data indicate "feelings and perceptions" regarding informants' illness.
3. This study used a mixed method approach. The quantitative aspect is reflected in the use of an intervention, the home-based exercise program. The qualitative aspect is reflected in the follow-up interviews to better understand parent–child experiences with the exercise program.
4. The study used only a quantitative approach to measure the effects of an educational strategy (independent variable) on attitudes and knowledge base (dependent variables) about organ donation.

TEST-TAKING TIP: The key word in the question stem is "mixed," which indicates two approaches—quantitative and a qualitative—in the study. Read each option carefully and identify the approach based on information you know about quantitative and qualitative studies.

Content Area: *Activities and Processes in Qualitative Studies;* ***Cognitive Level:*** *Analysis;* ***Question Type:*** *Multiple Choice*
CRITICAL THINKING FACILITATOR:
What is the purpose of doing a mixed methods study? Identify research activities consistent with the study's quantitative approach and its qualitative approach.

18 Understanding Qualitative Approaches

KEY WORDS

The following words include English vocabulary, nursing/medical terminology, concepts, principles, or information relevant to content specifically addressed in the chapter or associated with topics presented in it. English dictionaries, your nursing textbooks, and medical dictionaries such as *Taber's Cyclopedic Medical Dictionary* are resources that can be used to expand your knowledge and understanding of these words and related information.

Case study
Core variable
Emic approach
Etic approach
Ethnography
Feminist research
Grounded theory
Historical research
Participatory action research
Phenomenology
Symbolic interaction

QUESTIONS

Characteristics and Design Features of Qualitative Approaches

1. What characteristics do all qualitative approaches share? **Select all that apply.**
   Qualitative approaches
   1. "make the world of the individual visible to the rest of us" (Barroso, 2010, p. 86).
   2. "tend to be holistic, striving for an understanding of the whole" (Polit & Beck, 2014, p. 266).
   3. "make comparisons to provide a context for interpreting results" (p. 151).
   4. aim for accuracy, which means "all aspects of a study systematically and logically flow from the research question or hypothesis" (LoBiondo-Wood, 2010, p. 160).
   5. are concerned with the belief that the "discovery of meaning is the basis for knowledge" (Barroso, 2010, p. 88).

2. What are the specific design features of qualitative approaches? **Select all that apply.**
   Qualitative approaches
   1. have a variable of interest called the dependent variable.
   2. use naturalistic settings for the collection of data.
   3. facilitate understanding of phenomena.
   4. have no specified time dimensions.
   5. use reliable and valid research instruments

Major Types of Qualitative Approaches

3. Which of the following statements applies to the phenomenologic approach? In the phenomenologic approach, the researcher
   1. "views the person as integrated with the environment. The world shapes the self, and the self shapes the world" (Burns & Grove, 2010, p. 76).
   2. "seeks to understand the interaction between self and group from the perspective of those involved" (p. 78).
   3. "is able to determine the degree or strength and type (positive or negative) of a relationship between two variables" (p. 35).
   4. has as a goal "to test [a] theory and validate its usefulness in clinical practice" (p. 37).

4. Of the following research information, which one indicates the study is phenomenological?
   1. The researchers interviewed faculty teaching second-degree baccalaureate nursing students to understand their how "experiences helped or hindered their teaching and learning practices with these students" (Cangelosi & Moss, 2010, p. 137).
   2. The researchers used theoretical and purposive sampling in their study. "A basic social process of how nurse anesthetists practice 'Keeping Vigil over the Patient' was identified" (Schreiber & MacDonald, 2010, p. 352).
   3. "The purposes of the study were to "describe the perceptions of Armenian child-bearing women about the meaning of giving birth and to conduct an outcome evaluation of the Erebuni Women's Wellness Center" (Amoros, Callister, & Sarkisyan, 2010, p. 135).
   4. "The specific aim of the study was to explore the decision-making of medical-surgical nurses who use charting-by-exception (CBE) as their method of documentation" (Kerr, 2013, p. 111).

5. The grounded theory approach "explores how people define reality and how their beliefs are related to their actions. Reality is created by attaching meanings to situations" (Burns & Grove, 2010, p. 77). People use words and a variety of objects to express meaning. These roots of the grounded theory approach are based on ________________________.

6. Grounded theory researchers have as a goal the understanding of people's behavior that reflects how they address concerns, issues, or problems. The manner in which people resolve this main concern is called the ________________________.

7. Which of the following research information suggests a grounded theory study?
   1. The researchers examined the "Complex decisions: Theorizing women's infant feeding decisions in the first 6 weeks after birth" (Sheehan, Schmied, & Barclay, 2010, p. 371).
   2. The purpose was to "describe intentions to prevent another fall as discerned during a study with older homebound women" (Porter, Matsuda, & Lindbloom, 2010, p. 101).
   3. Bolas and Holloway's 2012 study had an aim to "gain insight into patients' experience of negative pressure wound therapy (NPWT) to assist practitioners to better prepare them for this therapy" (p. 531).
   4. Using a focus groups methodology, the researchers studied the "perspectives of female adolescents on dating relationships and dating violence (DV)" (Haglund, Belknap, & Garcia, 2012, p. 215).

8. Which of the following information indicates that the study is an ethnographic one?
   1. A study on the life-limiting illnesses of persons receiving palliative care identified themes that included "life review, current situation, and legacy principles" (Keall, Butow, Steinhauser, & Clayton, 2011, p. 454).
   2. Lindy and Schaefer (2010) studied bullying encountered by staff on their unit. Some themes identified from the data included "They just take it," "That's just how she is," and "There are three sides to a story" (p. 285).
   3. The aim of the study was to "explore the meaning of the nursing culture within an Australian prison hospital and the migration of the culture over a 12-month period" (Cashin, Newman, Eason, Thorpe, & O'Discoll, 2010, p. 39).
   4. "The aim of the study was to explore the feelings and experiences of hospice-at-home nurses when providing palliative nursing care for patients in the community" (Tunnah, Jones, & Johnstone, 2012, p. 284).

9. Which of the following statements describes the "etic" approach in ethnographic study? The etic approach
   1. "refers to the way the members of the culture regard their world—the insiders' view" (Polit & Beck, 2014, p. 269).
   2. "is the outsider's interpretation of the experiences of that culture" (p. 269).
   3. "includes the process by which the ethnographer comes to understand a culture" (p. 269).
   4. has as its focus the study of the ethnographer's own culture (Polit & Beck, 2014).

10. Which of the following ethnographic studies indicate the use of the "emic" approach? **Select all that apply.**
    1. The researchers used observation, in-depth interviews, and focus groups to provide the data that generated themes about the culture of vascular access cannulation (Wilson, Harwood, Oudshoorn, & Thompson, 2010).
    2. Cashin, Newman, Eason, Thorpe, and O'Discoll (2010) used observational data, semistructured interviews, and cultural artifacts to understand forensic nursing culture in an Australian prison.
    3. The researchers concluded that "women's feeding decisions cannot be viewed in isolation from other post-natal experiences and needs" (Sheehan, Schmied, & Barclay, 2009, p. 171).
    4. Cangelosi and Moss (2010) identified themes including "At the Top of My Game" and "Teaching to Think Like a Nurse" (p. 137) in their study of faculty teaching second-degree baccalaureate nursing students.
    5. Noble and Jones (2010) came to understand spirituality among oncology nurses through identification of themes that included "constraints and barriers to providing spiritual care, skills required, and education and support needs" (p. 565).

11. Which of the following topics would be best studied using an ethnographic approach?
    1. The lived experience of losing a parent to HIV/AIDS
    2. Transitioning into a life without a spouse
    3. The past decade of diploma nursing programs
    4. Tenured academic faculty: A formidable group

12. For which of the following situations would a historical approach be appropriate?
    1. The early years of NLN accreditation
    2. A community's fight against drug addiction
    3. Asian Americans: Integrating into mainstream United States
    4. Nurse practitioners: Nurses or junior doctors?

13. Which of the following information indicates the study is a historical one?
    1. The researchers explored the work of forensic nurses in custodial settings. They concluded that "custodial settings are dominated by personally diminishing prison architecture where forensic nurses have to contend with oppressive security controls and overcrowding" (Cashin, Newman, Eason, Thorpe, & O'Discoll, 2010, p. 39).
    2. During the 1918 flu epidemic, "New York City nurses provided care to thousands of patients. They did so with minimal federal support, relying on local community agencies to establish makeshift hospitals and provide soup kitchens" (Keeling, 2009, p. 2732).
    3. "Participants described how they lived with what they described as an 'unknown cancer', and talked about their feelings of loss. They reported having an altered body image as a result of alopecia and fatigue" (Kelly & Dowling, 2011, p. 38).
    4. The researcher sought to discuss the physical and mental burden of family caregivers who provide long-term at-home support for a family member with chronic kidney disease or other illness" (Schrauf, 2011, p. 395).

Other Types of Qualitative Approaches

14. When is a qualitative case study method appropriate? This approach is appropriate when the researcher's goal is to
    1. "discover the main concern and the basic social process that explains how people resolve it" (Polit & Beck, 2014, p. 272).
    2. "understand fully the lived experience and the perceptions to which it gives rise" (p. 270).
    3. "analyze and understand issues that are important to the history, development, or circumstances of the entity under study" (p. 273).
    4. direct questions toward "exploring, describing, and analyzing a process or event during a specific time period" (Burns & Grove, 2010, p. 82).

15. Which of the following research information would indicate that the study is feminist research?
    1. Phillips (2010) studied the stressors faced by students in nurse anesthetist programs. Data analysis indicated that coping with stressors was related to how participants viewed the stressors. The students' coping mechanisms included how they integrated their programs into their personal lives. For some, coping meant focusing more on the future.
    2. Liu, F., Williams, Liu, H., and Chien (2010) studied the lived experience of persons with lower extremity amputations. "Participants described suffering in physical, psychological, and sociocultural realms and the ways they strived to cope with these challenges" (p. 2152).
    3. Noble and Jones (2010) did a qualitative study to explore oncology nurses' understanding of spirituality. "Five major themes were identified: understanding of spirituality, the nurses' own spirituality, skills required, constraints and barriers to providing spiritual care, and education and support needs" (p. 565).
    4. The study explored the mentoring relationships between nurses in the intrapartum setting. "The theme, relational learning, highlights how perinatal nurses engage with each other and engage with birthing women on a journey of learning in perinatal nursing" (Ryan, Goldberg, & Evans, 2010, p. 181).

16. **Research Study Information:** The researchers' objective was to "develop an action plan based on asthma management challenges identified by Head Start teachers in a multi-site program" (Garwick, Seppelt, & Riesgraf, 2010, p. 329). The study can be identified as a(n)
    1. ethnographic approach.
    2. grounded theory study.
    3. participatory action research (PAR).
    4. historical research.

17. What statements are true about a descriptive qualitative study? **Select all that apply.**
    1. The researchers will not claim a particular "disciplinary or methodologic root" (Polit & Beck, 2014, pp. 274).
    2. The title of the study specifies the qualitative approach used.
    3. References used indicate the type of approach used.
    4. The researchers will state that themes and patterns were analyzed.
    5. "Descriptive qualitative studies tend to be more eclectic in their designs and methods" (p. 275).

The correct answer number and rationale for why it is the correct answer are given in **boldface blue type**. Rationales for why the other possible answer options are incorrect also are given, but they are not in boldface type.

1. **1. The statement is a characteristic of qualitative approaches. Because qualitative approaches are descriptive and explanatory, they provide a view of an individual's world.**
   2. The statement is a characteristic of qualitative approaches. The experience of the individual shared with the researcher yields data about the experience of the research participant. The researcher collects, analyzes, and interprets the data simultaneously, constructing a whole as the perceived reality of the participant.
   3. The statement does not describe a characteristic of qualitative approaches. In a quantitative approach, groups are compared relative to some outcome or effect (dependent variable) produced by a cause (independent variable).
   4. The statement does not describe a characteristic of qualitative approaches. The research question formulated at the beginning of a quantitative study guides all subsequent steps.
   5. The statement is a characteristic of qualitative approaches. The understanding of the meaning of people's experiences is the goal of most approaches. This understanding is facilitated by the narrative descriptions of the participant's experience.

   TEST-TAKING TIP: Recall the assumptions and beliefs of the naturalistic paradigm for research. Phenomenology, grounded theory, ethnography, and historical research incorporate these assumptions and beliefs,

   Content Area: *Characteristics and Design Features of Qualitative Approaches;* ***Cognitive Level:*** *Knowledge;* ***Question Type:*** *Multiple Response*
   CRITICAL THINKING FACILITATOR: Although the qualitative approaches share common characteristics, each has a specific purpose. Identify these purposes to facilitate understanding of the different processes in each approach.

2. 1. Qualitative approaches are used to explore a phenomenon that could be a lived experience or a social process. The phenomenon is not called a dependent variable. Qualitative approaches do not deal with variables.
   2. The world of the research participants is the setting for qualitative approaches, and these are naturalistic.
   3. Data in qualitative approaches are not subjected to statistical analyses; rather, the themes and patterns that emerge are analyzed in order to understand the phenomena of interest.
   4. Qualitative approaches use both cross-sectional and longitudinal designs to fully understand the experience of the research participants. Time dimensions do not produce any type of bias in the study.
   5. Data collection instruments used in qualitative approaches are not subjected to reliability and validity tests similar to those in quantitative approaches. However, through a review of available literature, the qualitative researcher might create a comprehensive questionnaire to use during an interview. Questions may be added to the questionnaire as data collection progresses to provide an in-depth knowledge of the phenomenon under investigation.

   TEST-TAKING TIP: Recall the design features of quantitative approaches. Compare and contract these with the design features of the qualitative approaches to help in selecting the correct options.

   Content Area: *Characteristics and Design Features of Qualitative Approaches;* ***Cognitive Level:*** *Knowledge;* ***Question Type:*** *Multiple Response*
   CRITICAL THINKING FACILITATOR: Look at a sample phenomenologic study and identify the design features of this qualitative approach.

3. **1. The statement describes the phenomenologic approach. In phenomenology, the researcher's interactions with the research participant facilitate the construction of reality as it is perceived through the lived experience.**
   2. The statement describes the researcher who does a grounded theory study.
   3. The statement does not describe the phenomenologic researcher. The statement describes the researcher who does correlational research.
   4. The statement describes the goal of a researcher who does applied research.

   TEST-TAKING TIP: The key word in the question stem is *phenomenologic*. This type of study focuses on the lived

experience of a person in relation to some phenomenon.

Content Area: *Major Types of Qualitative Approaches;* ***Cognitive Level:*** *Comprehension;* ***Question Type:*** *Multiple Choice*
CRITICAL THINKING FACILITATOR: What are some research topics that can be studied using a phenomenologic approach?

4. **1. The study is phenomenologic because it focuses on the understanding of an experience.**
2. The study is a grounded theory one because its focus is a basic social process, "keeping vigil."
3. The study is a descriptive qualitative one. There are some aspects of phenomenology as well as evaluation research.
4. The study is a grounded theory one because its focus was a process of decision making.

TEST-TAKING TIP: Remember that the focus of phenomenology is the study of the lived experience. The correct option includes the term "experience."

Content Area: *Types of Qualitative Approaches;* ***Cognitive Level:*** *Application;* ***Question Type:*** *Multiple Choice*
CRITICAL THINKING FACILITATOR: What is the purpose of doing a phenomenologic study? Why is the "lived experience" the focus?

5. symbolic interaction

TEST-TAKING TIP: The key phrase in the statement is "attaching meanings to situations." The meanings people attach to situations would be something that represents that situation (i.e., a symbol). For instance, the color red symbolizes courage. Note how this symbol, red, gives added meaning to the insignia of the American Red Cross.

Content Area: *Types of Qualitative Approaches;* ***Cognitive Level:*** *Comprehension;* ***Question Type:*** *Fill-in-the-Blank*
CRITICAL THINKING FACILITATOR: What is the purpose of the researcher who does a grounded theory study? Does the name of the approach suggest its purpose?

6. core variable

TEST-TAKING TIP: What holds together the themes that emerge from the analysis of the data? The center, or "core," of the process is the focus of the study.

Content Area: *Types of Qualitative Approaches;* ***Cognitive Level:*** *Knowledge;* ***Question Type:*** *Fill-in-the-Blank*
CRITICAL THINKING FACILITATOR: Think of theories you know. How might these theories have come about if the researcher had studied the core variable using a grounded theory approach?

7. **1. The information indicates the study is grounded theory. A clue in the statement is "infant feeding decisions," which indicates a process. The grounded theory method uses "a systematic set of procedures to arrive at a theory about a basic social process" (LoBiondo-Wood & Haber, 2010, p. 579).**
2. The information indicates the study is a phenomenologic one. Phenomenology focuses on the lived experience. In the study, an experience with a previous fall was the phenomenon of interest.
3. The information indicates the study is a phenomenologic one. The focus is the lived experience of persons undergoing negative-pressure wound therapy.
4. The information indicates the study used a qualitative descriptive approach. The study did not focus on a lived experience (phenomenology), a culture (ethnography), a basic social process (grounded theory), or past events (historical).

TEST-TAKING TIP: The key phrase in the question stem is "grounded theory." Recall that the focus of this approach is to describe a process.

Content Area: *Types of Qualitative Approaches;* ***Cognitive Level:*** *Analysis;* ***Question Type:*** *Multiple Choice*
CRITICAL THINKING FACILITATOR: To facilitate understanding of the other approaches, examine the incorrect options and see whether these can be studied from a grounded theory approach.

8. 1. The information does not indicate the study was ethnographic. The qualitative analysis identified themes that are the data in either phenomenology or grounded theory.
2. The information indicates that the study is a phenomenologic one and not an ethnographic study. Note the term "themes" in the statement.
3. The information indicates the study is ethnographic. An ethnographic study focuses on "the culture of a group of people, with an effort to understand the world view and customs of those under study" (Polit & Beck, 2014, p. 380).
4. The information indicates the study is qualitative with elements of the phenomenologic approach. Note the term "experiences," which is consistent with the focus in phenomenology.

TEST-TAKING TIP: The key word in the question stem is "ethnographic." Relate this term to the term "ethnic," which is used to denote a sharing of something such as a culture.

Content Area: *Types of Qualitative Approaches;* ***Cognitive Level:*** *Analysis;* ***Question Type:*** *Multiple Choice*
CRITICAL THINKING FACILITATOR:
What are groups you know of that share a common culture in an academic or clinical setting?

9. 1. The statement refers to the "emic" approach.
   2. The outsider's view of a culture is the "etic" approach.
   3. The statement refers to field work.
   4. The statement refers to autoethnography.

TEST-TAKING TIP: The key word in the question stem is "etic." This is the outsider's view of a culture. It is considered looking into the culture from the outside, such as observing the interaction of a group with an observer who is not part of the group.

Content Area: *Types of Qualitative Approaches;* ***Cognitive Level:*** *Comprehension;* ***Question Type:*** *Multiple Choice*
CRITICAL THINKING FACILITATOR:
What are the advantages and disadvantages of using an "etic" approach in studying a group? A researcher is studying the culture of nurses who work in hospice settings. Will the findings be different if the researcher interacted with these nurses during their work time?

10. **1. The information indicates that the researchers used an emic approach because of the use of multiple methods to collect data from the research participants. "Ethnographers can begin to access the emic view by interviewing group members, observing their behavior, and collecting cultural artifacts" (Streubert & Carpenter, 2011, p. 172).**
    2. The information indicates that the researchers used an emic approach because of the use of multiple methods to collect data.
    3. The research information does not indicate an emic perspective because this study is not an ethnographic study. It is a grounded theory study.
    4. The research information does not indicate the emic approach because the study is phenomenological, not ethnographic.
    5. The research information does not indicate the emic approach. This is a qualitative study with some elements of grounded theory.

TEST-TAKING TIP: The key word in the question stem is "emic," which means the insider's view. The emic view "refers to the way members of a culture themselves view their world" (Polit & Beck, 2014, p. 380).

Content Area: *Types of Qualitative Approaches;* ***Cognitive Level:*** *Analysis;* ***Question Type:*** *Multiple Response*
CRITICAL THINKING FACILITATOR: What are the advantages of using an "emic" perspective in an ethnographic study?

11. 1. A phenomenologic approach is appropriate to study the lived experience.
    2. A grounded theory approach is appropriate to study a basic social process.
    3. A historical study would be appropriate to look at this past event.
    4. An ethnographic study would be appropriate to look at the culture of this group.

TEST-TAKING TIP: The key phrase in the question stem is "ethnographic approach." The phrase indicates the study of the "culture" of a group.

Content Area: *Types of Qualitative Approaches;* ***Cognitive Level:*** *Application;* ***Question Type:*** *Multiple Choice*
CRITICAL THINKING FACILITATOR:
What are some common situations that could be studied by using an ethnographic approach?

12. **1. This topic could be studied using a historical approach because the study would be "designed to discover facts and relationships about past events" (Polit & Beck, 2014, p. 382).**
    2. This topic can be studied appropriately using PAR because this approach is "based on the premise that the use and production of knowledge can be political and used to exert power" (p. 382).
    3. This topic can be studied by a grounded theory approach because its focus is a social process, integrating.
    4. The topic can be studied by using an ethnographic approach to study the "culture" of nurse practitioners whose practice entails nursing care and some medical aspects.

TEST-TAKING TIP: The key phrase in the question stem is "historical approach." The phrase indicates a study of past events.

Content Area: *Types of Qualitative Approaches;* ***Cognitive Level:*** *Application;* ***Question Type:*** *Multiple Choice*

CRITICAL THINKING FACILITATOR: If you have a copy of a historical study, read and analyze the impact of the findings on nursing.

13. 1. The information indicates that the study is an ethnographic one. The information implies an exploration of the "culture" of nurses working in a forensic setting.
    2. **The information indicates that the study is a historical one. The study looked at and analyzed a past event that was a milestone in the practice of nursing.**
    3. The information indicates the study is a phenomenologic one because it focused on a lived experience.
    4. The statements indicate that this is a case study. A case study is "a method involving a thorough, in-depth analysis of an individual, group, or other social unit" (Polit & Beck, 2014, p. 375).

TEST-TAKING TIP: The key word in the question stem is "historical." Look for an indication of a past event in the information provided. Only option 2 mentions a date.

Content Area: *Types of Qualitative Approaches;* ***Cognitive Level:*** *Application;* ***Question Type:*** *Multiple Choice*

CRITICAL THINKING FACILITATOR: What are some major events that have influenced nursing? Take one of these events and determine the impact it has made on nursing.

14. 1. The statement describes the grounded theory approach.
    2. The statement describes the phenomenological approach.
    3. **The statement describes the case study approach.**
    4. The statement describes historical research.

TEST-TAKING TIP: The key words in the question stem are "case study." The information mentions an "entity." This is typical of a case study that is a "method involving a thorough, in-depth analysis of an individual, group, or other social unit" (Poli & Beck, 2014, p. 375).

Content Area: *Other Types of Qualitative Approaches;* ***Cognitive Level:*** *Application;* ***Question Type:*** *Multiple Choice*

CRITICAL THINKING FACILITATOR: You are familiar with case studies as a way to learn. You read the situation thoroughly, analyze and understand what is going on, and then make informed conclusions about the situation. What are examples of clinical situations that can be studied through a case study approach?

15. 1. The information indicates the study used a grounded theory approach.
    2. The information indicates the study used a phenomenological approach.
    3. The information indicates the study used a grounded theory approach.
    4. **The information indicates the study is feminist research. "Feminist investigators seek to understand how gender and a gendered social order have shaped women's lives and their consciousness" (Polit & Beck, 2014, p. 276). The study focused on the relationships of nurses with each other and how they in turn relate to women undergoing the birthing process.**

TEST-TAKING TIP: First, note that the study focused on women and their relationships with each other. Then look at the situation under study, the birthing process, which is primarily a feminine concern.

Content Area: *Other Types of Qualitative Approaches;* ***Cognitive Level:*** *Analysis;* ***Question Type:*** *Multiple Choice*

CRITICAL THINKING FACILITATOR: Why are feminist research studies important in evidence-based practice?

16. 1. The information is not indicative of an ethnographic study because an ethnographic study focuses on culture.
    2. The information does not indicate that the study is grounded theory because the aim of this approach is to "develop theories about psychosocial processes grounded in real-world observations" (Polit & Beck, 2014, p. 381).
    3. **The information indicates the study is PAR. PAR aims "to produce an impetus that is directly used to make improvements through education and sociopolitical action" (p. 277).**
    4. The information does not indicate the study was a historical one. Historical studies are designed to "discover facts and relationships about past events" (p. 382).

TEST-TAKING TIP: The key phrase in the question stem is "action plan." Also note the inclusion of a community-type program in the research information.

Content Area: *Other Types of Qualitative Approaches;* ***Cognitive Level:*** *Analysis;* ***Question Type:*** *Multiple Choice*

CRITICAL THINKING FACILITATOR: What are some topics that can be studied using participatory action research? If you have any community health experience, think of issues or concerns that can be studied using this approach.

17. 1. **This is a true statement. Researchers who identify their study as a descriptive qualitative study do not describe it as phenomenologic, grounded theory, or ethnographic.**
2. The study title does not often indicate the type of qualitative approach particularly if it is a descriptive qualitative one.
3. The literature used and listed as references does not indicate the type of study because these references come from a variety of sources.
4. **This is a true statement about descriptive qualitative studies. In the data analysis section of the published study report, the researcher would describe content analysis and the themes and patterns that emerged from the data.**
5. **This is a true statement of descriptive qualitative studies. Because the researcher doe not specify the roots of the approach, he or she could combine aspects of different approaches. A descriptive qualitative approach might have aspects of phenomenology as well as ethnography.**

TEST-TAKING TIP: The key words in the question stem are "descriptive qualitative study." This study does not use any specific aspects of the qualitative approaches (phenomenology, grounded theory, or ethnography). Participant data are descriptive in nature, and these are analyzed from a qualitative perspective as opposed to quantitative approach.

Content Area: *Other Types of Qualitative Approaches;* ***Cognitive Level:*** *Application;* ***Question Type:*** *Multiple Choice*

CRITICAL THINKING FACILITATOR:
Create a grid on the types of qualitative approaches to enhance understanding of these.

19 Linking Qualitative Processes with Evidence-Based Practice

KEY WORDS

The following words include English vocabulary, nursing/medical terminology, concepts, principles, or information relevant to content specifically addressed in the chapter or associated with topics presented in it. English dictionaries, your nursing textbooks, and medical dictionaries such as *Taber's Cyclopedic Medical Dictionary* are resources that can be used to expand your knowledge and understanding of these words and related information.

Bracketing
Codes
Confirmability
Constant comparative method
Credibility
Data reduction
Focus groups
Immersion
Metaphor
Narrative analyses
Participant observation
Stories
Themes
Theoretical sampling
Transferability
Trustworthiness

QUESTIONS

Sampling, Data Collection, and Analysis in Qualitative Studies

1. What question is appropriate to ask in selecting a sample for a qualitative study?
   1. Who will meet the eligibility criteria in order to obtain a representative sample?
   2. What limitations must be imposed on the sample to prevent bias?
   3. What measures should be taken to ensure an adequate sample?
   4. Who will be the source for the richest information for the phenomenon under study?

2. Which of the following studies would use purposive sampling appropriately?
   1. Liu, F., Williams, Liu, H., and Chien (2010) want to study the lived experience of persons having a lower extremity amputation.
   2. Garwick, Seppelt, and Riesgraf (2010) did a study that focused on "addressing asthma management challenges in a multi-site, urban, Head Start Program" (p. 329).
   3. Schrauf (2011) investigated ways "nephrology nurses may help families learn about state or federal programs to assist with their families" (p. 395).
   4. Wilson, Harwood, Oudshoorn, and Thompson (2010) studied "the culture of vascular access cannulation among nurses in a chronic hemodialysis unit" (p. 35).

3. A qualitative researcher wanted to look at the adjustment process of older widowed immigrant women. The researcher identified a neighbor who could possibly be a potential research participant. The researcher plans to ask her whether she could recommend any of her friends. This type of sample selection is called
   1. convenience.
   2. quota.
   3. snowball.
   4. systematic.

4. Which of the following statements describes bracketing in qualitative research? Bracketing is a process of
   1. "transforming raw data into standardized form for data processing and analysis" (Polit & Beck, 2014, p. 376).
   2. "identifying and holding in abeyance any preconceived beliefs and opinions about the phenomena under study" (p. 375).
   3. "organizing and integrating narrative, qualitative information according to emerging themes and concepts" (p. 377).
   4. "gaining access to study participants through the cooperation of key actors in the selected community or site" (p. 381).

5. ________________________ is described as "the collection of different kinds of data about a single complex phenomenon to bring clarity to the phenomenon that cannot be achieved with only one method." It "provides an opportunity to more fully address the complex nature of the human experience" (Barroso, 2010, p. 119).

6. In ____________________________, qualitative researchers "take part in functioning of the group under study and strive to observe, ask questions, and record information within the contexts and structures that are relevant to group members" (Polit & Beck, 2014, p. 292).

7. What secondary materials serve as major sources of data for historical research? **Select all that apply.**
   1. Oral histories
   2. Personal diaries
   3. Autobiographies
   4. Recount of an eyewitness's story
   5. Minutes of organizational meetings

8. Which of the following is an appropriate data collection method for a qualitative study?
   1. Q sort
   2. Likert scale
   3. Open-ended questionnaire
   4. Visual analog scale

9. The use of _________________________ is a way to collect qualitative data on a specific topic. One of its assumptions is that it can "help people to express and clarify their views in ways that are less likely to occur in a one-to-one interview" (Burns & Grove, 2010, p. 87).

10. In the analysis of qualitative data, researchers "search for broad categories." A broad category is called a(n) ____________________. It is "an abstract entity that brings meaning and identity to a current experience and its variant manifestations" (Polit & Beck, 2014, p. 305).

11. Noble and Jones (2010) did a qualitative study to explore nurses' understanding of spirituality. Which of the following statements from the study is a theme?
    1. "The study identified a view that patients might wish to be left alone in order to cope and that not all patients may want spiritual care from nurses" (p. 568).
    2. "However, more experienced nurses working at a higher grade had greater understanding of spirituality, related ethical considerations, and the individual responsibility of spiritual care-giving" (p. 568).
    3. "This study has demonstrated that spirituality is a highly subjective, complex topic that is difficult to define" (p. 569).
    4. "I am not a spiritual person" and "I have always been spiritual" are statements indicating the "wide variety in participants' reports of their own spirituality" (p. 567).

12. One of the processes in qualitative data analysis is dwelling with the data, or immersion. Which of these statements describes immersion? It is a process that
    1. entails creating codes that "may result in themes, processes, or exemplars of the phenomenon being studied" (Burns & Grove, 2010, p. 95).
    2. enables the researcher to "simultaneously gather, manage, and interpret a growing number of data" (p. 93) in the study.
    3. facilitates the placing of the "findings in a larger context and may link different themes or factors in the findings to each other" (p. 97).
    4. includes reading and rereading notes, transcripts of interviews, recalling observations and experiences, and looking at or listening to recordings (Burns & Grove, 2010).

13. To analyze the high volume of qualitative data, the researcher must perform ____________________ to effectively manage the data. It is a process wherein the qualitative researcher "begins to tentatively attach meaning to elements in the data" (Burns & Grove, 2010, p. 94).

14. ____________________ are labels that "provide a way for the researcher to identify patterns in the data" (Burns & Grove, 2010, p. 95).

15. An aspect of data analysis in the grounded theory method is theoretical sampling. Which of the following statements describes theoretical sampling? It is a process
    1. "that is used to select experiences that will help the researcher test ideas and gather complete information about developing concepts" (Barroso, 2010, p. 108).
    2. that looks for the levels of complexity in the data and assures that the data are "grounded in the informant's reality and synthesized by the researcher" (p. 111).
    3. whereby "meaning is pursued through a dialogic process, which extends beyond a single interview and requires thoughtful presence on the part of the researcher" (p. 102).
    4. whereby the researcher "will do what is needed to get a sense of the environment and relationships that provide the context for the case" (p. 113).

16. In a grounded theory study, data are continuously examined for differences and similarities. Theory is constructed through the clustering of codes into categories that are "expanded and developed or collapsed into one another" (Barroso, 2010, p. 108). This systematic process is called ____________________.

17. A type of qualitative approach is narrative analyses in which "people most effectively make sense of their world—and communicate these meanings" (Polit & Beck, 2014, p. 274). The foci of these narrative analyses are ____________________.

18. A metaphor, a qualitative analytic strategy, is a "symbolic comparison, using figurative language to evoke a visual analogy" (Polit & Beck, 2014, p. 305). Which of the following is a metaphor?
    1. Schreiber and MacDonald (2010) explored the role and practice of nurse anesthesia. The basic social process of the practice was called "Keeping Vigil over the Patient" (p. 552).
    2. Kelly and Dowling (2011) reported the following statement from a participant: "I was told I had myeloma, now I never hear of myeloma. . . . I did not think it was cancer and I did get a shock when I realized that it was cancer" (p. 20).
    3. Cangelosi and Moss (2010) explored the voices of faculty teaching second degree students in a baccalaureate nursing program. "Teaching to think like a nurse" (p. 140) was identified as a theme in the data.
    4. Lindy and Schaefer (2010) studied workplace behaviors and found that the bully is an expert clinician with several years of experience. The researchers called the theme a "management perspective" (p. 289).

19. What are the challenges of analyzing qualitative data? (Polit & Beck, 2014). **Select all that apply.**
    1. Lack of universal standards for analysis
    2. Voluminous amount of data to organize
    3. Need for skills in reducing the data for dissemination
    4. Complex statistical procedures
    5. Preciseness and accuracy of the data

Critiquing a Qualitative Study

20. What questions can be asked to critique a qualitative study? **Select all that apply.**
    1. "Is the design appropriate, given the research question?" (Polit & Beck, 2014, p. 278).
    2. "What steps did the researcher take in designing the study to enhance statistical validity?" (p. 170).
    3. "Does the design lend itself to a thorough, in-depth, intensive examination of the phenomenon of interest?" (p. 278).
    4. "Is there evidence that the researcher's interpretation captured the participant's meaning?" (Barroso, 2010, p. 122).
    5. If the research hypotheses were not supported, "might data quality play a role in the failure to confirm the hypotheses?" (Polit & Beck, 2014, p. 209).

21. In appraising qualitative data, the research consumer looks for trustworthiness of the data. What does this include? **Select all that apply.**
    1. Credibility
    2. Confirmability
    3. External validity
    4. Transferability
    5. Internal validity

22. Which of the following research information indicates a concern for trustworthiness of qualitative data?
    1. "Representative excerpts from field notes and quotes from focus group discussions are used to illustrate the findings in the data presented" (Carlson, Philhammar, & Wann-Hansson, 2009, p. 435).
    2. "There is a need to increase professional understanding of the complex and diverse circumstances within which women make infant feeding decisions, with an emphasis placed on requirements for effective communication and sensitive care practices in professional educational programmes" (Sheehan, Schmied, & Barclay, 2010, p. 378).
    3. "Four themes emerged from the participant's stories and through researcher interpretation and analysis: the meaning of nurse-to-nurse mentoring, mentoring as relational learning, and mentoring as embodied learning, and a contextual understanding of nurse-to-nurse mentoring" (Ryan, Goldbery, & Evans, 2010, p. 186).
    4. Hemodialysis nurses "reported willingness to help out their peers when there were problems with cannulation and identified the good cannulators as those nurses routinely asked for help. . . . Well, if you can't get it, then you get one of the other nurses to help" (Wilson, Harwood, Oudshoorn, & Thompson, 2010, p. 40).

A Qualitative Study's Contribution to EBP

23. What is the contribution of a case study to evidence-based practice (EBP)? The study
    1. "is an important approach to accumulating evidence when studying a new topic about which little is known" (Barroso, 2010, p. 106).
    2. provides "in-depth evidence-based discussion of clinical topics that can be used to guide practice" (p. 113).
    3. "will answer questions about how cultural knowledge, norms, and values, and other cultural variables influence the health experience of a particular patient population in a specific setting" (p. 111).
    4. provides evidence generated by the method that can explain, interpret, or predict the phenomenon of interest (Barroso, 2010).

ANSWERS AND RATIONALES

The correct answer number and rationale for why it is the correct answer are given in **boldface blue type.** Rationales for why the other possible answer options are incorrect also are given, but they are not in boldface type.

1. 1. This question is not appropriate to ask in selecting a sample for a qualitative study. Qualitative studies are not concerned about a representative sample as a strategy to control extraneous variables.
2. Imposing limitations on a sample to control bias is not an issue with qualitative research. Qualitative research is concerned with the trustworthiness of the data.
3. This is not an appropriate question to ask. An adequate sample is a requirement in quantitative studies because data are subjected to statistical analysis. An adequate sample has to do with power. Power is the "ability of a design or strategy to detect true relationships that exist among variables" (Polit & Beck, 2014, p. 388).
4. **This question is most appropriate to ask when selecting the sample in qualitative studies. Qualitative studies focus on the human experience, and the richness and depth of the data depend on having a research participant who will share her or his experience with the researcher.**

TEST-TAKING TIP: The key phrase in the question stem is "sample for a qualitative study." Recall the purpose and focus of qualitative approaches and the type of data collected to answer this question.

Content Area: *Data Collection Concepts and Processes in Qualitative Approaches;* ***Cognitive Level:*** *Analysis;* ***Question Type:*** *Multiple Choice*
CRITICAL THINKING FACILITATOR: Review the requirements for a quantitative study and contrast these with the requirements of qualitative studies.

2. 1. **This is a phenomenologic study that used a purposive sampling procedure because the participants shared a lived experience. Purposive sampling is a "non-probability sampling method in which the researcher selects participants based on personal judgment about who will be most informative" (Polit & Beck, 2014, p. 389).**
2. The study is participatory action research (PAR) and uses different members of a community. PAR is a "research approach based on the premise that the use and production of knowledge can be political and used to exert power" (p. 387).
3. The study is classified as a case study and used multiple sources of data to achieve its goals. A case study is a method "involving a thorough in-depth analysis of an individual, group, or other social unit" (p. 325).
4. The study is an ethnographic one. Key informants and other methods of data collection are used to study the group's culture.

TEST-TAKING TIP: The key phrase in the question stem is "purposive sampling." This type of sampling would be most appropriate when a researcher wants to explore the lived experience and purposely selects those who have had the experience.

Content Area: *Data Collection Concepts and Processes in Qualitative Approaches;* ***Cognitive Level:*** *Analysis;* ***Question Type:*** *Multiple Choice*
CRITICAL THINKING FACILITATOR: What are the additional types of sampling procedures for other qualitative approaches? How does a researcher determine which one to use?

3. 1. Convenience sampling is a type of nonprobability sampling procedure that entails "selection of the most readily available persons as participants in a study" (Polit & Beck, 2014, p. 372). This type of sampling would not be appropriate because the information indicates the study is a grounded theory one.
2. Quota sampling will not be appropriate for this study. Quota sampling is a "nonprobability sampling strategy that identifies the strata of the population and proportionately represents the strata in the sample" (LoBiondo-Wood & Haber, 2010, p. 584). Certain characteristics must be present in the person to be considered a participant.
3. **The sampling procedure described is snowball sampling, or networking. In snowball sampling, "subjects who meet the eligibility criteria are asked for assistance in getting in touch with others who meet the same criteria" (p. 586).**
4. Systematic sampling is a probability sampling procedure and is not appropriate to use in qualitative studies.

TEST-TAKING TIP: The key clause in the question stem is "recommend any of her friends." This implies making a contact with others, that is, networking.

Content Area: *Data Collection Concepts and Processes in Qualitative Approaches;* ***Cognitive Level:*** *Analysis;* ***Question Type:*** *Multiple Choice*
CRITICAL THINKING FACILITATOR: What are the characteristics of a sample that was recruited by the snowball technique?

4. 1. This statement describes the process of coding.
2. This statement describes bracketing. "Researchers strive to bracket out presuppositions in an effort to confront their data in pure form" (Polit & Beck, 2014, p. 270).
3. This statement describes content analysis of qualitative information.
4. This statement describes gaining entrée that is common procedure in ethnographic studies.

TEST-TAKING TIP: The key word in the question stem is "bracketing." Think of the use of brackets when you are writing. When you use a pair of brackets, you set a word, phrase, or clause apart from the rest of the sentence. Use this same idea with bracketing in qualitative research.

Content Area: *Data Collection Concepts and Processes in Qualitative Approaches;* ***Cognitive Level:*** *Comprehension;* ***Question Type:*** *Multiple Choice*
CRITICAL THINKING FACILITATOR: What do you suppose happens when a researcher does not use bracketing as he or she collects and analyzes qualitative data? Recall that the goal of qualitative research is to understand the experience or phenomenon from the perspective of the participants.

5. Triangulation

TEST-TAKING TIP: The key phrase in the question stem is "collection of different kinds of data about a single phenomenon." Think of a triangle, the three points of which converge, or join together, from different locations.

Content Area: *Data Collection Concepts and Processes in Qualitative Approaches;* ***Cognitive Level:*** *Knowledge;* ***Question Type:*** *Fill-in-the-Blank*
CRITICAL THINKING FACILITATOR: Think of triangulation as a process similar to the one used before making a nursing diagnosis. You collect multiple sources of data, and when they converge, you will easily see what the data are telling you (nursing diagnosis).

6. participant observation

TEST-TAKING TIP: The key phrase in the question stem is "take part." Recall that observation is a major strategy to collect data in ethnographic studies. Add the involvement, or participation, of the researcher.

Content Area: *Activities and Processes in Qualitative Approaches;* ***Cognitive Level:*** *Comprehension;* ***Question Type:*** *Fill-in-the-Blank*
CRITICAL THINKING FACILITATOR: What are the advantages of participant observation? Consider the ethical implications of this process.

7. 1. Oral histories are primary sources. These are accounts of events related by a person to the researcher.
2. Personal diaries are primary sources because they are written by the person who has experienced the event or situation.
3. Autobiographies are written by the person herself or himself. Therefore, these are considered primary sources.
4. A recount of an eyewitness' story is a secondary source because it is written by another person concerning an event or person.
5. Minutes of organizational meetings are considered secondary sources if they are used by a researcher who was not present at the meeting.

TEST-TAKING TIP: The key words in the question stem are "secondary materials." Recall that secondary sources are "second-hand accounts of events or facts" (Polit & Beck, 2014, p. 391).

Content Area: *Data Collection Activities and Processes in Qualitative Approaches;* ***Cognitive Level:*** *Comprehension;* ***Question Type:*** *Multiple Response*
CRITICAL THINKING FACILITATOR: If you have a sample historical study, identify secondary sources from its references.

8. 1. The Q sort is used "to characterize opinions, attitudes, or judgments of individuals through comparative ranking ordering" (Stephenson, 1975, as cited in Fain, 2009, p. 139). This tool is used in quantitative studies.
2. Likert scales are used in quantitative studies. They "require subjects to respond to a series of statements to express a viewpoint. Subjects read each statement and select an appropriately ranked response" (Fain, 2009, p. 132).
3. An open-ended questionnaire is an appropriate method to collect qualitative data. "Open-ended questions allow more varied information to be collected and require a qualitative or content analysis method to analyze responses" (Sullivan-Bolyai & Bova, 2010, p. 275).
4. The visual analog scale is "useful for measuring subjective phenomena (e.g., pain, fatigue, shortness of breath, anxiety). The scale is unidimensional, quantifying intensity only" (Fain, 2009, p. 138). This tool is used in quantitative studies.

TEST-TAKING TIP: The key phrase in the question stem is "appropriate data collection methods." Look at the options and decide which of the tools would elicit narrative, descriptive statements from research participants.

Content Area: *Data Collection Activities and Processes in Qualitative Approaches;* ***Cognitive Level:*** *Comprehension;* ***Question Type:*** *Multiple Choice*
CRITICAL THINKING FACILITATOR: Identify all types of data collection methods for qualitative approaches and compare them with those used in quantitative approaches.

9. focus groups

TEST-TAKING TIP: The key word in the second statement is "people." Also, the verbs "express" and "clarify" require focusing on something.

Content Area: *Data Collection Activities and Processes in Qualitative Approaches;* ***Cognitive Level:*** *Knowledge;* ***Question Type:*** *Fill-in-the-Blank*
CRITICAL THINKING FACILITATOR: Focus groups are an excellent way to obtain information. For instance, a focus group could be used to evaluate a nursing program. In this instance, would findings be different if individuals were interviewed instead?

10. theme

TEST-TAKING TIP: The key words in the question stem include "abstract" and "current experience and its variant manifestations." What is an abstract concept that expresses the commonalities between one experience and its variants? It is a theme. A theme is a unifying concept. Proms and other formal dances or parties often have themes. The colors and decorations, even the menus that are chosen, all support the theme of the event.

Content Area: *Activities and Processes in Qualitative Approaches;* ***Cognitive Level:*** *Comprehension;* ***Question Type:*** *Fill-in-the-Blank*
CRITICAL THINKING FACILITATOR: Look at a sample qualitative study and identify themes as described by the researcher. These will be found under the results or data section. How do the themes relate to the researcher's observations?

11. 1. This statement is a conclusion of the researchers.
    2. This statement is also a concluding statement.
    3. This statement is part of the conclusions of this study.
    4. **The statements indicate a theme in the study. The statements are reflective of the theme of the "nurse's own spirituality."**

TEST-TAKING TIP: A theme would include verbatim statements from participants that give meaning to the theme. Only option 4 has such statements.

Content Area: *Activities and Processes in Qualitative Approaches;* ***Cognitive Level:*** *Application;* ***Question Type:*** *Multiple Choice*
CRITICAL THINKING FACILITATOR: When identifying the themes from a qualitative study, are you able to visualize the phenomenon as described by the themes?

12. 1. The process described is called coding.
    2. The process described is data management in qualitative research.
    3. The process described is interpretation of the data.
    4. **The process described is immersion in the data.**

TEST-TAKING TIP: The key phrase in the question stem is "dwelling with the data." This literally means "living with the data" and figuratively means being deeply involved (immersed) in the data. Only option 4 shows the deep involvement of the researcher with the data.

Content Area: *Activities and Processes in Qualitative Approaches;* ***Cognitive Level:*** *Comprehension;* ***Question Type:*** *Multiple Choice*
CRITICAL THINKING FACILITATOR: Why is immersion an important process in the analysis of qualitative data?

13. data reduction

TEST-TAKING TIP: Key phrases in the question stem include "analyze the high volume of qualitative data" and "attach meaning to elements in the data." This process is a way of organizing data analogous to sorting large volumes of material, taking out certain pieces, and categorizing them in order to reduce the material to a manageable amount.

Content Area: *Activities and Processes in Qualitative Approaches;* ***Cognitive Level:*** *Comprehension;* ***Question Type:*** *Fill-in-the-Blank*
CRITICAL THINKING FACILITATOR: Compare the qualitative approaches' strategies to manage data with the strategies for quantitative approaches.

14. codes

TEST-TAKING TIP: The key word in the statement is "labels." A label is a name of something. For example, with the aid of

technology, things are identified or named by "bar codes."

Content Area: *Activities and Processes in Qualitative Approaches;* ***Cognitive Level:*** *Knowledge;* ***Question Type:*** *Fill-in-the-Blank*
CRITICAL THINKING FACILITATOR: Locate the codes used by the qualitative researcher in a sample phenomenologic study. How did the researcher come up with the codes used?

15. 1. **This statement describes theoretical sampling.**
 2. This statement describes the data analysis process in an ethnographic study.
 3. This statement describes the phenomenologic method.
 4. This statement describes the process of data gathering in a case study.

TEST-TAKING TIP: The key phrase in the question stem is "theoretical sampling." A clue in option 1 is "concepts." Recall that concepts are the building blocks of theories. Also realize that "grounded theory researchers generate conceptual categories and integrate them into a substantive theory grounded in the data" (Polit & Beck, 2014, p. 272).

Content Area: *Activities and Processes in Qualitative Approaches;* ***Cognitive Level:*** *Comprehension* ***Question Type:*** *Multiple Choice*
CRITICAL THINKING FACILITATOR: Look at a sample grounded theory study and identify the theoretical sampling process.

16. **constant comparative method**

TEST-TAKING TIP: The key phrase is "continuously examined for differences and similarities." This implies a constant process of comparison.

Content Area: *Activities and Processes in Qualitative Approaches;* ***Cognitive Level:*** *Comprehension;* ***Question Type:*** *Fill-in-the-Blank*
CRITICAL THINKING FACILITATOR: Look at a sample grounded theory study and identify the constant comparative process that was undertaken by the researcher.

17. **stories**

TEST-TAKING TIP: The key word in the question stem is "narrative," derived from the verb "narrate," which means to tell a story. Recall that in qualitative research, participants share their perceptions and views of their world and experiences. These data are told as stories.

Content Area: *Activities and Processes in Qualitative Approaches;* ***Cognitive Level:*** *Knowledge;* ***Question Type:*** *Fill-in-the-Blank*
CRITICAL THINKING FACILITATOR: What are stories made of? What makes a story unique to the person telling it? If a researcher were to ask you to relate your first experience of caring for a patient in clinicals, you would relate your story with the meaning and significance that you attach to that experience.

18. 1. **This statement indicates use of a metaphor. The nurse anesthesia students compare their role in the care of patients undergoing surgery with that of religious observers keeping a solemn watch ("vigil") over a dead body. Patients who are receiving anesthesia are nonfunctional ("dead"), and nurse anesthesia students are keeping vigil by closely watching over them.**
 2. The information describes s participant statement that supports a theme identified by the researcher.
 3. The information describes a theme and an example of a statement that supports the theme in the data.
 4. Management perspective is a theme identified by the researcher from the analysis of the data.

TEST-TAKING TIP: The key phrase in the question stem is "figurative language to evoke a visual analogy." A metaphor is not literally true, but it is a descriptive use of language to depict a situation. An example is a description of pain as "a thousand needles sticking into my body."

Content Area: *Activities and Processes in Qualitative Approaches;* ***Cognitive Level:*** *Analysis;* ***Question Type:*** *Multiple Choice*
CRITICAL THINKING FACILITATOR: What are some other familiar metaphors, and how do they convey information and help you understand someone else's experience?

19. 1. **There is an "absence of standard procedures" (Polit & Beck, 2014, p. 300) for analyzing qualitative data. With quantitative data, researchers can use statistical packages to manage and analyze the data.**
 2. **The data in qualitative research are narrative descriptions of research participants, and these are gathered through multiple sources. These multiple sources yield many pages of information that need to be organized and analyzed.**
 3. **The researchers have a particularly difficult task of looking over the data many times to "search for meanings**

and understanding" (Polit & Beck, 2014, p. 300). The process requires skills and patience.

4. Qualitative researchers collect narrative information, not numerical data. Therefore, they do not face the challenge of using complex statistical procedures.
5. Precision and accuracy are not challenges of qualitative researchers. They are most concerned with true understanding of the experiences of research participants. Trustworthiness is the goal of the qualitative researcher. Trustworthiness is the "degree of confidence qualitative researchers have in their data and analyses" (Polit & Beck, 2014, p. 394).

TEST-TAKING TIP: A key word in the question stem is "challenge." Recall all you know about qualitative research to identify the challenges of analyzing data gathered from a qualitative study.

Content Area: *Activities and Processes in Qualitative Approaches;* ***Cognitive Level:*** *Comprehension;* ***Question Type:*** *Multiple Choice*

CRITICAL THINKING FACILITATOR:
Although there are many challenges in analyzing qualitative data, there are also many rewards. Can you think of some?

20. **1. The question is appropriate to ask because the research question guides the specific qualitative approach to be used. For example, if the researcher is interested in the lived experience of participants, then a phenomenologic approach will be used. Qualitative designs are emergent designs. As questions about the data are asked, the researcher might use an additional qualitative approach to fully understand the phenomenon of interest.**

2. The question is not appropriate to ask in analyzing a qualitative study because the question focuses on statistical analysis, a process in quantitative approaches.
3. **The question is appropriate to ask because it addresses an appraisal of the phenomenon's depth and intensity, which are the foci of the qualitative researcher.**
4. **The question is appropriate to ask because it ascertains the meaning of the phenomenon within the perspective of the research participant.**
5. The question is appropriate to ask in critiquing a quantitative study. The question addresses a hypothesis which is a part of a quantitative study.

TEST-TAKING TIP: Key words are found in the options. Option 1 contains the clue words "design" and "question." Option 2 contains the words "statistical validity." Option 3 includes the clue words "phenomenon of interest." Option 4 has the clue words "participant's meaning." Finally, option 5 has the clue word "hypotheses." Based on what you know about the goals and purposes of qualitative approaches, pick the correct options.

Content Area: *Activities and Processes in Qualitative Approaches;* ***Cognitive Level:*** *Analysis;* ***Question Type:*** *Multiple Response*

CRITICAL THINKING FACILITATOR:
Think of other questions that could be asked to critically appraise a qualitative study.

21. **1. Credibility has to do with "confidence in the truth of the data" (Polit & Beck, 2014, p. 328). The researcher asks whether the data truly represent the participant's experience.**

2. **Confirmability refers to the "objectivity or neutrality of the data and interpretations" (p. 377). The researcher asks whether the data have congruence among participants.**
3. External validity is applicable to quantitative studies. Recall that it means the "degree to which study results can be generalized to settings or samples other than the one studied" (p. 380).
4. **Transferability means the "extent to which qualitative findings can be transferred to other settings or groups" (p. 393).**
5. Internal validity is applicable to quantitative studies. Recall that it means "the degree to which it can be inferred that the experimental treatment (independent variable), rather than confounding factors, is responsible for observed effects on the outcome" (p. 383).

TEST-TAKING TIP: The key word in the question stem is "trustworthiness," a combination of two words, *trust,* which involves integrity and *worthy,* which means valuable. In looking at the options, options 1, 2 and 4 embody trustworthiness.

Content Area: *Critical Appraisal of Qualitative Approaches;* ***Cognitive Level:*** *Comprehension;* ***Question Type:*** *Multiple Response*

CRITICAL THINKING FACILITATOR: Look at any qualitative study in the Appendix of your core textbook. Then select an aspect of trustworthiness and determine how it was achieved in the study.

22. 1. The information indicates that the researcher attempted to meet data trustworthiness by using multiple sources of data (i.e., field notes and quotes from focus groups) to validate findings.

2. The information presents the implications of the study findings for practice. The clue in the statement is "there is a need."
3. The information identifies the themes that emerged from the analysis of the data.
4. The information is an identified theme, and the statement in italics is an example of a participant's statement that reflects the theme.

TEST-TAKING TIP: The key word in the question stem is "trustworthiness." Look for words in the options that indicate attempts of the researcher to validate or confirm data.

Content Area: *Critical Appraisal of Qualitative Approaches;* ***Cognitive Level:*** *Analysis;* ***Question Type:*** *Multiple Choice*

CRITICAL THINKING FACILITATOR: Compare how quantitative researchers and qualitative researchers meet the criteria of rigor in their studies.

23. 1. This statement is about the contribution of a phenomenological study to EBP.

2. This statement indicates the contribution of a case study to EBP.

3. This statement describes the contribution of an ethnographic study to EBP.
4. This statement describes the contribution of grounded theory to EBP.

TEST-TAKING TIP: The key phrase in the questions stem is "case study." Think of a clinical example of a patient and her or his health issues. Often doctors and nurses use a particularly memorable patient, diagnosis, or situation as a teaching strategy. The in-depth study of this clinical situation is often referred to as a case study.

Content Area: *Activities and Processes in Qualitative Approaches;* ***Cognitive Level:*** *Knowledge;* ***Question Type:*** *Multiple Choice*

CRITICAL THINKING FACILITATOR: Read one of the qualitative studies in the Appendix of your core textbook and identify its potential contributions to EBP.

20 Comprehensive Final Examination

QUESTIONS

Research Case Study: A faculty researcher did a study to determine the effectiveness of an educational program on students' success in the first clinical course of the baccalaureate program in nursing. This educational program's main emphasis is to strengthen critical thinking, which is vital for success. The program strategies have been refined and implemented in the past 5 years on previous groups of students who were not successful in their first attempt at the first clinical course. The current study sample consists of 24 BSN students who were unsuccessful in the first clinical course.

Questions 1 to 4 refer to the study.

1. The study's purpose was to determine the effectiveness of an educational program on students' success in the first clinical course of the baccalaureate program. What is the level of the study's purpose?
   1. Description
   2. Exploration
   3. Prediction
   4. Identification

2. What type of sampling was used in the study?
   1. Probability, random assignment
   2. Nonprobability, convenience
   3. Probability, systematic
   4. Nonprobability, purposive

3. What would be a possible design of the study?
   1. Phenomenological
   2. Quasi-experimental
   3. Longitudinal
   4. Descriptive

4. The appropriate research question for the above case study is as follows: What is the relationship of a remedial educational program on the subsequent success of students who were unsuccessful in their first attempt at a clinical nursing course? What is the independent variable?
   1. Success of students
   2. Educational program
   3. Unsuccessful students
   4. Relationship

Research Study Information: Chan, Wong, Onishi, and Thayala (2011) did a study to determine the effects of music on depression in older people. The 52 eligible and willing older adults were randomly assigned to the music (experimental) group or the nonmusic (control) group. Participants' personal information was identified only by case number.

Questions 5 to 7 refer to the study.

5. What is the level of purpose communicated in the study information?
   1. Description
   2. Prediction
   3. Exploration
   4. Identification

6. What ethical aspect is evident when participant information was identified only by case number?
   1. Freedom from harm and discomfort
   2. Right to privacy
   3. Right to fair treatment
   4. Right to protection from exploitation.

7. The researchers identified their study as a randomized clinical trial (RCT). What requirements of an RCT are evident in the study information? **Select all that apply.**
   1. The independent variable was manipulated.
   2. The sample was randomly assigned to groups.
   3. Power was evident with the large sample.
   4. There is evidence of adherence to ethical guidelines.
   5. The data collection method was appropriate.

Research Study Information: Chan, Wong, Onishi, and Thayala (2011) did a study to determine the effects of music on depression in older people. They hypothesized that "there is a statistically significant lower depression level in older adults in the music group than those in the non-music group" (p. 777). Depression was measured using a scale that had a Cronbach's alpha ranging from 0.88 to 0.91.

Questions 8 and 9 refer to the study information.

8. What statements are true about the study tool's Cronbach's alpha? **Select all that apply**.
   1. Cronbach's alpha is test of instrument validity.
   2. Cronbach's alpha is a test of instrument stability.
   3. The range is acceptable since it is over 0.70.
   4. Internal consistency is established by Cronbach's alpha.
   5. Cronbach's alpha is a test for reliability.

9. What type of hypothesis was proposed in the study? **Select all that apply.**
   1. Simple
   2. Nondirectional
   3. Null
   4. Complex
   5. Directional

Research Study Information: The vice president of nursing at a large tertiary facility wants to determine the relationship of leadership style and job satisfaction among nurse managers. During the course of the study, a generous tuition reimbursement was added to the benefit package of all employees.

10. What does this process represent?
    1. Threat to external validity, sampling plan
    2. Threat to internal validity, history
    3. Threat to internal validity, selection
    4. Threat to external validity, Hawthorne effect

Research Study Information: Thornton, Parrish, and Swords (2011) did a systematic review to "determine best practices for the use of systemic antibiotics compared to topical treatment of acute otitis media (AOM)" (p. 263). Their question was: "In children age 6 months to 17 years with AOM, is symptom resolution similar for topical treatment (antibiotic eardrops and/or analgesic eardrops) compared to systemic antibiotics?" (p. 263).

11. Using the PICO format, the O in the question is __________.

Research Study Information: Zhuang, An, and Ziao (2013) did a study to determine the "yoga effects on mood and quality of life in Chinese women undergoing heroin detoxification" (p. 260). Under the discussion section, the researchers stated that "the participants could not be blinded by the intervention. Only the outcome assessor was blinded to group allocation" (p. 267).

12. What is true about the process of blinding?
1. The process entails participants not know the identity of the researcher.
2. Only the researcher knows the identities of the research participants.
3. A research team member does not know which participant belongs to the experimental or control group.
4. The research team member does not know what potential outcome can be expected as a result of the intervention.

Research Case Study: A nurse in an outpatient diabetic clinic sees clients who are able to manage their therapeutic regimens effectively. He identified these clients as demonstrating self-efficacy. He would like to do a study to describe factors that influence self-efficacy.

Questions 13-15 refer to the situation.

13. What type of study should he do?
1. Correlation
2. Exploratory
3. Quasi-experimental
4. Ethnography

14. What would be the next study to do as a follow-up?
1. Correlation
2. Quasi-experimental
3. Descriptive
4. Phenomenological

15. In the follow-up study above, what type of hypothesis would the researcher propose? **Select all that apply.**
1. Simple
2. Directional
3. Nondirectional
4. Complex
5. None

Research Case Study: A faculty researcher wants to determine the effectiveness of a new teaching approach on students' ability to do parenteral medication administration. One group of students participated in a simulation exercise in addition to the faculty demonstration and skill practice sessions. The other group of students participated only in the faculty demonstration and the practice sessions.

Questions 16 and 17 refer to the case study.

16. What process is evident in the situation?
1. Random assignment to groups
2. Manipulation of the independent variable
3. Observation of the dependent variable
4. Designing the intervention

17. Because the researcher was not able to use a probability sampling procedure, she will use a(n) __________ design for the study.

Research Study Information: "Continuing research is needed to determine the effectiveness of topical antibiotics compared to systemic antibiotics in resolving acute otitis media (AOM) versus palliative treatments to decrease pain" (Thornton, Parrish, & Swords, 2011, p. 242).

18. What part of the research study is the information included?
    1. Implication for practice
    2. Recommendation
    3. Limitation
    4. Conclusion

Research Study Information: George and Thomas (2010) studied the lived experience of diabetes among older, rural people. During the data analysis "the principal investigator revisited two participants and asked them if the thematic structure was accurate. Both were able to recognize their own experiences in the findings" (p. 1095).

19. What do these statements indicate in this phenomenological study?
    1. Data saturation
    2. Accurate theme identification
    3. Rigor of the analysis
    4. Objectivity of analysis

Research Study Information: Simon, Klaus, Gajewski, and Dunton (2013) investigated "the agreement of fall classifications among staff in U.S. hospitals." The researchers stated that "results indicate that the National Quality Forum fall definition needs further refinement to classify all scenarios properly" (p. 74).

20. What does the statement represent?
    1. Recommendation
    2. Limitation
    3. Conclusion
    4. Data analysis

Research Study Information: "Participants were self-referred, by accepting the invitation to one of the information meetings. This procedure of self-selection presumably involves a systematic bias in the sample as motivated persons, with a wish to reduce the effects of their disease, will dominate" (Jacobsen et al., 2011, p. 772).

21. What does this statement from the researchers indicate?
    1. The study information indicates an ethical issue with self-selection.
    2. This study information reflects the difficulty in recruiting research participants.
    3. The study information is an identified limitation of the study.
    4. The study information describes quota sampling.

Research Study Information: In the analysis of data, Jacobsen et al. (2011) stated that "An independent *t* test was used to analyze the difference between groups at baseline and also to analyze the difference between groups in improvement from 0-10 weeks" (p. 769).

22. What does the information indicate? **Select all that apply.**
    1. There were at least two groups compared at baseline and at 10 weeks.
    2. The test used is an inferential parametric test.
    3. The difference analyzed between the two groups refers to the study outcome.
    4. The design of the study is nonexperimental.
    5. No data were collected before the intervention.

Research Study Information: Dowling (2011) did a study on patients' lived experience with myeloma. The researcher described some of the findings as follows: "Lived body: a changing body. All participants commented on changes in their bodily function and appearance" (p. 39). These changes included alopecia and fatigue.

23. The findings in this study are called __________.

Research Study Information: The purpose of the researchers was "to provide a current synthesis of all controlled and uncontrolled studies examining the effectiveness of renal transplant (RT) on specific domains of quality of life compared to the most frequently used renal replacement therapy, which is hemodialysis" (Landreneau, K., Lee, K. & Landereneau, M. D., 2010, p. 37).

24. What does the information indicate?
   1. Clinical practice guidelines
   2. Review of literature
   3. Metasynthesis
   4. Meta-analysis

Research Study Information: The researchers stated that "in addition to interviewing the pioneers in the women's health practitioner role, we conducted a search of the literature on educational programs. We consulted the literature on the conduct of oral histories and based our approach on the recommendations of that literature" (Fontenot & Hawkins, 2011, pp. 315-316).

25. What does the information indicate?
   1. The information indicates the phenomenological study's data collection methods.
   2. The information indicates a grounded theory study's data sources.
   3. The information indicates a historical study's method of data collection.
   4. The information indicates an ethnographic study's methodology.

Research Study Information: "Critical thinking skills, in combination with a strong foundational knowledge and its application to patient care, are essential to administer safe anesthesia. Failure in a provider's critical thinking ability or deficiencies in knowledge base may set the stage for negative patient outcomes" (McClain, Biddle, & Cotter, 2012, p. 12).

26. What does the information represent?
   1. The information is the study's research question.
   2. The information is the study's conclusion.
   3. The information is the significance of the study.
   4. The information is the study's purpose.

Research Study Information: Ward, Wiltshire, Detry, and Brown (2013) did a study on "African American men and women's attitudes toward mental illness, perceptions of stigma, and preferred coping behaviors" (p. 185). One of their guiding statements was: "Individuals have common sense beliefs and representations about illnesses that guide how they cope with health threats and illness" (p. 186).

27. The second sentence above is the study's
   1. hypothesis.
   2. conclusion.
   3. conceptual model.
   4. significance to practice.

Research Study Information: A review of the literature on African Americans' attitudes toward mental illness revealed that mental illness was viewed as stigmatizing. However, other studies found African Americans to have positive health beliefs and attitudes toward seeking services but not necessarily treatment (Ward et al., 2013).

28. What does the information indicate?
   1. The information indicates a gap in the knowledge base on the topic.
   2. The information is an inconsistency of findings in literature reviewed.
   3. The information is the conclusion of the study.
   4. The statements indicate the statement of the problem on the topic.

Research Study Information: The study had a "sample size of 34 to detect a large interaction effect (Cohen's f = 0.55) in traditional repeated measures, assuming a power of .80, an alpha of .05 and standard error rates in the literature" (Norris et al., 2013).

29. What is described here is ________.

Research Study Information: "A randomized longitudinal intervention trial was designed to test the effects of a psychoeducational intervention on persons receiving their initial implantable cardioverter defibrillator (ICD)" (Berg, Higgins, Reilly, Langberg, & Dunbar, 2012, p. 431).

30. What statements are applicable to the study? **Select all that apply.**
    1. There would be an intervention and one or more dependent variables.
    2. At least two groups, a control and an experimental group, would be used.
    3. There would be more than one data collection period after the intervention.
    4. The sampling procedure would be convenience sampling.
    5. The primary data collection methods would be interviews.

Research Study Information: "Delivering care to children with diabetes involves more than controlling glucose and food intake and physical exercise. Understanding the nature and development of these problems in family functioning is critical to formulate effective interventions" (de Oliveira, Nascif-Junior, & Rocha, 2010, p. 106).

31. What does the information indicate?
    1. The information is a study's aim or purpose.
    2. The information is the research question.
    3. The information is a theme in the study.
    4. The information is a statement of the need for the study.

Research Study Information: The study focused on families with diabetic children. It emphasized the identification of social supports and networks to strengthen interventions aimed at health promotion. "The results presented the families' characterization and testimonies grouped in the following categories: social support, social networks, and family roles" (de Oliveira, Nascif-Junior, & Rocha, 2010, p. 106).

32. What type of qualitative approach is evident in the information?
    1. Participatory action research
    2. Ethnography
    3. Case study
    4. Phenomenology

Hypothetical Study: The researcher studied the lived experience of teenagers who have lost a parent to HIV/AIDS. The researcher interviewed eight teenagers and stopped data collection after the ninth teenager.

Questions 33 and 34 refer to the situation above.

33. What type of study did the researcher do as indicated by the information?
    1. Historical
    2. Ethnography
    3. Phenomenology
    4. Grounded theory

34. What statements are true regarding the sample of the study? **Select all that apply.**
    1. The sample is obtained by using a probability method.
    2. A convenience sample would be appropriate for the study.
    3. A purposive sample would be appropriate for this study.
    4. The research participants are referred to as subjects.
    5. The sample will share narrative data with the researcher.

35. A baccalaureate program in nursing eliminated the use of the SATs as a criterion to predict success in the program because a large percentage of those who did not meet the required score were successful in the program. What statement might explain elimination of the SATs?
    1. The SATs are not stable and reliable..
    2. The SATs have not been tested adequately as an admission requirement.
    3. The SATs have not demonstrated validity in predicting success in the program.
    4. The SATs have not met interrater reliability.

36. Hypothetical Study: A researcher/epidemiologist wants to find out the rate of urinary tract infections (UTIs) among men with paraplegia who self-catheterize. The researcher would recruit potential participants from six outpatient clinics in a metropolitan area. What type of population would the study come from?
   1. Total
   2. Target
   3. Quota
   4. Accessible

37. Hypothetical Study: A faculty researcher wants to do a study in which a program to strengthen critical thinking skills would be implemented. After the study was explained, several students opted not to participate. An informed consent was signed by the participants. Which ethical principle was addressed when students opted not to participate in the program?
   1. Right to self-determination
   2. Right to freedom from harm and discomfort
   3. Right to privacy
   4. Right to fair treatment

38. Hypothetical Study: A researcher was doing a phenomenological study on the lived experience of adolescents undergoing drug rehabilitation. Why did the researcher stop collecting data after interviewing and analyzing the data provided by the ninth teenager?
   1. Nine teenagers were deemed to be an adequate sample for the study.
   2. Data saturation was achieved after the ninth teenager.
   3. No other research participant could be recruited.
   4. The researcher used other studies as guidelines for the number of participants.

39. Formulating a clinical question is the first step in the development of an evidence-based research project. In this process, a format known as PICO can be used to facilitate the development of researchable questions. The C in PICO stands for __________.

40. Hypothetical Study: A researcher wants to study the emergence of nurse midwifery as an area of advanced nursing practice. What would be an appropriate design for this study?
   1. Ethnography
   2. Case study
   3. Historical
   4. Grounded theory

41. Hypothetical Study: A retired nurse sees the potential to establish parish nursing in her underserved community. She approached key individuals to obtain funding to start a small clinic staffed by volunteers. The community group would have to do a participatory action research (PAR) for the project to materialize. Which statements are true about PAR? **Select all that apply.**
   1. Both qualitative and quantitative data collection methods are used.
   2. Research participants are selected based on their experience with the political machinery.
   3. The goal of the research is improved knowledge that can be instrumental for sociopolitical activism.
   4. The community as a group serves as the study's principal investigator.
   5. PAR mobilizes the community to work as a group to solve problems.

42. Hypothetical Study: A nurse practitioner noted lowered cholesterol levels in outpatient clinic patients who were not taking any antilipidemic medications. The nurse is interested in possible "causes" of this situation. What would be an appropriate design for the study?
   1. Retrospective
   2. Descriptive
   3. Correlation
   4. Prospective

43. Hypothetical Study: A nurse researcher published a meta-analysis of research studies on pressure ulcer treatments. What types and sources of literature are used in a meta-analysis? **Select all that apply.**
    1. Primary source
    2. Secondary source
    3. Theoretical literature
    4. Journal literature
    5. Data-based literature

44. What are the purposes of a literature review in a quantitative study? **Select all that apply**. A literature review
    1. identifies gaps in the existing literature on the topic.
    2. discovers reliable and valid research instruments.
    3. provides the rationale for funding.
    4. discovers conceptual traditions used to examine problems.
    5. identifies impressions on the topic by various researchers.

45. The researcher stipulated that students who have had a negative health care–related experience be considered ineligible to participate in the study. What is the researcher trying to do in imposing this stipulation? The researcher is
    1. establishing reliability of measurement.
    2. controlling extraneous variables.
    3. controlling for history as a threat.
    4. making sure there is an adequate sample.

46. The researcher carefully developed the protocols for the teaching, trained the research assistants, and observed the research assistants at least twice when they were implementing the protocols for teaching. This action of the researcher ensures __________.

47. Anxiety is an overall feeling state as measured by the Smith Anxiety Trait Scale. What does this statement describe?
    1. Independent variable
    2. Dependent variable
    3. Operational definition
    4. Conceptual definition

48. Hypothetical Study: A home care nurse wants to do a study to determine the most efficient, low-cost glucometer on the market. What type of research is this?
    1. Basic
    2. Applied
    3. Experimental
    4. Correlation

49. A nurse researcher observed psychiatric patients as they interacted during group therapy. The patients were not told about the researcher's intent. What ethical principle was violated?
    1. Right of confidentiality
    2. Right of anonymity
    3. Right to self-determination
    4. Right to fair treatment

50. Hypothetical Study: A woman relived a very traumatic event in her life (a rape) when she was interviewed by a researcher about her experience. Caution must be exercised by the researcher as the subject shares her pain and trauma. What right can potentially be violated in this situation?
    1. Freedom from harm and discomfort
    2. Right to fair treatment
    3. Anonymity and confidentiality
    4. Right to self-determination

51. A researcher did her study in a patient unit within a tertiary care facility. If the researcher failed to extend the benefits of the study to those patients who refused to participate in the study, what principle of research ethics was violated?
1. Informed consent
2. Right to fair treatment
3. Freedom from harm
4. Right to self-determination

52. Hypothetical Study: A faculty researcher wants to investigate how new graduates undergo the transition from senior nursing student to graduate nurse in the first 2 years of practice. What would be the most appropriate design for this study?
1. Survey
2. Ethnography
3. Phenomenology
4. Grounded theory

53. During the data collection process, unbeknownst to the researcher, several subjects were experiencing discomfort from gastric hyperacidity. What type of measurement error could be produced by physical discomfort of the subjects during the data collection period?
1. Consistent
2. Random
3. Systematic
4. Bias

54. What essential research activity is done by the researcher who espouses the beliefs proposed by the naturalistic paradigm? The researcher
1. uses inferential statistics to analyze data.
2. imposes controls on identified biases and extraneous variables.
3. collects descriptive, narrative data from participants.
4. reports data in tables to protect anonymity.

55. In 1989, a historical researcher investigated the contributions of Dorothea Dix (1802–1887) on mental health reform. What type of data sources would this researcher most likely use?
1. Data-based
2. Secondary
3. Theoretical literature
4. Primary

56. Which of the following hypothetical titles is suggestive of an ethnographic study? *(Note: Study titles are hypothetical)*
1. The assimilation and acculturation of Mexican-Americans in Queens
2. The lived experience of adults with HIV/AIDS
3. Florence Nightingale: The first nurse researcher
4. The relationship of health beliefs and health-seeking behaviors of adolescents

57. A factor analysis was done on the Attitudes Toward Older People Scale (ATOP). Data indicated that the items clustered around one to two factors. What is the researcher's interest when doing a factor analysis test?
1. Stability
2. Internal consistency
3. Validity
4. Equivalence

58. Which of the following hypothetical study titles suggests a phenomenological study? *(Note: Study titles are hypothetical)*
1. The culture of a clinical nursing group
2. The meaning of grief among mothers of SIDS babies
3. Linda Richards: The first trained nurse
4. Attitudes of first-time mothers toward breast-feeding

59. A comprehensive examination on maternal–child health omitted some relevant topical areas. What did the examination fail to fulfill?
   1. Test–retest reliability
   2. Alternate form reliability
   3. Construct validity
   4. Content validity

60. A researcher wants to study life satisfaction in elderly adults. One of the beginning steps is to do a literature review on life satisfaction. Which of the following hypothetical titles would the researcher consider as a secondary source for this topic? *(Note: Study titles are hypothetical)*
   1. Smith, E. (2012). Life satisfaction among African American elders: A survey. *Journal of Black Studies, 12*(5), 24-39.
   2. Jones, J. (2011). Life satisfaction: A reliability and validity study. *Journal of Psychometrics, 2*(4), 29-31.
   3. Adams, C. (2013). Predictors of life satisfaction among older women. *Journal of Women's Health, 6*(2), 46-51.
   4. Knoll, T. (2010). Life satisfaction: A critique of tools and instruments 2004-2009. *Psychometrics,* 7(3), 83-85.

61. What aspects of the literature review would a researcher be ***least*** interested in doing?
   1. Noting the availability of reliable and valid instruments to measure life satisfaction
   2. Understanding the detailed impressions of various researchers' on the topic
   3. Noting the recommendations and suggestions for future studies by previous researchers
   4. Getting familiar with approaches and designs used in studying the topic

62. Which of the following hypothetical works would the researcher consider as a primary source for the topic of life satisfaction in the elderly? *(Note: Study titles are hypothetical)*
   1. Arthurs, C. (2010). A review of conceptual models of life satisfaction. *Journal of Psychology of Aging, 2*(6), 125-129.
   2. Jolles, T. (2011). An analysis of 25 years of research on life satisfaction. *Journal of the Humanities, 3*(1), 6-10.
   3. Troll, F. (2013) (Ed.). *A Collection of Essays on Social Aspects of Aging.* Philadelphia: J. B. Lippincott.
   4. White, W. (2013). Health and life satisfaction among nursing home residents: A correlation study. *Journal of Aging, 2*(5), 69-73.

63. The researcher used both conceptual and data-based literature. Which of the following hypothetical titles would be considered theoretical literature? *(Note: Study titles are hypothetical)*
   1. Life satisfaction: The core concept in the developmental model of adulthood
   2. The relationship between social support and life satisfaction among community dwelling elders
   3. A meta-analysis of 25 years of research on life satisfaction among older adults
   4. A reliability and validity study of the center on aging life satisfaction scale

64. Which of the following activities suggests a retrospective study? The researcher
   1. looked at factors that may have contributed to the outbreak of influenza.
   2. examined the relationship between self-efficacy and adherence to the diabetic regimen.
   3. surveyed the attitudes of RN applicants to the AIDS unit.
   4. did a reliability and validity study on the Quality of Sleep Tool.

65. Which of the following meets the criteria for a cross-sectional study? The researcher
   1. expects trends in the data during the course of the study.
   2. collects data several times during the duration of the study.
   3. expects attrition due to loss of subjects as a major threat.
   4. does a single data collection period for all subjects.

66. Hypothetical Study: A researcher wants to determine whether continuing education should be made mandatory as a requirement for license renewal. The researcher asked attendees at an organizational convention to participate. What is the source for potential threat to the study?
1. Reactivity of participants
2. Sampling plan
3. History
4. Maturation

67. In a study of psychomotor ability, the researcher did not use subjects who have had physical training. This process was done to control for physical training as a(n)
1. independent variable.
2. extraneous variable.
3. dependent variable.
4. dichotomous variable.

68. A researcher wants to use quota sampling in her study. What will she do to get her sample?
1. Go to a senior center and ask for volunteers.
2. Recruit subgroups of 50 persons with specific characteristics.
3. Ask colleagues to recommend potential participants from their network.
4. From a list, randomly select numbers of persons.

69. A researcher wants to determine whether a new antihypertensive medication produces a significant decrease in the blood pressure of adults with moderate hypertension. What type of data measurement is blood pressure assessment?
1. In vivo
2. Invasive
3. In vitro
4. Intrusive

70. A researcher wants to determine the degree of pain experienced by persons who are not able to articulate their pain because of language limitations. What would be the most effective tool to use?
1. Questionnaire
2. Closed-ended scale
3. Visual analog
4. Likert-type scale

71. Which of the following studies would be considered an evaluation study? The researcher
1. looked at the relationship between age and level of critical thinking.
2. determined the effectiveness of a documentation protocol on quality of team cooperation.
3. studied the feasibility of establishing a day care program at a college.
4. explored the attitudes of long-term care residents toward nurses from different cultures.

72. Which of the following statements would be applicable to meta-analysis research?
1. The researcher collects data from a randomly selected sample.
2. Tools and instruments to collect data have high reliability coefficients.
3. Both primary and secondary sources are used in the literature review.
4. No new data are collected by the researcher who does the analysis.

73. Which of the following hypothetical titles suggests a methodological study? *(Note: Study titles are hypothetical)*
1. The relationship of breast-feeding and maternal-infant bonding in mothers with pre-term infants
2. The attitude towards older people scale: A reliability and validity study
3. Health control perception and health seeking behaviors: A pilot study
4. Domestic violence: A review of the literature

74. Which of the following statements is true regarding nonexperimental designs?
 1. They are strong designs to infer cause and effect.
 2. The researcher cannot actively manipulate the independent variable.
 3. They are seldom used in nursing research, particularly in clinical studies.
 4. Ethical dilemmas are not a serious concern of the researcher.

75. Hypothetical Study: A researcher wants to determine whether a new diuretic severely depletes the potassium levels of hypertensive patients. To determine K levels, blood was drawn from subjects. What type of in vitro measurement is this?
 1. Microbiologic
 2. Chemical
 3. Cytologic
 4. Physical

76. The following statement was made by researchers who investigated the agreement on falls classification: "Considering the expert classifications including all unambiguous scenarios, the sensitivity was 0.90 (SD = 0.16, n = 6,342)" (Simon et al., 2013, p. 77). What does the sensitivity number indicate?
 1. The proportion of patients who fell but did not exhibit any signs of having fallen (false negative)
 2. The proportion of patients who fell and had signs of having fallen (true positive)
 3. The proportion of patients who did not fall and had no signs of having fallen
 4. The proportion of patients who did not fall but had signs of falling

77. In a study, Kerr (2013) stated: "No previously published work has focused primarily on the perspectives or reflected an in-depth examination of decision-making from the perspective of registered nurses (RN) who use the method" (p. 110). What does this statement represent?
 1. Limitation of the study
 2. Conclusion of the study
 3. Problem statement
 4. Gap in the literature

78. "Creating a protective picture describes the three-step process that registered nurses use in deciding whether to follow a charting-by-exception policy" (Kerr, 2013, p. 110). In a grounded theory study, "creating a protective picture" is known as the __________.

79. Beeber et al. (2013) investigated "parenting enhancement, interpersonal psychotherapy to reduce depression in low-income mothers of infants and toddlers" (p. 82). The researchers stated: "Rigorous clinical depressive symptom and depression assessments and videotaped and coded interactions were used as baseline and 14-, 22-, and 26-week post-intervention measures" (p. 82). This randomized clinical trial was also a(n) __________ (type of design) as indicated by the second statement.

80. "Mothers have to be the biological parent and primary caretaker of an enrolled EHS child, speak English as their primary language, be at least 15 years of age, and be at least 6 weeks postpartum" (Beeber et al., 2013, p. 83). What does the information represent?
 1. Descriptive statistics of the sample
 2. Accessible population
 3. Sample inclusion criteria
 4. Comparison group

81. __________ judges whether the data source in historical studies is authentic. For instance, is the voice on the tape recorder really that of the person who has been identified as the one speaking?

82. What statements are correct regarding the Solomon four-group experimental design? **Select all that apply.**
1. There are two experimental and two control groups.
2. All groups are measured at baseline.
3. All groups are measured postintervention.
4. One control group is not measured at baseline, and the other control group is measured at baseline.
5. Both experimental groups are measured at baseline.

83. In a study using observation, the researcher is not concealed when assessing the effect(s) of an intervention. In this type of observation, ethical issues are not a concern, but __________ is a major issue.

84. A novice researcher asked an experienced faculty researcher to collaborate with her on a study. The novice is concerned whether he has the experience and skills to complete the project. The novice's concern is with the __________ of the study.

85. A research instrument was subjected to psychometric testing and had a Kuder-Richardson coefficient of 0.60 when it was used in a pilot study. What does the statement indicate? **Select all that apply.**
1. The coefficient results from a test of stability, an aspect of reliability.
2. The reliability coefficient is not acceptable.
3. The test is one of homogeneity, an aspect of reliability.
4. The test is used for Likert-type scales.
5. The test is used for dichotomous scales.

86. Hypothetical Study: A community health nurse wants to find out the current walking routines of the elders in a senior center. How should the nurse organize the initial data so that these are useful in planning a structured walking program? The nurse will first
1. focus on the lived experience of walking as an exercise.
2. analyze the demographic data using descriptive statistics.
3. correlate the relationship of exercise with the elders' attitudes.
4. compare the walking routines of everyone to determine which is best.

87. Which of the following hypothetical research questions is worded appropriately according to the PICO format?
1. What is the relationship of a self-efficacy building program and management of therapeutic regimen compliance by adolescents who have type 1 diabetes?
2. What is the effectiveness of a standardized educational program and success on the NCLEX-RN examination?
3. What outcomes can be expected in implementing a new method of documentation?
4. What structured program of exercise will be effective among young men with paraplegia and spinal cord injuries?

88. Which of the following hypothetical research report titles would be most useful in determining the design of the study?
1. Advanced practice roles in nursing: Nurses or junior doctors?
2. Solving the shortage of academic nurse educators
3. Lillian Wald: A pioneer in public health nursing
4. Obesity and its comorbidities

89. __________ is a process in qualitative research wherein the researcher uses one or more studies to clarify and enhance understanding of a phenomenon. Sometimes the researcher uses two sources to find another source.

90. In systematic sampling, a type of probability sampling, the researcher must calculate a(n) __________ to determine the number of elements that must be included as part of the sample.

91. A researcher wanted to determine the relationship between 24-hour lights in a newborn nursery and infants' sleep behaviors. The researcher randomly assigned 25 newborns to the experimental group or control group. This process fulfills which criteria for an experimental design? **Select all that apply.**
1. Control
2. Order
3. Generalization
4. Consistency
5. Randomization

92. The advancement of nursing through research was made possible by earlier studies such as the Lysaught Report, which was published in 1970. What recommendation from this report had a significant impact on nursing?
1. Advanced preparation is essential for the profession of nursing.
2. Professional nursing education should take place in the university setting.
3. Research focusing on clinical problems as well as nursing education is essential.
4. Research should be integrated into graduate nursing curricula.

93. Which of the following data are at the interval level of measurement?
1. Scoring on a scale: 3 = unable to feed self; 2 = needs some assistance; 1 = able to feed self
2. Information on a marital status checklist: Single, married, divorced/separated
3. Data on test scores: 90% = A; 80% = B; 70% = C. Each grade reflects a 10-point difference
4. Data: Time required to walk 1 mile: Person A = 20 minutes; person B = 40 minutes. (Person B took twice as long as person A.)

94. An inferential test known as analysis of variance (ANOVA) tests the difference among three or more groups (relative to the outcome measure or dependent variable). A researcher then looks at the variation between groups and contrasts this with variation within groups. The researcher compares the data with the _________ table to determine whether the differences are significant.

95. Which of the following are appropriate questions to ask in critiquing a qualitative study? **Select all that apply.**
1. What are the potential biases in the sampling method used?
2. How was the framework used in inking the purposes, variables, and findings of the study?
3. "Were the selected subjects able to provide data relevant to the study purpose and research questions?" (Burns & Grove, 2011, p. 444).
4. "Were the readers able to hear the voice of the participants and gain an understanding of the phenomenon studied?" (p. 446).
5. "Were the statistically significant findings also examined for clinical significance?" (p. 427).

96. Researchers who do ethnographic studies use two different approaches. The "_________" approach is the "outsider's" interpretation of the experiences of that culture—the words and concepts they use to refer to the same phenomena, (Polit & Beck, 2014, p. 269).

97. In their review of literature, Chan, Wong, Onishi, and Thayala (2011) indicated that several studies support the effects of music on depression. However, they also cited studies that found no significant relationship between music and reduction of depression. What does the second statement describe?
1. There is a gap in the research literature on the phenomenon of interest.
2. There are inconsistencies in the body of knowledge about the relationship between music and depression.
3. The research on these variables has clinical significance in health care.
4. The numbers of depressed persons who become nonfunctional deem this study a priority.

98. The researchers based their music intervention on the knowledge that music has the potential for altering mood, resulting in improved health outcomes. They also indicated that the use of the right type of music could help achieve therapeutic outcomes such as lowering levels of depression (Chan et al., 2011). What do these statements by the researchers reflect?

1. The statements reflect the aim or purpose of the proposed study.
2. The statements are part of the review of the literature.
3. The statements provide the background of the study.
4. The statements are part of the theoretical framework for the study.

99. Which of the following questions are appropriate to ask in critiquing the data analysis of a quantitative study? **Select all that apply.**

1. "Are the results for each of the research questions or hypotheses presented clearly and appropriately?" (Sullivan-Bolyai & Bova, 2011, p. 330).
2. Were the level of data measurement and sample size appropriate for the type of statistics used?
3. Did the researcher select a sample that could provide the best data on the phenomenon of interest?
4. "Is there evidence that the researcher's interpretation captured the participants' meaning?" (Barroso, 2011, p. 122).
5. "Are examples provided to guide the reader from the raw data to the researcher's synthesis?" (p. 122).

100. As a nursing student, what evidence from research would you consider important to evidence-based practice (EBP)? **Select all that apply.**

1. The study adds to the body of knowledge on a topic on which there is a dearth of information.
2. The study provides the rationale that strengthens the image of nursing as a scientific discipline.
3. The study further builds on a theory that facilitates understanding of human phenomena.
4. The study confirms the importance of research in testing interventions that could improve patient care outcomes.
5. The study provides the building blocks for more advanced research on a topic significant to practice.

ANSWERS AND RATIONALES

The correct answer number and rationale for why it is the correct answer are given in **boldface blue type**. Rationales for why the other possible answer options are incorrect also are given, but they are not in boldface type.

1. 1. The purpose statement does not indicate description as the level of purpose. Description focuses on looking at characteristics of research subjects or of a phenomenon.
2. The purpose statement does not indicate exploration as the level of purpose. Exploration involves focusing on a phenomenon and looking at factors that are relevant to it.
3. Prediction is the level of purpose expressed in the study information. Given another group of students, a researcher would anticipate a similar outcome based on previous experience. The faculty researcher had positive outcomes with the educational program and therefore can predict that the same outcomes will be seen with a new group.
4. Identification is not indicated in the level of purpose. Identification entails asking, for instance, "What is this phenomenon?" or "What will this phenomenon be called?"

TEST-TAKING TIP: The key phrase in the question stem is "to determine the effectiveness." The phrase indicates "doing something" and observing its "effects."

Content Area: *Research Purposes;* ***Cognitive Level:*** *Application;* ***Question Type:*** *Multiple Choice*
CRITICAL THINKING FACILITATOR: What are the contributions of prediction studies to EBP?

2. 1. There is no evidence that a probability sampling procedure and random assignment to groups were used.
2. Although a nonprobability sampling procedure was used, it was not convenience sampling. A convenience sample is accessible but might lack the necessary characteristics.
3. There is no evidence that a probability, systematic sampling procedure, was used. Systematic sampling involves finding a sampling interval (kth) and using this to select the research participants.
4. The study information indicates that a nonprobability, purposive sampling procedure was used. In purposive sampling, the researcher selects participants who would be the most appropriate to provide the data. In the study, the selected students were those who were unsuccessful in the course and who will participate in the educational program.

TEST-TAKING TIP: Read the statement in the study information about the sample and note how the students were selected.

Content Area: *Sampling;* ***Cognitive Level:*** *Application;* ***Question Type:*** *Multiple Choice*
CRITICAL THINKING FACILITATOR: What are the possible biases in the sampling procedure used in the study?

3. 1. The study information does not indicate a phenomenological approach as an appropriate possible design. This study is not about the lived experience, which is the focus of a phenomenological study.
2. A "before and after" quasi-experimental design is possible. Students' course outcomes before they come into the course will be compared with the outcomes after their participation in the educational program. In addition, the sample was selected using a nonprobability approach, which precludes an experimental design.
3. Although a longitudinal design can be added, this was not indicated in the study information.
4. A descriptive design is not possible because there is an intervention (cause) and an expected outcome, the dependent variable (effect).

TEST-TAKING TIP: Reread the first statement of the research case study. After you identify an independent variable and a dependent variable, then you know that the design is some type of an experimental design. You can eliminate a true experimental design when you see that the study does not meet the three requirements of an experimental design.

Content Area: *Research Design;* ***Cognitive Level:*** *Application;* ***Question Type:*** *Multiple Choice*
CRITICAL THINKING FACILITATOR: What are the common action words (verbs) used in experimental and quasi-experimental designs? Knowing these words will help you determine a study's design from its abstract or title.

4. 1. The success of students is the outcome, or the dependent variable, because it is the variable the researcher is interested in predicting. The success of students *depends* on the manipulated, or independent, variable.
2. The educational program is the independent variable because this is "the

variable that is believed to cause or influence the dependent variable" (Polit & Beck, 2014, p. 382).
3. The unsuccessful students are the study sample.
4. The relationship is "the bond or connection of two or more variables" (p. 390).

TEST-TAKING TIP: The key phrase in the question stem is "educational program." This is an intervention, program, or approach—a type of independent variable.

Content Area: *Quantitative Studies;* ***Cognitive Level:*** *Application;* ***Question Type:*** *Multiple Choice*
CRITICAL THINKING FACILITATOR: Think of potential research studies based on your clinical experience. Write a sample research question and identify your variables. If you have a study partner, share this exercise.

5. 1. Description is not indicated in the study information. Studies that have description as a level of purpose focus on looking at "characteristics or circumstances and/or the frequency with which certain phenomena occur" (Polit & Beck, 2014, p. 379).
2. **Prediction is the level of purpose of the study. Prediction means "estimation of the probability of a specific outcome in a given situation that can be achieved through research" (Burns & Grove, 2011, p. 544). The researchers hypothesized the effect of the independent variable (music) on the dependent variable (depression).**
3. Exploration as the level of purpose is not indicated by the study information. Exploration entails "examining the data descriptively to become as familiar as possible" (p. 538).
4. Identification is not the level of purpose communicated in the study information. Identification is a level of purpose used by qualitative researchers to "study phenomena about which little is known. In some cases, so little is known that the phenomenon has yet to be clearly identified or named or has been inadequately defined" (Polit & Beck, 2014, pp. 11–12).

TEST-TAKING TIP: The key phrase in the study information is "to determine the effects." The phrase suggests a study with independent and dependent variables. The researchers would do something to (manipulate) the independent variable and try to anticipate (predict) the outcome.

Content Area: *Quantitative Studies;* ***Cognitive Level:*** *Analysis;* ***Question Type:*** *Multiple Choice*
CRITICAL THINKING FACILITATOR: What contributions to EBP do predictive studies make?

6. 1. The right to freedom from harm and discomfort is not evident in the study information.
2. **The right to privacy was addressed and is in evidence in the study information.**
3. The right to fair treatment is not described in the study information.
4. The right to protection from exploitation is only implied in the study information.

TEST-TAKING TIP: The key statement in the study information is "participant information is identified only by case number." This means that the identity of the research participants is not revealed, and this protects their privacy.

Content Area: *Ethics in Research;* ***Cognitive Level:*** *Comprehension;* ***Question Type:*** *Multiple Choice*
CRITICAL THINKING FACILITATOR: What are the other ways of protecting the identity of research participants?

7. 1. **In an RCT, the independent variable is manipulated to see its effect on the dependent variable. One group gets a variation of the independent variable, and the other group gets another variation. Group data are then compared to determine differences that can be attributed to the independent variable.**
2. **An RCT has the most stringent requirements to control biases of every kind. Controls are also imposed so that study findings are valid. Random assignment eliminates sample bias by ensuring homogeneity of subjects in comparison groups.**
3. Power is defined as "the ability of a design or analysis strategy to detect true relationships that exist among variables" (Polit & Beck, 2014, p. 388). An RCT would aim to have this, but the study information does not provide this information.
4. The study information did not include information on all the requirements for a research instrument.

TEST-TAKING TIP: The key phrase in the question stem is "randomized clinical trial." RCTs are high up in the hierarchy of research designs; therefore, they must meet all the requirements for the study to have validity.

Content Area: *Quantitative Studies;* ***Cognitive Level:*** *Analysis;* ***Question Type:*** *Multiple Response*
CRITICAL THINKING FACILITATOR: What are the contributions of randomized clinical trials to EBP?

8. 1. This statement is not true. Cronbach's alpha is not a test of validity. It is a test for establishing reliability. Cronbach's alpha "estimates the internal consistency of a measure composed of several subparts" (Polit & Beck, 2014, p. 379).
   2. This statement is not true. Cronbach's alpha is a test of internal consistency, an aspect of reliability.
   3. **This statement is true because the range is acceptable. "A level of 0.70 or higher is considered to be an acceptable level of reliability" (Sullivan-Bolyai & Bova, 2011, p. 295).**
   4. **This statement is true because Cronbach's alpha is a test of internal consistency, an aspect of reliability.**
   5. **The statement is true. Reliability means "the degree to which a measurement is free from measurement error—its accuracy and consistency" (Polit & Beck, 2014, p. 391).**

TEST-TAKING TIP: A clue in the research study information is "0.88 to 0.91." Additionally, the statement describes a research instrument. These details indicate a characteristic, and the number is the coefficient.

Content Area: *Quantitative Studies;* ***Cognitive Level:*** *Analysis;* ***Question Type:*** *Multiple Response*

CRITICAL THINKING FACILITATOR:
Recall the different tests for reliability.

9. 1. **The hypothesis is simple because it has one independent variable, music, and one dependent variable, depression levels.**
   2. The proposed hypothesis is not nondirectional. A nondirectional hypothesis only states that there is a relationship between two variables, but it does not specify the direction of the relationship.
   3. The proposed hypothesis is not a null hypothesis because a null hypothesis proposes that there is no relationship between the two variables.
   4. The proposed hypothesis is not complex because a complex hypothesis has more than one independent or dependent variable.
   5. **The proposed hypothesis is a directional one because the relationship of the two variables is specified.**

TEST-TAKING TIP: A clue in the research study information is "lower depression levels," which indicates a direction.

Content Area: *Research Hypothesis;* ***Cognitive Level:*** *Application;* ***Question Type:*** *Multiple Response*

CRITICAL THINKING FACILITATOR:
How do directional hypotheses emerge? What is a study's level of purpose when a directional hypothesis is proposed?

10. 1. The situation described is not a threat to external validity, specifically the sampling plan. Such a threat relates to the generalizability of findings. If the sampling plan does not yield a representative sample, then generalizability becomes an issue.
    2. **The situation described is a threat to internal validity. Internal validity is the "extent to which it can be inferred that the independent variable is truly causing the outcome" (Polit & Beck, 2014, p. 167). A threat to internal validity is history. This can be any event or situation occurring at the same time that can influence the outcome.**
    3. The situation described is not a selection threat. A selection threat to internal validity "reflects biases stemming from preexisting differences between groups. When people are not assigned randomly to groups, the groups being compared may not be equivalent" (p. 168). Differences between the groups might account for the difference in the outcome and not the independent variable.
    4. The Hawthorne effect, a threat to external validity, is not the threat described. The Hawthorne effect is "the effect on the dependent variable resulting from subjects' awareness that they are participants under study" (p. 381).

TEST-TAKING TIP: The key phrase in the question stem is "during the course of the study." This implies an event or situation occurring at the same time as the study.

Content Area: *Internal and External Validity;* ***Cognitive Level:*** *Analysis;* ***Question Type:*** *Multiple Choice*

CRITICAL THINKING FACILITATOR:
Let's say there is a study in progress in your facility regarding the effectiveness of a program on breastfeeding. During the course of this study, what could be potential threats to internal validity?

11. symptom resolution

TEST-TAKING TIP: Recall what the acronym PICO stands for. The outcome is a symptom resolution from AOM.

Content Area: *PICO Format;* ***Cognitive Level:*** *Application;* ***Question Type:*** *Fill-in-the-Blank*

CRITICAL THINKING FACILITATOR:
Identify the PIC in the study.

12. 1. The statement does not describe blinding.
2. The statement refers to confidentiality.
3. **The statement describes blinding. The research team member implements the intervention, the independent variable, to the participants without knowing the group assignment of each participant.**
4. The statement does not describe blinding. The statement might indicate lack of knowledge of the research hypothesis.

TEST-TAKING TIP: The key word in the question stem is "blinding." *Blinding* is derived from the word *blind*, which means "unable to see" or "hidden."

Content Area: *Research Controls;* ***Cognitive Level:*** *Comprehension;* ***Question Type:*** *Multiple Choice*
CRITICAL THINKING FACILITATOR:
What potential bias can be prevented by using a blinding procedure in implementing the research intervention?

13. 1. A correlation is not appropriate at this time because the researcher is not ready to look at the relationship between variables.
2. **The researcher could appropriately do an exploratory study to find out what influences self-efficacy behaviors.**
3. A quasi-experimental study would not be appropriate at this time because there is no intervention, or independent variable, to be manipulated. In addition, the level of purpose is exploration and not prediction.
4. An ethnographic study is not appropriate because the purpose of the researcher is to explore and not to study the culture of diabetics.

TEST-TAKING TIP: The key word in the question stem is "factors." A factor is an element or situation that may produce an "outcome" such as self-efficacy.

Content Area: *Exploratory Research;* ***Cognitive Level:*** *Application;* ***Question Type:*** *Multiple Choice*
CRITICAL THINKING FACILITATOR:
Why are there factors and not variables in exploratory studies?

14. 1. **A next follow-up study would be a correlation. The researcher could do one or more correlational studies to determine the presence of a relationship between an identified factor with self-efficacy.**
2. The researcher cannot do a quasi-experimental study because there needs to be an intervention (an independent variable) for this type of study.
3. A descriptive study is not appropriate as a follow up study because the researcher needs to find relationship of each factor to the phenomenon of interest, self-efficacy.
4. A phenomenological study is not appropriate because the researcher is not focusing on the lived experience of the diabetics.

TEST-TAKING TIP: The key word in the question stem is "follow-up." As the researcher learns more about the phenomenon of interest, he or she focuses on gaining even more knowledge. The researcher's level of purpose and study designs become more complex.

Content Area: *Correlational Research;* ***Cognitive Level:*** *Application;* ***Question Type:*** *Multiple Choice*
CRITICAL THINKING FACILITATOR:
What are the different relationships between variables that can be studied using a correlation?

15. 1. **A simple hypothesis would be appropriate. It would state a relationship between two variables.**
2. A directional hypothesis would not be appropriate because there is still only preliminary knowledge and variables have not been identified.
3. **In this first follow-up study, the hypothesis would be nondirectional. Not enough is known about the variables to predict the direction of the hypothesis.**
4. **A complex hypothesis could be appropriate based on the findings of the exploratory study (multiple factors influencing self-efficacy).**
5. It would not be appropriate to have no hypothesis because there is some knowledge about the relationship between variables.

TEST-TAKING TIP: The key word in the question stem is "hypothesis." A hypothesis is a statement of relationship between two or more variables.

Content Area: *Research Hypothesis;* ***Cognitive Level:*** *Application;* ***Question Type:*** *Multiple Response*
CRITICAL THINKING FACILITATOR:
How are hypotheses deduced from a theory?

16. 1. Random assignment to groups is a measure to eliminate bias. Random assignment is not reflected in the situation.
2. **Manipulation is defined as the process whereby the experimenter does something (some type of intervention) to some subjects.**
3. Observation of the dependent variable is measurement.

4. Designing the intervention is part of preparing for the study to ensure intervention fidelity.

TEST-TAKING TIP: The second and third statements of the situation indicate that the two groups of research participants got something different. These statements mean that something was changed.

Content Area: *Quantitative Studies;* ***Cognitive Level:*** *Application;* ***Question Type:*** *Multiple Choice*
CRITICAL THINKING FACILITATOR:
What are the different ways of manipulating the independent variable?

17. quasi-experimental

TEST-TAKING TIP: The key phrase in the question stem is "not able to use a probability sampling procedure." This means that this requirement for a true experimental design would be missing.

Content Area: *Quantitative Studies;* ***Cognitive Level:*** *Comprehension;* ***Question Type:*** *Fill-in-the-Blank*
CRITICAL THINKING FACILITATOR:
Compare the inference of causality between experimental and quasi-experimental designs.

18. 1. The research information is not an implication for practice. An implication is "the meaning of research conclusions for the body of knowledge, theory, and practice" (Burns & Grove, 2011, p. 539).
2. **The research information is considered a recommendation. A recommendation is a "suggestion provided by a study's researcher for ways to design a better study next time" (p. 346).**
3. The information does not indicate a limitation. Limitations include "theoretical or methodological restrictions in a study that may decrease the generalizability of the findings" (p. 541).
4. The study information is not a conclusion. Conclusions are "syntheses and clarifications of the meanings of the study findings" (p. 534).

TEST-TAKING TIP: The key phrase in the study information is "continuing research." The phrase implies something that needs to be done for future studies.

Content Area: *Discussion of Findings;* ***Cognitive Level:*** *Application;* ***Question Type:*** *Multiple Choice*
CRITICAL THINKING FACILITATOR:
What benefits do researchers gain from the discussion section of a study?

19. 1. Data saturation is not indicated by the statement. Data saturation is the "point when data collection can cease" (LoBiondo-Wood & Haber, 2010, p. 576).
2. A theme is not indicated in the statement. "A theme is a label that represents a way of describing large quantities of data in a condensed manner" (p. 587).
3. **Rigor in qualitative research consists of credibility, dependability, confirmability, and transferability (Polit & Beck, 2014). In the study information, credibility was established when the researcher asked the participants about the identified themes in the analysis.**
4. A qualitative researcher must consider and acknowledge her or his own feelings, thoughts, and perceptions. However, this is not what is indicated in the information

TEST-TAKING TIP: The second statement is a key one. The process of asking participants about the theme is an act of confirming the data. This process is part of establishing rigor in qualitative studies.

Content Area: *Rigor in Qualitative Research;* ***Cognitive Level:*** *Analysis;* ***Question Type:*** *Multiple Choice*
CRITICAL THINKING FACILITATOR:
What are the other ways of establishing rigor in qualitative studies?

20. 1. The statement is not a recommendation. A recommendation is a suggestion for "ways to design a better study next time" (Burns & Grove, 2011, p. 546).
2. The statement is not a limitation. Limitations are "theoretical or methodological restrictions in a study that may decrease the generalizability of the findings" (p. 541).
3. **The statement is part of the conclusion. Conclusions are "syntheses and clarifications of meanings of study findings" (p. 534).**
4. The statement is not data analysis which includes the "technique to reduce, organize, and give meaning to the data" (p. 535).

TEST-TAKING TIP: The key word in the research information is "indicate," which means to make known. In this instance, it is to make known the judgment of the researchers based on evidence.

Content Area: *Study Discussion;* ***Cognitive Level:*** *Application;* ***Question Type:*** *Multiple Choice*
CRITICAL THINKING FACILITATOR:
How do research consumers use the conclusions of researchers in relation to EBP?

21. 1. Self-selection would not be considered an ethical issue because the persons involved

are exercising their right to self-determination by opting to participate.
2. The information does not indicate there is difficulty in recruiting subjects.
3. The information describes a limitation of the study, and there is mention of systematic bias. Limitations are "theoretical or methodological restrictions in a study that may decrease the generalizability of the findings" (Burns & Grove, 2011, p. 541).
4. The information is not descriptive of quota sampling, which is a "non-random sampling method in which 'quotas' for certain subgroups based on sample characteristics are established to increase the representativeness of the sample" (Polit & Beck, 2014, p. 389).

TEST-TAKING TIP: The key phrase in the second statement is "will dominate." This implies the limited applicability of the findings to other persons.

Content Area: *Sampling Concepts;* ***Cognitive Level:*** *Analysis;* ***Question Type:*** *Multiple Choice*
CRITICAL THINKING FACILITATOR:
What is the value of identifying a study's limitations?

22. **1. The study information indicates that there were at least two comparison groups.**
2. The test performed is a parametric one. The t test is used to "determine significant differences between measures of two samples" (Burns & Grove, 2011, p. 552).
3. The outcome, or dependent variable, is the data analyzed from the groups.
4. The design of the study is not nonexperimental because the study information indicated that there was an outcome that was measured.
5. The statement is not indicated by the information. Groups were compared at baseline, which means before the intervention.

TEST-TAKING TIP: The key phrase in the statement is "t test." Recall the rationale for using this test.

Content Area: *Inferential Analysis;* ***Cognitive Level:*** *Analysis;* ***Question Type:*** *Multiple Response*
CRITICAL THINKING FACILITATOR:
What are the other statistical procedures that can test for differences in groups?

23. **themes**

TEST-TAKING TIP: The key phrase in the research study information is "lived experience of myeloma." Recall the process of analyzing qualitative data in phenomenological and grounded theory studies.

Content Area: *Data in Qualitative Studies;* ***Cognitive Level:*** *Application;* ***Question Type:*** *Fill-in-the-Blank*
CRITICAL THINKING FACILITATOR:
How does the qualitative researcher come up with themes, and how are these supported by the data?

24. 1. The study information is not indicative of clinical practice guidelines. Practice guidelines are "evidence-based; combining a synthesis and an appraisal of research evidence with specific recommendations for clinical decisions" (Polit & Beck, 2014, p. 376).
2. The study information does not indicate a review of literature, which is a "summary of theoretical and empirical sources to generate a picture of what is known and not known about a particular problem" (Burns & Grove, 2011, p. 547).
3. The study information is not indicative of a meta-synthesis, which is a "synthesis of qualitative research involving the critical analysis of primary qualitative studies and synthesis of findings into a new theory or framework for the topic of interest" (p. 541).
4. A meta-analysis is indicated in the study information. A meta-analysis focuses on "performing statistical analyses to integrate and synthesize findings from completed studies to determine what is known or not known about a particular research area" (p. 541).

TEST-TAKING TIP: The key phrase in the research study information is "synthesis of all controlled and uncontrolled studies." This phrase focuses on quantitative studies. Also look at key words in the options. Option 1 is a practice guideline, option 2 is a summary, and option 3 is focused on qualitative studies.

Content Area: *Meta-analysis;* ***Cognitive Level:*** *Application;* ***Question Type:*** *Multiple Choice*
CRITICAL THINKING FACILITATOR:
Why is a meta-analysis study placed close to the top of the hierarchy of evidence for EBP?

25. 1. The statement is incorrect because the study is not a phenomenological one.
2. The statement is incorrect because the study is not a grounded theory study.
3. The statement is correct because the study is a historical one. Interviews and

oral histories are methods of obtaining data from sources.

4. The statement is incorrect because the study is not an ethnographic one.

TEST-TAKING TIP: The key word in the research study information is "pioneers," which means people who are first in doing something. The pioneers made their contributions in the past.

Content Area: *Historical Method;* ***Cognitive Level:*** *Application;* ***Question Type:*** *Multiple Choice*
CRITICAL THINKING FACILITATOR:
What are the contributions of historical studies to EBP?

26. 1. The information is not the question of the study. An interrogative statement, or research question, includes the variables and the population to be studied, and it "implies possibility of empirical testing" (Haber, 2010, p. 34).
2. The information is not the study's conclusion. Conclusions are "syntheses and the meanings of the study's findings" (Burns & Grove, 2011, p. 534).
3. The information describes the significance of the study. Significance "indicates the importance of the problem to nursing and health care and to the health of individuals, families and communities" (p. 549).
4. The information is not the study's purpose. A purpose is a "clear, concise statement of the specific goal or focus of a study" (p. 146).

TEST-TAKING TIP: The key word in the research study information is "essential," which means highly important.

Content Area: *Significance of a Study;* ***Cognitive Level:*** *Comprehension;* ***Question Type:*** *Multiple Choice*
CRITICAL THINKING FACILITATOR:
When you read the introduction of a research study report, where do you focus your initial attention and why?

27. 1. The statement is not a hypothesis. A hypothesis states a relationship between two or more variables.
2. The statement is not a conclusion. Conclusions are "syntheses and clarifications of the meanings of study data" (Burns & Grove, 2011, p. 534).
3. The statement is part of the study's conceptual model. A conceptual model "broadly explains phenomena of interest, expresses assumptions, and reflects a philosophical stance" (p. 228).
4. The statement does not indicate the significance of the study because *significance* means the importance of the study.

TEST-TAKING TIP: The key phrase in the statement is "guiding statements." Researchers would use the conceptual model to propose a hypothesis about the phenomenon of interest.

Content Area: *Conceptual Models;* ***Cognitive Level:*** *Application;* ***Question Type:*** *Multiple Choice*
CRITICAL THINKING FACILITATOR:
What are the components of a conceptual model, and how are they used in a study?

28. 1. The information is not a gap. A gap is an interruption or something missing on the topic.
2. The information is an inconsistency in the literature reviewed for a study. An inconsistency is a finding that is different from findings of other studies. The researcher who does an objective review must present gaps, consistencies, and inconsistencies.
3. The information is not a conclusion because a conclusion gives the study findings meaning in relation to current knowledge on the topic.
4. The information is not the statement of the problem. The statement of the problem is a basis for the study.

TEST-TAKING TIP: The key phrase in the statement is "however, other studies found," which means other findings are not the same as the previously mentioned ones.

Content Area: *Review of the Literature;* ***Cognitive Level:*** *Comprehension;* ***Question Type:*** *Multiple Choice*
CRITICAL THINKING FACILITATOR:
Relative to EBP, how are inconsistencies in study findings addressed?

29. power analysis

TEST-TAKING TIP: The key phrase in the statement is "a sample of 34 to detect a large interaction effect."

Content Area: *Analysis of Quantitative Findings;* ***Cognitive Level:*** *Comprehension;* ***Question Type:*** *Fill-in-the-Blank*
CRITICAL THINKING FACILITATOR:
Review the concept of a type II error and its relation to effect size.

30. **1. The statement is applicable because one of the designs of the study is an**

RCT. One of the requirements of this design is the manipulation of an independent variable and the observation of its effects on a dependent variable.

2. **There would be at least two groups to compare. Even in a one-group pre- and post-RCT, there will be "two" groups, in which the experimental group acts as its own control (preintervention).**
3. **The statement is applicable because the study is also a longitudinal design; this means multiple data collection periods are needed to observe the duration of the effects of the intervention.**
4. The statement is not applicable because in randomized clinical trials, the sampling is probability.
5. The design of the study calls for multiple methods of data collection and not just interviews. Quantitative measurements will be appropriate data collection methods.

TEST-TAKING TIP: The key phrase in the information is "randomized longitudinal intervention trial." Recall requirements of a randomized clinical trial and a longitudinal study.

Content Area: *Quantitative Research Designs;* ***Cognitive Level:*** *Analysis;* ***Question Type:*** *Multiple Response*

CRITICAL THINKING FACILITATOR:

What is the purpose of combining two designs in one study?

31. 1. The information is not the study's aim or purpose. The purpose states the "researcher's summary of the overall goal" (Polit & Beck, 2014, p. 100).

2. The information is not the research question. Research questions are "specific queries researchers want to answer, which guide the types of data to be collected in a study" (p. 100).
3. The information is not a theme. A theme is a "recurring regularity emerging from the analysis of qualitative data" (p. 393).
4. **The information is a statement of the need for the study because it provides the rationale for the doing the study.**

TEST-TAKING TIP: The key word in the study information is "critical," which means pressing or urgent.

Content Area: *Research Introductory Concepts;* ***Cognitive Level:*** *Application;* ***Question Type:*** *Multiple Choice*

CRITICAL THINKING FACILITATOR:

Think of a clinical problem and the rationale for studying it.

32. 1. The study information does not indicate participatory action research. This is a type of research that is "based on the premise that the use and production of knowledge can be political and used to exert power" (Polit & Beck, 2014, p. 387).

2. The study information does not indicate the study is an ethnographic one. Ethnography "focuses on the culture of a group of people, with an effort to understand the world view and customs of those under study" (p. 380).
3. **The study information indicates this is a case study. The case study is a "method involving a thorough, in-depth analysis of an individual, group, or other social unit" (p. 375).**
4. The information is not indicative of a phenomenological study because it is not about people's lived experience.

TEST-TAKING TIP: The key phrase in the study information is "focused on families."

Content Area: *Qualitative Designs;* ***Cognitive Level:*** *Application;* ***Question Type:*** *Multiple Choice*

CRITICAL THINKING FACILITATOR:

What are the contributions of case studies to EBP?

33. 1. The statement does not indicate the study was historical. A historical study looks at past events and their relationships to the present.

2. The statement does not indicate the study was an ethnographic one. An ethnographic study looks at the culture of a group in order to understand the perspectives, customs, and traditions of that group.
3. **The statement indicates that this study is a phenomenological one. The lived experience is the focus of phenomenology.**
4. A grounded theory study is not indicated in the statement. A grounded theory study focuses on a psychological or social process.

TEST-TAKING TIP: The key phrase in the question stem is "lived experience," which is a focus of phenomenology.

Content Area: *Qualitative Studies;* ***Cognitive Level:*** *Application;* ***Question Type:*** *Multiple Choice*

CRITICAL THINKING FACILITATOR:

What is the end product of a study that focuses on the lived experience?

34. 1. The study is a qualitative one, and therefore a probability sampling procedure is not appropriate. Probability sampling procedures ensure a representative sample;

representativeness is not a concern in qualitative study. A qualitative study has other requirements to meet validity.

2. A convenience sample is not appropriate because it consists of those who are ready and available. These persons might not have the lived experience that is the focus of the study.
3. **A purposive sample would be appropriate because the selection of the subjects would be based on who can provide information about the lived experience.**
4. Research participants in the study are not called subjects. The term is more appropriate in quantitative studies when something is done to cause something or "subjecting the person to an intervention."
5. **The participants selected will share their experiences with the researcher through in-depth descriptions of their lived experience.**

TEST-TAKING TIP: Think of the focus of the study and determine how to best answer the research question.

Content Area: *Qualitative Studies;* ***Cognitive Level:*** *Comprehension;* ***Question Type:*** *Multiple Response*

CRITICAL THINKING FACILITATOR:
Review all the different types of sampling procedures for qualitative studies. If you were a researcher, where could you recruit participants for different types of studies?

35. 1. The stability and reliability of the SATs are not the issues. Reliability has to do with consistency, and stability is an aspect of reliability.

2. The SATs have been the standardized test (well-established reliability and validity) used as an admission criterion for other programs. The program used it for lack of other standardized examinations.
3. **The statement was the rationale given for discontinuing use of the SATs. The program administration and faculty deemed the examination as an inappropriate (not valid) measure to predict success in the doctoral program.**
4. The statement was not the rationale because the SATs are reliable tests.

TEST-TAKING TIP: The key word in the situation is "criterion." This term is relevant to validity. The validity of a research instrument is "the degree to which an instrument measures what it is supposed to measure" (Polit & Beck, 2014, p. 394). One type of validity is called criterion-related validity defined as "the degree to which scores on an instrument are correlated with an external criterion" (p. 378). In the situation given, the external criterion is success in the program.

Content Area: *Validity of Research Instruments;* ***Cognitive Level:*** *Application;* ***Question Type:*** *Multiple Choice*

CRITICAL THINKING FACILITATOR:
What is the relationship between an instrument's reliability and its validity?

36. 1. Use of the total population is not implied in the situation. The total population would include all members.

2. Use of the target population is not implied in the situation. The target population is "the entire population in which a researcher is interested and to which he or she would like to generalize the study results" (Polit & Beck, 2014, p. 393).
3. The term *quota* is relevant to the sample, not the population.
4. **An accessible population is described in the situation. An accessible population is "the population available for a study, often a nonrandom subset of the target population" (Polit & Beck, 2014, p. 374).**

TEST-TAKING TIP: The key phrase in the situation is "recruit from six outpatient clinics." This phrase indicates those settings where the researcher can have access to patients who report to the clinic.

Content Area: *Concepts in Sampling;* ***Cognitive Level:*** *Application;* ***Question Type:*** *Multiple Choice*

CRITICAL THINKING FACILITATOR:
What effects would using an accessible population have on the validity of study findings?

37. 1. **The person's right to self-determination is evident in the statement. This right protects a person's ability to decide whether to participate or not.**

2. This right is not indicated in the statement. This right prevents or minimizes harm to research participants.
3. This right is not evident in the statement. This right includes protection of the individual's identity and information about him or her.
4. The right to fair treatment is not evident in the statement. This right has to do with "equitable distribution of benefits and burdens" (Polit & Beck, 2014, p. 85).

TEST-TAKING TIP: The key word in the question stem is "opted." To opt means to decide.

Content Area:** Ethics in Research;* ***Cognitive Level: *Application;* ***Question Type:*** *Multiple Choice*
CRITICAL THINKING FACILITATOR:
What other actions of participants indicate the exercise of the right to self-determination?

38. 1. The concept of an adequate sample is not consistent in a phenomenological study because this is a type of qualitative study.
2. The statement explains why the researcher stopped data collection. Data saturation "occurs when the information being shared with the researcher becomes repetitive. Ideas conveyed by the participant have been shared before by other participants; inclusion of additional participants does not result in new ideas" (LoBiondo-Wood & Haber, 2010, pp. 575-576).
3. This is not the correct rationale for stopping data collection.
4. The statement is not applicable in the study. The depth and quality of the information collected are possible by asking relevant questions about the experience regarding the phenomenon of interest.

TEST-TAKING TIP: The key phrase in the study information is "phenomenological study." Recall that this study is qualitative and that the naturalistic paradigm guides the research.

Content Area:** Qualitative Studies;* ***Cognitive Level: *Application;* ***Question Type:*** *Multiple Choice*
CRITICAL THINKING FACILITATOR:
Compare and contrast data collection and analysis between qualitative and quantitative approaches to research.

39. comparison

TEST-TAKING TIP: Recall the initial steps in a study. The research question asked in a quantitative study has similar components to the PICO format.

Content Area:** PICO Format;* ***Cognitive Level: *Knowledge;* ***Question Type:*** *Fill-in-the-Blank*
CRITICAL THINKING FACILITATOR:
Look at a sample research question and see whether you can identify its PICO.

40. 1. The study information does not indicate the study is ethnographic because its focus is not the culture of a group.
2. The study information does not indicate that it is a case study. A case study is "a method involving a thorough, in-depth analysis of an individual, group, or other social unit" (Polit & Beck, 2014, p. 375).
3. The study information indicates that the study is a historical one. The beginning of midwifery as an area of nursing practice is a past event. The study and analysis of a past event is the focus of historical studies.
4. The study information does not indicate the study is a grounded theory one. A grounded theory study focuses on a social process.

TEST-TAKING TIP: The key word in the statement is "emergence," which means the beginning or rise of something in the past.

Content Area:** Historical Study;* ***Cognitive Level: *Application;* ***Question Type:*** *Multiple Choice*
CRITICAL THINKING FACILITATOR:
What are the contributions of historical studies to nursing and EBP?

41. **1. The statement is accurate. Data collection strategies include "interviewing and observations" (Polit & Beck, 2014, p. 277). Other methods include "storytelling, socio-drama, photography, drawing, skits, and other activities designed to encourage people to find creative ways to explore their lives, tell their stories, and recognize their own strengths" (p. 277).**
2. Groups in the community are the research participants and not just individuals familiar with the political machinery.
3. This is an accurate statement about PAR.
4. The principal investigator(s) might not always be member(s) of the community. He or she could be an individual outside the community who has a commitment to the community (e.g., a nurse researcher who has health-related ties with the community).
5. This is an accurate statement about PAR.

TEST-TAKING TIP: The key phrase in the question stem is "participatory action research." ***Participatory,*** **derived from "participate," means to work with others. The work might be a project or activity that would benefit the group.** ***Action,*** **as its used here, indicates doing something to energize and mobilize.**

Content Area:** Participatory Action Research;* ***Cognitive Level: *Comprehension;* ***Question Type:*** *Multiple Response*
CRITICAL THINKING FACILITATOR: In your community, what potential health-related issues can be addressed using PAR? Some examples

are substance abuse, obesity, and lack of health-care resources.

42. **1. A retrospective design would be appropriate. A retrospective design is a "study design that begins with the manifestations of the outcome variable in the present (e.g., lung cancer) followed by a search for a presumed cause occurring in the past (e.g., cigarette smoking)." In the situation, lowered cholesterol levels are seen in the present. The nurse practitioner will have to look at possible factors that caused these lowered levels (Polit & Beck, 2014, p. 391).**
2. A descriptive study would not be appropriate. A descriptive study would focus on an "accurate portrayal of people's characteristics or circumstances and/or the frequency with which certain phenomena occur" (p. 379).
3. A correlation would not be used because the two variables to be correlated have not been identified.
4. A prospective study would not be appropriate at this time. A prospective design is a "study design that begins with an examination of a presumed cause (e.g., cigarette smoking) and then goes forward in time to observe presumed effects (e.g., lung cancer)" (p. 389).

TEST-TAKING TIP: The key phrases in the situation are "has noted" and "lowered cholesterol levels." Note the referral to the past in these two phrases.

Content Area: *Retrospective Research;* ***Cognitive Level:*** *Application;* ***Question Type:*** *Multiple Choice*
CRITICAL THINKING FACILITATOR:
What are possible biases in doing a retrospective study? When is it a design of choice?

43. **1. A primary source includes "scholarly literature that is written by person(s) who developed the theory or conducted the research" (LoBiondo-Wood & Haber, 2011, p. 583). A meta-analysis synthesizes the findings of many studies and presents a conclusion of these studies. Studies used are primary sources.**
2. The meta-analysis does not use secondary sources because it has to look at the results of primary sources in order to synthesize these and write a conclusion about the topic that is the focus of all the studies included.
3. Theoretical literature is not included because the focus is on synthesizing the results of multiple studies on the same topic.
4. Not all journals publish research studies. Only publications that present research studies can be used.
5. **Data-based literature includes "reports of completed research studies" (p. 576). These studies are the foci of the meta-analysis article.**

TEST-TAKING TIP: The key word in the question stem is "meta-analysis." The prefix *meta-* means "beyond." In this instance, meta-analysis means beyond one study.

Content Area: *Meta-analysis;* ***Cognitive Level:*** *Comprehension;* ***Question Type:*** *Multiple Response*
CRITICAL THINKING FACILITATOR:
What are the contributions of meta-analysis articles to EBP?

44. **1. A literature review identifies gaps in the topic. These gaps are essential in identifying what needs to be done to continue building the knowledge base on the topic.**
2. Reliable and valid instruments can be discovered through a literature review. Why reinvent the wheel? Continued use of research instruments strengthens their positive properties.
3. The literature review does not provide the rationale for funding. The significance and potential contributions of the study to the profession and its clientele are most important for funding.
4. Conceptual traditions used by other researchers are identified in a literature review. Research studies further strengthen the conceptual models that in turn refine the models in understanding phenomena of interest to nursing.
5. Impressions are not purposes in a literature review because they present subjective information.

TEST-TAKING TIP: The key phrase in the question stem is "literature review." Recall that the researcher who plans to do a study must go through the conceptual phase (conceiving the study). A literature review will provide information on the current state of the phenomenon of interest.

Content Area: *Phases in a Quantitative Study;* ***Cognitive Level:*** *Knowledge;* ***Question Type:*** *Multiple Response*

CRITICAL THINKING FACILITATOR:
How does a researcher present a useful literature review in her or his study?

45. 1. Establishing reliability of measurement is not indicated in the statement. This process entails looking at the characteristics of the data collection tools.

2. Controlling extraneous variables is indicated by the statement. If the groups in the study are not equal with regards to specified criteria, a potential bias from the difference would result. This bias would be considered an extraneous variable.

3. The statement does not indicate that there is a threat to internal validity.

4. The statement does not relate to the adequacy of the sample.

TEST-TAKING TIP: The key phrase in the statement is "be considered ineligible." Recall the reasons for using eligibility criteria or inclusion criteria in selecting a sample.

Content Area: *Sampling in Quantitative Studies;* ***Cognitive Level:*** *Application;* ***Question Type:*** *Multiple Choice*

CRITICAL THINKING FACILITATOR:
What are the other sources of extraneous variables in sampling?

46. intervention fidelity

TEST-TAKING TIP: The key phrase the statement is "carefully developed, trained, and observed." All of these actions relate to the intervention.

Content Area: *Intervention Fidelity in Quantitative Studies;* ***Cognitive Level:*** *Application;* ***Question Type:*** *Fill-in-the-Blank.*

CRITICAL THINKING FACILITATOR:
How is validity of study findings affected by intervention fidelity?

47. 1. The statement does not describe an independent variable. An independent variable is "the treatment or experimental activity that is manipulated or varied by the researcher to cause an effect on the dependent variable" (Burns & Grove, 2011, p. 539).

2. The statement does not describe the dependent variable. A dependent variable is "the response, behavior, or outcome that is predicted or explained in research" (p. 536).

3. The statement is an operational definition. An operational definition is a "description of how variables or concepts will be measured or manipulated in a study" (p. 543).

4. The statement is not a conceptual definition. A conceptual definition "provides a variable or concept with connotative (abstract, comprehensive, theoretical) meaning" (p. 534).

TEST-TAKING TIP: The key phrase in the statement is "as measured," which refers to a data collection tool.

Content Area: *Operational Definitions;* ***Cognitive Level:*** *Comprehension;* ***Question Type:*** *Multiple Choice*

CRITICAL THINKING FACILITATOR:
Do all variables in different studies use the same operational definitions?

48. 1. The information does not indicate that the study is basic. Basic research is "research designed to extend the knowledge base in a discipline for the sake of knowledge production or theory construction, rather than solving an immediate problem" (Polit & Beck, 2014, p. 375).

2. The information indicates the study is applied. Applied research is "research designed to find a solution to an immediate practical problem" (p. 374).

3. The information does not indicate that the study is an experimental one. There is no independent variable that can be actively manipulated to see its effects on a dependent variable.

4. The information does not indicate a correlational study. A correlational study looks at the relationship between two variables. There are no variables in the study.

TEST-TAKING TIP: You know that people with diabetes should test their blood glucose levels regularly. Would having an efficient, easy-to-use, low-cost glucometer increase the likelihood that they will monitor their blood glucose regularly?

Content Area: *Applied Research;* ***Cognitive Level:*** *Application;* ***Question Type:*** *Multiple Choice*

CRITICAL THINKING FACILITATOR:
Why are most nursing studies applied? What contributions to nursing and health care can be expected from applied research?

49. 1. This right was not the one violated. Confidentiality means "management of private data in such a way that only the researcher knows the subjects' identities and can link them with their responses" (Burns & Grove, 2011, p. 535).

2. This right was not the one violated. Anonymity is in evidence when even the researcher cannot link data with the specific research participant.

3. **The right of self-determination was violated because there is no mention of a process whereby those being observed gave their permission.**
4. The right to fair treatment was not the one violated. This right protects persons who refuse to participate or who withdraw from a study. This right means they should not receive prejudicial treatment.

TEST-TAKING TIP: The key phrase in the question stem is "were not told." This means no permission was sought, and those being observed did not have the opportunity to agree or refuse.

Content Area: *Ethics in Research;* ***Cognitive Level:*** *Analysis;* ***Question Type:*** *Multiple Choice*
CRITICAL THINKING FACILITATOR:
Would the health problem of a research participant allow a researcher to ignore ethical guidelines? What provisions are made for vulnerable persons such as those with a psychiatric problem?

50. 1. **The researcher can potentially violate the subject's right to freedom from harm and discomfort. Mental and physical discomfort, if experienced by the subject, would violate this right.**
2. The right to fair treatment is not violated in the situation. The right to fair treatment means that a person who refused to participate must not receive prejudicial treatment and must be respected at all times.
3. Breach of anonymity and confidentiality is not evident in the situation.
4. Violation of the right of self-determination is not evident in the situation.

TEST-TAKING TIP: The key phrase in the information is "shares her pain and trauma." This is indicative of potential emotional pain in reliving the experience.

Content Area: *Ethics in Research;* ***Cognitive Level:*** *Analysis;* ***Question Type:*** *Multiple Choice*
CRITICAL THINKING FACILITATOR:
What other phenomena, if studied, could potentially cause harm and discomfort to a research participant?

51. 1. Informed consent was not violated as indicated in the situation. Informed consent is "an ethical principle that requires researchers to obtain people's voluntary participation in a study, after informing them of possible risks and benefits" (Polit & Beck, 2014, p. 382).
2. **The right to fair treatment was violated. "Researchers must treat people who decline to participate in a study or who withdraw from it in a non-prejudicial manner" (p. 85).**
3. Freedom from harm was not violated as indicated in the study information.
4. The right to self-determination was not violated. This right means that research participants "have the right to ask questions, to refuse to participate, or to withdraw from the study" (Polit & Beck, 2014, p. 84).

TEST-TAKING TIP: The key phrase in the question stem is "failed to extend the benefits." This implies prejudicial treatment of those who refused to participate.

Content Area: *Ethics in Research;* ***Cognitive Level:*** *Analysis;* ***Question Type:*** *Multiple Choice*
CRITICAL THINKING FACILITATOR:
How should a researcher deal with persons who refuse to participate or who withdraw from a study without compromising ethics and integrity of the study?

52. 1. A survey would not be appropriate because only descriptive data will emerge.
2. An ethnographic approach would not appropriate because the study is not focusing on culture.
3. A phenomenological approach would not be appropriate because the focus is not on the lived experience.
4. **A grounded theory approach is appropriate because its focus would be a social process, the transition from student to practicing nurse.**

TEST-TAKING TIP: The key phrase in the question stem is "transition," which implies a process of passing from one phase to another.

Content Area: *Qualitative Studies;* ***Cognitive Level:*** *Application;* ***Question Type:*** *Multiple Choice*
CRITICAL THINKING FACILITATOR:
What are some patient-related processes that can be studied using a grounded theory approach?

53. 1. Errors that are consistent are systematic. An example is a blood pressure apparatus that gives false high readings at each use.
2. **Random errors are those that cause "individual subjects' observed scores to vary haphazardly around their true scores" (Burns & Grove, 2011, p. 546). Some examples of subject-related situations that can cause random errors include fatigue or discomfort during data collection.**

3. Systematic errors occur consistently and are due to flaws in the measurement tool.
4. Errors produce bias in the data.

TEST-TAKING TIP: The key phrase in the question stem is "discomfort from gastric hyperacidity." This situation in research participants is transient and unpredictable.

Content Area: *Errors in Measurement;* ***Cognitive Level:*** *Application;* ***Question Type:*** *Multiple Choice*
CRITICAL THINKING FACILITATOR: A disciplined, well-trained athlete might not perform at optimum levels at certain times. How would you explain this? On the other hand, what would you observe in an athlete who has not reached her or his peak performance level?

54. 1. Inferential statistics are used to analyze data in quantitative studies and are not used by qualitative researchers.
2. Control of biases and extraneous variables are not a concern of qualitative researchers.
3. **The qualitative researcher collects in-depth narrative data from research participants, and together they construct the phenomenon of interest.**
4. Data reported in tables are usually quantitative. The data in qualitative research could be presented as diagrams or illustrations of the study phenomena.

TEST-TAKING TIP: The key phrase in the questions stem is "naturalistic paradigm." Recall that this is the paradigm for qualitative research.

Content Area: *The Naturalistic Paradigm for Research;* ***Cognitive Level:*** *Comprehension;* ***Question Type:*** *Multiple Choice*
CRITICAL THINKING FACILITATOR: Think of all the activities in qualitative research and how they flow from the assumptions and beliefs in the naturalistic paradigm.

55. 1. Data-based literature consists of "research reports, both published reports and journals and books and unpublished reports such as theses and dissertations" (Burns & Grove, 2011, p. 535). These are types of literature and not sources.
2. **Secondary sources would be most likely used. A secondary source is one "whose author summarizes or quotes content from primary sources" (p. 548). The researcher would have to use the works of people who knew Dorothea Dix, who lived from 1802 to 1887.**
3. Theoretical literature includes "concept analyses, maps, theories, conceptual frameworks that support a selected problem or purpose" (p. 551). Theoretical literature is a type of literature and not a source.
4. A primary source is a "source whose author originated or is responsible for generating the ideas published" (p. 544). Primary sources can be used but might not be available because of the time period.

TEST-TAKING TIP: The keys in the question stem are the dates 1989 and 1802 to 1887. The study was done almost 100 years after the death of the subject of the investigation. Many of the primary sources might not be accessible.

Content Area: *Literature Sources;* ***Cognitive Level:*** *Application;* ***Question Type:*** *Multiple Choice*
CRITICAL THINKING FACILITATOR: What are specific sources of data for historical research?

56. 1. **The study title suggests an ethnographic study because assimilation and acculturation are processes that are relevant to immigrant groups.**
2. The study title suggests a phenomenological study as evidenced by the words "lived experience."
3. The study title suggests a historical study on the life of a nurse who lived in the past.
4. The study title suggests a quantitative study, specifically a correlation that looks at the relationship between two variables.

TEST-TAKING TIP: The key word in the question stem is "ethnographic," which relates to culture. Also each of the incorrect options have clue words. Option 2 has the words "lived experience," option 3 has the name of a nurse who lived in the past, and option 4 has the word "relationship."

Content Area: *Qualitative Studies;* ***Cognitive Level:*** *Application;* ***Question Type:*** *Multiple Choice*
CRITICAL THINKING FACILITATOR: What are the contributions of the different qualitative approaches to EBP?

57. 1. Stability is an aspect of reliability. "Stability is the degree to which similar results are obtained on separate occasions" (Polit & Beck, 2014, p. 202). Factor analysis is not a test of stability.
2. Internal consistency is an aspect of reliability. "An instrument is internally consistent to the extent that its items measure the same trait" (p. 203). Factor analysis is not a procedure to establish internal consistency.
3. **Validity is the "degree to which an instrument measures what it is supposed**

to measure." Factor analysis is a "method for identifying clusters of related items for a scale." It "identifies and groups together different measures into a unitary scale based on how participants reacted to the items, rather than based on the researcher's preconceptions" (p. 207).

4. Equivalence is an aspect of reliability. Equivalence is the "degree to which two or more independent observes or coders agree about scoring on an instrument" (p. 204).

TEST-TAKING TIP: The key phrase is "items clustered around one to two factors." The clustering process reduces the number of items by grouping them according to the larger categories where most items cluster.

Content Area: *Reliability and Validity;* ***Cognitive Level:*** *Comprehension;* ***Question Type:*** *Multiple Choice*

CRITICAL THINKING FACILITATOR:
Are you familiar with the Glasgow Coma Scale (GCS) with its three indicators of neurologic status? How might a factor analysis have contributed to the development of the GCS?

58. 1. The title suggests an ethnographic study with the words "culture" and "group."

2. The title suggests a phenomenological study. The feeling of grief is a lived experience that has personal meaning for each research participant.

3. The title suggests historical research. Linda Richards is a considered a nurse leader in the past.

4. The title suggests a survey that has the purpose of describing characteristics and frequency of a phenomenon. A quantitative approach is indicated in the question.

TEST-TAKING TIP: Look at each option carefully and eliminate those that do not indicate a phenomenological approach. Option 1 contains the words "culture" and "group." Option 3 names a nurse leader in the past. Option 4 suggests looking into attitudes that can be ascertained through a survey.

Content Area: *Types of Research Studies;* ***Cognitive Level:*** *Application;* ***Question Type:*** *Multiple Choice*

CRITICAL THINKING FACILITATOR:
What are some clue words you can use to identify each type of research study when you are looking at the title of a study?

59. 1. This is not indicated in the question. Test–retest reliability addresses the consistency between two sets of scores obtained on two separate occasions.

2. This is not indicated in the question. Alternate form reliability addresses the consistency between two sets of scores on two alternate forms of a test.

3. Construct validity is not indicated in the question. Construct validity has to do with the appropriateness of a research instrument to measure the construct under investigation.

4. Content validity is indicated in the question. Content validity is the "degree to which the items in an instrument adequately represent the universe of content for the concept being measured" (Polit & Beck, 2014, p. 377).

TEST-TAKING TIP: The key phrase in the question stem is "relevant topical areas." Topical areas are also called content.

Content Area: *Research Instruments;* ***Cognitive Level:*** *Application;* ***Question Type:*** *Multiple Choice*

CRITICAL THINKING FACILITATOR:
What is the purpose of test blueprints in courses you take?

60. 1. The title suggests a primary source, a data-based article, because the "author originated or is responsible for generating the ideas published" (Burns & Grove, 2011, p. 544).

2. The title suggests a primary source, a data-based article published by the author who did the study.

3. The title suggests a primary source, a data-based article published by the author who did the study.

4. The title suggests a secondary source. The author who did the critique used someone else's primary work.

TEST-TAKING TIP: The key word in the question stem is "secondary." A secondary source is written by an "author who summarizes or quotes content from primary sources." Note the word "critique" in option 4.

Content Area: *Sources of Literature;* ***Cognitive Level:*** *Application;* ***Question Type:*** *Multiple Choice*

CRITICAL THINKING FACILITATOR:
Think of clue words that you could use to determine whether a source is primary or secondary just based on the title of the work.

61. 1. Noting available reliable and valid research instruments is part of doing a literature review.

2. A literature review is not about the impressions of others. This activity should not be part of the literature review process.

3. The recommendations and suggestions of previous researchers are critical to prevent mistakes and facilitate the conduct of the current study.
4. Approaches and designs used by others can assist in making decisions and facilitate many aspects of the current study.

TEST-TAKING TIP: The key phrase in the question stem is "least interested." This implies information that would not be useful to the person doing the review.

Content Area: *Sources of Literature;* ***Cognitive Level:*** *Knowledge;* ***Question Type:*** *Multiple Choice*
CRITICAL THINKING FACILITATOR:
How should the literature review be organized and written?

62. 1. The title suggests a secondary source as indicated by the term "review." The author used several primary sources to do this article.
2. The title suggests a secondary source because of the word "analysis." To do the analysis article, the author looked at 25 years of literature on the topic.
3. The title suggests a secondary source. The publication, edited by one person, is a collection of multiple publications by different authors.
4. The title suggests a primary source. It is a study done and then reported by the researcher.

TEST-TAKING TIP: There is a key word in every option. Option 1 contains the word "review," option 2 contains the word "analysis," and option 3 contains the word "collection."

Content Area: *Sources of Literature;* ***Cognitive Level:*** *Application;* ***Question Type:*** *Multiple Choice*
CRITICAL THINKING FACILITATOR:
Why do researchers rely more on primary sources than on secondary ones?

63. **1. The title suggests theoretical literature. The title is about a conceptual or theoretical model.**
2. The title suggests data-based literature.
3. The title suggests data-based literature.
4. The title suggests data-based literature.

TEST-TAKING TIP: There is a key word in every option. Eliminate the options that are data based. Option 2 contains the word "relationship," option 3 contains the word "meta-analysis," and option 4 contains the word "study."

Content Area: *Sources of Literature;* ***Cognitive Level:*** *Application;* ***Question Type:*** *Multiple Choice*
CRITICAL THINKING FACILITATOR:
What are terms used in titles that could help in identifying theoretical literature? From among a list of resources, try identifying theoretical literature by eliminating the data-based resources because these are easier to spot.

64. **1. This suggests a retrospective study because the phenomenon, an "outbreak of influenza" has already manifested itself. The researcher would go back and trace the events or situations that might have "caused" it.**
2. This suggests a correlational study because the focus is the relationship between two variables.
3. This is a survey that is used to "describe a phenomenon by collecting data using questionnaires or personal interviews" (Burns & Grove, 2011, p. 550).
4. A reliability and validity study is not a retrospective study. It is a methodological study.

TEST-TAKING TIP: The key word in the question stem is "retrospective." The prefix *retro-* means backward; the root *spec* means to look.

Content Area: *Retrospective Study;* ***Cognitive Level:*** *Application;* ***Question Type:*** *Multiple Choice*
CRITICAL THINKING FACILITATOR:
What are the contributions of retrospective studies to EBP?

65. 1. Trends are not expected in a cross-sectional study. Trends are changes seen over time. Trends are observed in longitudinal studies.
2. The statement is not true in cross-sectional studies. Studies that have multiple data collection periods are longitudinal studies.
3. Attrition is not major threat in cross-sectional studies because research participants have a one-time participation. There are no follow-up collection data periods.
4. The statement is true for a study with a cross-sectional design.

TEST-TAKING TIP: Think of the two designs that have a temporal aspect, that is, cross-sectional designs and longitudinal designs. The "long" in longitudinal indicates something that is extended.

Content Area: *Cross-Sectional Study;* ***Cognitive Level:*** *Application;* ***Question Type:*** *Multiple Choice*
CRITICAL THINKING FACILITATOR:
What phenomenon could be studied using a cross-sectional design?

66. 1. Reactivity is not the threat described in the situation. Reactivity is "a measurement distortion arising from the study participant's awareness of being observed, or, more generally, from the effect of the measurement procedure itself" (Polit & Beck, 2014, p. 390).

2. The sampling plan can be the source of a threat to the study. If the sample is not representative of the population, then the ability to generalize is reduced. Attendees at a convention are not representative of all those who need to renew a license. Also, attendees to a convention have preexisting biases in relation to the research question because they inherently support mandatory continuing education by their attendance at a convention that awards continuing education credits.

3. History is not a source of a threat. A history threat is seen when there is a concurrent event that can affect the outcome.

4. Maturation is not a source of threat. This threat occurs as a result of the passage of time that can influence the outcome.

TEST-TAKING TIP: The key word in the question stem is "threat," which is something that can negatively affect the outcome of the study.

Content Area: *Threats to Study Validity;* ***Cognitive Level:*** *Application;* ***Question Type:*** *Multiple Choice*

CRITICAL THINKING FACILITATOR:
What measures can be implemented to resolve threats to the validity of a study?

67. 1. An independent variable is not indicated in the statement. The independent variable is "the treatment or experimental activity that is manipulated or varied by the researcher to cause an effect on the dependent variable" (Burns & Grove, 2011, p. 539).

2. Physical training would serve as an extraneous variable because those who have had it might perform differently from those who have not had it. The groups tested would not be equal at the outset of the study. Therefore, any difference between the groups cannot be attributed to the independent variable.

3. A dependent variable is not indicated in the statement. A dependent variable is the "response, behavior, or outcome that is predicted or explained; changes in the dependent variable are presumed to be caused by the independent variable" (Burns & Grove, 2011, p. 536).

4. A dichotomous variable is not indicated in the statement. A dichotomous variable is one with only two values such as smoker or nonsmoker.

TEST-TAKING TIP: The key word in the question stem is "control," which means "the process of holding constant confounding influences on the dependent variable (the outcome) under study" (Polit & Beck, 2014, p. 377).

Content Area: *Controls in Quantitative Studies;* ***Cognitive Level:*** *Application;* ***Question Type:*** *Multiple Choice*

CRITICAL THINKING FACILITATOR:
Suggest a study with an independent and a dependent variable. Then think of possible influences that could interfere with the outcome.

68. 1. The action will yield a convenience sample or persons who are readily accessible.

2. The action will yield a sample obtained by quota sampling.

3. The action refers to snowball, or network sampling.

4. The process refers to random selection.

TEST-TAKING TIP: The key word in the question stem is "quota," which means a specified number or amount.

Content Area: *Sampling;* ***Cognitive Level:*** *Application;* ***Question Type:*** *Multiple Choice*

CRITICAL THINKING FACILITATOR:
What kinds of biases could emerge in a quota sampling procedure?

69. **1. Blood pressure assessment is considered an in vivo biophysiologic measure. "In vivo measures are those performed directly within or on living organisms" (Polit & Beck, 2014, p. 182).**

2. Blood pressure measurements are not considered invasive from a data collection measurement perspective.

3. In vitro measurements require some type of specimen from the research participant.

4. A blood pressure assessment is not considered intrusive from a data collection perspective.

TEST-TAKING TIP: The key phrase in the question stem is "blood pressure." The assessment is done on the outside of the person, and no specimen is required.

Content Area: *Data Collection;* ***Cognitive Level:*** *Comprehension;* ***Question Type:*** *Multiple Choice*

CRITICAL THINKING FACILITATOR: What are some of the issues in using biophysiologic data collection methods?

70. 1. A questionnaire would not be the most effective because it would require the subject to answer verbally.
2. A closed-ended scale would not be the best tool because the subject would have to respond verbally.
3. A visual analog scale would be the most effective tool. For instance, a visual analog scale on pain would be used, and the person could just specify a point on a line indicating the degree of pain.
4. A Likert-type scale would not be effective because the subject would need to read statements and indicate her or his responses. For someone with a language limitation, the scale would not be useful.

TEST-TAKING TIP: The key phrase the question stem is "language limitations." Eliminate options that require reading or speaking.

Content Area: *Data Collection Methods;* ***Cognitive Level:*** *Application;* ***Question Type:*** *Multiple Choice*
CRITICAL THINKING FACILITATOR: What other data collection strategies can be used when subjects have language limitations?

71. 1. The approach does not suggest an evaluation study. It suggests a correlation because the purpose of a correlation is to discover the relationship between two variables.
2. The approach suggests an evaluation study because there is a procedure or strategy whose impact on another variable is to be evaluated.
3. The approach does not suggest an evaluation study. It suggests doing a survey to gather facts and other information to be used in making a decision.
4. The approach suggests a study that is descriptive, not evaluative.

TEST-TAKING TIP: Look for key words in each option. Option 1 contains the word "relationship," option 3 contains the word "feasibility," and option 4 contains the word "explored." Option 2 contains the word "effectiveness," which implies evaluation.

Content Area: *Evaluation Study;* ***Cognitive Level:*** *Application;* ***Question Type:*** *Multiple Choice*
CRITICAL THINKING FACILITATOR: What other clues can be used to determine whether a study is an evaluation one?

72. 1. In meta-analysis research, multiple studies are analyzed. The researcher does not collect new data.
2. The researcher who does meta-analysis research does not use the usual tools and instruments in doing a study but uses different processes to analyze the multiple studies selected according to a set of criteria.
3. Only completed research studies that are considered primary sources are selected according to established criteria.
4. The researcher who is doing the meta-analysis does not collect new information. The analysis is done on completed studies done by others.

TEST-TAKING TIP: The key word in the question stem is "meta-analysis." A meaning of the prefix, *meta-* is over or beyond. In this case, it means beyond just one study on a certain phenomenon. Therefore, the meta-analysis would include multiple studies that will be examined by the researcher.

Content Area: *Meta-Analysis;* ***Cognitive Level:*** *Comprehension;* ***Question Type:*** *Multiple Choice*
CRITICAL THINKING FACILITATOR: What are some criteria used by the researcher in selecting studies to be analyzed in a meta-analysis?

73. 1. The title suggests a correlational study that would look at the relationship between two variables.
2. The title suggests a methodological study. The word "scale" refers to a measurement instrument, and reliability and validity are instrument characteristics.
3. The title suggests a correlational study that would look at the relationship between two variables.
4. The title suggests an article on domestic violence. A review of the literature is part of doing an article.

TEST-TAKING TIP: The key word in the question stem is "methodological." It is derived from the term "method," which means some type of procedure or system. In a research study, the procedure refers to collecting data and therefore to data collection methods, or instruments.

Content Area: *Data Collection;* ***Cognitive Level:*** *Application;* ***Question Type:*** *Multiple Choice*
CRITICAL THINKING FACILITATOR: What are some clinical tools you use to collect data? How did these tools become part of accepted clinical practice?

74. 1. Nonexperimental designs are those that do not involve an intervention. Studies that are nonexperimental designs include descriptive, exploratory, and correlational studies and do not imply causality.
2. **This statement is true regarding nonexperimental designs. They do not have an independent variable that is actively manipulated.**
3. The statement is false. Nonexperimental studies are the foundation of future, more advanced studies.
4. The statement is false. Every study has ethical issues that must be addressed. Also, all research studies must adhere to ethical guidelines.

TEST-TAKING TIP: The key word in the question stem is "nonexperimental." "Experimental," derived from the word "experiment," means to test out something, so nonexperimental means not testing anything.

Content Area: *Research Design;* ***Cognitive Level:*** *Comprehension;* ***Question Type:*** *Multiple Choice*
CRITICAL THINKING FACILITATOR:
What are the contributions of nonexperimental studies to EBP?

75. 1. Potassium levels are not microbiologic measurements. Microbiologic assessments focus on microorganisms—bacteria, viruses, and so on—and their effects on the body.
2. **Potassium levels are chemical measurements. Potassium is an electrolyte normally found in body tissues and fluids. Its level is influenced by other substances in the body.**
3. Cytologic measurements are examinations of body tissues to detect any abnormal composition, such as cancer cells.
4. Potassium levels are not physical measurements, such as head circumference measurements of infants.

TEST-TAKING TIP: The key word in the question stem is "potassium." Recall what you have learned about fluids and electrolytes in the body.

Content Area: *Data Collection;* ***Cognitive Level:*** *Comprehension;* ***Question Type:*** *Multiple Choice*
CRITICAL THINKING FACILITATOR:
Give examples of tests in each category of in vitro measures.

76. 1. The statement is not consistent with the sensitivity number. The statement indicates a low sensitivity.
2. **The statement is consistent with the sensitivity number. This means that the classification system used had high sensitivity, that is, it was "very good in identifying the diseased patients" (Burns & Grove, 2011, p. 342).**
3. The statement refers to specificity, the "proportion of patients without the disease who have a negative test result or true negative" (p. 342) (did not fall and no signs of having fallen).
4. The statement refers to specificity.

TEST-TAKING TIP: The key word in the question stem is "sensitivity." It is derived from the word "sensitive," which means able to detect slight changes. With biophysiologic instruments, sensitivity would be a most desirable property in detecting true changes in a condition or situation.

Content Area: *Data Collection Methods;* ***Cognitive Level:*** *Application;* ***Question Type:*** *Multiple Choice*
CRITICAL THINKING FACILITATOR:
What are some familiar clinical measurement tools that you consider sensitive?

77. 1. The statement is not a limitation of the study because it does not express a restriction in the study.
2. The statement does not represent a conclusion because it is not a synthesis of the findings of the study.
3. The statement is not a problem statement. A problem statement addresses the issue that needs to be addressed by the study.
4. **The statement refers to a gap in the literature. A gap is an opening or an interruption that breaks the continuity of something. It could also mean something missing.**

TEST-TAKING TIP: The key phrase in the statement is "no previously published work." Recall the purpose of reviewing the literature for a study. The researcher would want to know the current state of knowledge about the topic and should know what research has and has not already been done.

Content Area: *Review of the Literature;* ***Cognitive Level:*** *Analysis;* ***Question Type:*** *Multiple Choice*
CRITICAL THINKING FACILITATOR:
Why is an awareness of any gaps in the body of knowledge about a phenomenon important for EBP?

78. **core variable**

TEST-TAKING TIP: The key phrase in the statement is "process." Recall that the

intent in a grounded theory study is to "use the data, grounded in reality, to describe or explain processes as they occur in reality, not as they have been conceptualized previously" (Polit & Beck, 2014, p. 140).

Content Area: *Grounded Theory Study;* ***Cognitive Level:*** *Comprehension;* ***Question Type:*** *Fill-in-the-Blank*

CRITICAL THINKING FACILITATOR:
Why are grounded theory studies important for EBP?

79. longitudinal study

TEST-TAKING TIP: The key phrase in the statement is "14-, 22-, and 26-week post-intervention measures." The phrase indicates continuing measurement of the effect of an independent variable over a period of time or multiple data collection periods.

Content Area: *Longitudinal Study;* ***Cognitive Level:*** *Application;* ***Question Type:*** *Fill-in-the-Blank*

CRITICAL THINKING FACILITATOR:
When an RCT has a longitudinal design as well, what advantages will be seen in the study?

80.
1. The statement is not a description of the sample. Descriptive statistics include measures of central tendency and frequency distributions.
2. The statement does not indicate an accessible population. No information was given as to where and how the sample was selected.
3. **The statement describes the inclusion criteria for the sample. The inclusion criteria are "sampling criteria or characteristics that the subjects or elements must possess to be considered part of the target population" (Burns & Grove, 2011, p. 539).**
4. The statement does not give information about any groups.

TEST-TAKING TIP: The key phrase in the statement is "have to be," which indicates a requirement.

Content Area: *Sampling Concepts;* ***Cognitive Level:*** *Comprehension;* ***Question Type:*** *Multiple Choice*

CRITICAL THINKING FACILITATOR:
How are inclusion criteria selected by the researcher?

81. external criticism

TEST-TAKING TIP: The key phrase in the research study information is "tape recorder." Data sources in historical studies include persons who are the direct sources. Sources outside (external) of the person would be any device that contains the information that must also be authenticated.

Content Area: *Historical Studies;* ***Cognitive Level:*** *Knowledge;* ***Question Type:*** *Fill-in-the-Blank*

CRITICAL THINKING FACILITATOR:
What other materials or devices must meet authenticity for a valid historical study?

82.
1. **The statement is correct because there are four groups.**
2. The statement is not correct because only two groups are measured at baseline.
3. **The statement is correct because all four groups will be measured relative to the outcome.**
4. **The statement is correct. There is a basis for comparing the two control groups.**
5. The statement is not correct because only one of the experimental groups is measured at baseline.

TEST-TAKING TIP: The key phrase in the question stem is "Solomon four-group design." A major advantage of this design is to control a threat to internal validity by removing the effects of pretesting.

Content Area: *Randomized Clinical Trials;* ***Cognitive Level:*** *Analysis;* ***Question Type:*** *Multiple Response*

CRITICAL THINKING FACILITATOR:
What are the advantages and disadvantages of the different variations in randomized clinical trials?

83. reactivity

TEST-TAKING TIP: The key phrase in the question stem is "not concealed." The researcher is present in the research setting, which could lead to "reactions" from the participants.

Content Area: *Observation in Data Collection;* ***Cognitive Level:*** *Comprehension;* ***Question Type:*** *Fill-in-the-Blank*

CRITICAL THINKING FACILITATOR:
What are the advantages and disadvantages of the different variations in observational research?

84. feasibility

TEST-TAKING TIP: The key phrase in the question stem is "novice researcher." The lack of experience of the novice researcher would be a concern relative to whether the study could be designed, conducted, and completed. The question that can be asked is: "Can the study be done?"

Content Area: Feasibility of a Study; Cognitive Level: Comprehension; Question Type: Fill-in-the-Blank
CRITICAL THINKING FACILITATOR: Recall another criterion for a study's feasibility and determine how it can be resolved.

85. 1. The Kuder-Richardson coefficient is not a test of stability.
 2. The reliability coefficient of an instrument should be 0.70 or above to be acceptable.
 3. The Kuder-Richardson coefficient is a test of internal consistency or homogeneity.
 4. The test is not used for Likert-type scales that consists of responses that include strongly agree, agree, neutral, disagree, and strongly disagree.
 5. The Kuder-Richardson coefficient is used for dichotomous scales that have only two possible responses.

TEST-TAKING TIP: The key word in the statement is "psychometric." Psychometrics is the theory and development of measurement instruments. Recall what you have learned about reliability and validity and about research studies that report reliability coefficients of instruments.

Content Area: Reliability of Measurements; Cognitive Level: Application; Question Type: Multiple Response
CRITICAL THINKING FACILITATOR: Review the different aspects of reliability and give an example of a test for it.

86. 1. The statement is a purpose of a study and not what a researcher would do first in relation to the situation.
 2. The statement is a correct one. Data about who elders are provide the start point in any program. Data are the bases for making decisions about the different aspects of the program.
 3. The statement is not an activity that is essential in the planning stage.
 4. The statement is an outcome. The outcomes are not the initial aspects that need to be considered.

TEST-TAKING TIP: The key phrase in the statement is "initial data." There needs to be some descriptive statistics first.

Content Area: Analysis of Quantitative Findings; Cognitive Level: Application; Question Type: Multiple Choice
CRITICAL THINKING FACILITATOR: In every type of study, demographic data are always reported. What purpose does this process serve?

87. **1. The question is appropriately worded. According to the PICO format, it has all the components.**
 2. The question is missing the population.
 3. The population is not included.
 4. The outcome is not included.

TEST-TAKING TIP: Recall the acronym PICO, which stands for patient, population, or problem; intervention; comparison; and outcome, and look at each option to see whether it contains all the elements.

Content Area: Research Questions; Cognitive Level: Application; Question Type: Multiple Choice
CRITICAL THINKING FACILITATOR: How would you reword the incorrect options in the question so that they are clearly worded research questions?

88. 1. The title is not specific enough for determining the design of the study. The study could be descriptive, ethnographic, or phenomenological.
 2. The title is not clear enough to indicate the design of study. It could be a survey focusing on different strategies for solving the nursing shortage or even a grounded theory study.
 3. The title suggests a historical study because it is about a leader in the past and her work.
 4. The title is not specific enough to indicate the design of the study. It could be a descriptive survey.

TEST-TAKING TIP: Eliminate each option when you cannot pinpoint the type of design using key words that you know.

Content Area: Research Design; Cognitive Level: Application; Question Type: Multiple Choice
CRITICAL THINKING FACILITATOR: Recall the key words you know to use when determining a study's design based on its title.

89. Triangulation

TEST-TAKING TIP: The key phrase is "uses two sources to find another source." You know that are three sides to a triangle and that any two points direct you to the third point so that you can "clearly" see the figure.

Content Area: Qualitative Research Processes; Cognitive Level: Knowledge; Question Type: Fill-in-the-Blank
CRITICAL THINKING FACILITATOR: What are other processes in qualitative research that help clarify the phenomenon of interest?

90. the kth or the sampling interval.

TEST-TAKING TIP: You can come up with the correct answer when you can recall the types of probability sampling procedures.

Content Area: *Probability Sampling;* ***Cognitive Level:*** *Knowledge;* ***Question Type:*** *Fill-in-the-Blank*
CRITICAL THINKING FACILITATOR: What are the advantages and disadvantages of systematic sampling?

91. 1. **The process described fulfills the criteria of control for an experimental design. Differences in the outcome can be attributed to the independent variable because the control group gets a variation of the independent variable. Control is imposed when groups are made homogenous with regards to specific criteria.**
2. Order is not evident in the study information. Order relates to a system and is not relevant in the situation.
3. Generalization is not a process evident in the information. A generalization is a wide application of something (as in generalizing from a specific situation to a larger one).
4. Consistency in relation to a process means doing it the same way each time. This is not evident in the information.
5. **Randomization is evident in the information. Random assignment means that research participants were put into control or experimental groups, not by a predetermined process but by chance.**

TEST-TAKING TIP: Recall the requirements for an experimental study to facilitate answering the question.

Content Area: *Experimental Designs;* ***Cognitive Level:*** *Application;* ***Question Type:*** *Multiple Response*
CRITICAL THINKING FACILITATOR: By now you are familiar with the requirements of an experimental design. Take a clinical topic and propose a study with an experimental design.

92. 1. The recommendation is not part of the study. The recommendation comes from many different sources.
2. **The statement is correct and gives strong support for moving nursing education into the academic setting.**
3. The recommendation comes from other sources such as studies conducted in the 1970s.
4. This is not a recommendation of the study. This statement comes from organizations that accredit nursing programs.

TEST-TAKING TIP: Recall the earlier studies that paved the way for the current status of nursing as a profession and were significant in advancing nursing research.

Content Area: *Nursing Historical Milestones;* ***Cognitive Level:*** *Knowledge;* ***Question Type:*** *Multiple Choice*
CRITICAL THINKING FACILITATOR: Consider this: With advances in research and EBP, what areas of nursing do you think will experience the greatest changes in the next 5 years?

93. 1. The data are at the ordinal level. The scoring ranked persons relative to their ability to feed themselves. Ordinal measurement is a "measurement level that rank orders phenomena along some dimension" (Polit & Beck, 2014, p. 386).
2. The data indicate measurement at the nominal level because it only categorized persons into single, married, and divorced or separated categories. Nominal measurement is measurement that simply assigns characteristics into categories.
3. **Data are at the interval level because the distance between each score is the same—20 points. Interval measurement is a "measurement level in which an attribute of a variable is rank ordered on a scale that has equal distance between points on that scale" (p. 383).**
4. The data are at the ratio level of measurement. Ratio measurement is "measurement level with equal distances between scores and a true meaningful zero point" (p. 390).

TEST-TAKING TIP: Look at each option to figure out the correct answer. Eliminate the incorrect options. Option 1 assigns a number or sequence (ordinal). You do not have a numerical measurement of the distance between someone with a score of 3 and someone with a score of 2. Option 2 is simply labeling categories (naming them). In option 4, you are able to determine the magnitude of the difference.

Content Area: *Levels of Measurement;* ***Cognitive Level:*** *Application;* ***Question Type:*** *Multiple Choice*
CRITICAL THINKING FACILITATOR: Think of attributes that can be measured and what level of measurements is appropriate to each.

94. F

TEST-TAKING TIP: Recall from your statistics class what you did after you finished calculating your ANOVA.

***Content Area:** Inferential Statistics; **Cognitive Level:** Comprehension; **Question Type:** Fill-in-the-Blank*

CRITICAL THINKING FACILITATOR:
How would you state your interpretation of ANOVA results after you consulted the F table?

95. 1. The question is not appropriate to ask in critiquing a qualitative study. Qualitative studies use nonprobability sampling procedures and select research participants based on who would be the best to provide the in-depth data to describe the phenomenon of interest.
2. The question is not appropriate to ask in critiquing a qualitative study because qualitative studies do not use frameworks and have no variables.
3. The question is appropriate to ask in critiquing a qualitative study. Research participants in a qualitative study are selected based on their experience and potential for sharing data about the phenomenon of interest.
4. The question is appropriate to ask in critiquing a qualitative study. Readers should get a clear, comprehensive understanding of the phenomenon because the reality of this is constructed by the researcher and the participant.
5. The question is not appropriate to ask in critiquing a quantitative study. The statement refers to statistics used to analyze findings in a quantitative study.

TEST-TAKING TIP: Look at each option and find a clue word that you can use to eliminate any question that is appropriate in critiquing a quantitative study. Option 1 contains the word "bias." Option 2 contains the words "framework" and "variables." Option 5 contains the words "statistically significant findings."

***Content Area:** Critiquing Qualitative Studies; **Cognitive Level:** Analysis; **Question Type:** Multiple Response*

CRITICAL THINKING FACILITATOR:
Recall the assumptions of the positivist and the naturalistic paradigms. Compare two areas where critiquing would be different for a qualitative study and a quantitative study.

96. etic

TEST-TAKING TIP: The key phrase in the question stem is "outsider's interpretation." Recall the mnemonic OuTsider = eTic; iNsider = eMic.

***Content Area:** Ethnographic Studies; **Cognitive Level:** Knowledge; **Question Type:** Fill-in-the-Blank*

CRITICAL THINKING FACILITATOR:
What is the value of the outsider's perspective when studying a culture?

97. 1. A gap is not described in the statement. A gap is a void or interruption.
2. The statement describes an inconsistency in the literature. An inconsistency is an incompatibility between two situations.
3. The topic's potential for clinical significance is not described in the statement.
4. The need for the study is not what is described in the statement.

TEST-TAKING TIP: The key phrase in the information is "found no relationship." Contrast the second statement with the first in the information.

***Content Area:** Review of the Literature; **Cognitive Level:** Comprehension; **Question Type:** Multiple Choice*

CRITICAL THINKING FACILITATOR:
How should a review of the literature be presented if the current study is intended to make a contribution to EBP?

98. 1. The statements do not reflect the aim or purpose of the study. The purpose is the goal of the study.
2. The statements are not part of the literature review because previous studies are not mentioned.
3. The background of the study is not reflected in the statements. The background of a study would include factual information about the phenomenon of interest.
4. The statements reflect the theory used by the researchers. The statements are derived from the theory and propose a relationship between the variables of the study.

TEST-TAKING TIP: The key phrase in the information is "based their music intervention." This indicates the use of a theory or framework from which hypotheses could be deduced.

***Content Area:** Use of Theory in Research; **Cognitive Level:** Analysis; **Question Type:** Multiple Choice*

CRITICAL THINKING FACILITATOR:
Where do theories come from? Name a few that you can use in clinical practice.

99. **1. The question would be appropriate to ask in critiquing a quantitative study. Quantitative studies propose hypotheses, which are tested in the study.**

2. **Level of data and sample size are concepts in quantitative studies, so the question is appropriate to ask.**
3. The question is appropriate to ask in critiquing a qualitative study that focuses on a phenomenon of interest. Those selected to participate should have experience relevant to the phenomenon.
4. The question is appropriate to ask in critiquing a qualitative study that focuses on in-depth description of the phenomenon of interest. The researcher validates with the participants her or his interpretation of the data.
5. The question is appropriate to ask in critiquing a qualitative study. The researcher identifies themes in the narrative descriptions. Each theme is supported by relevant narrative data, or examples.

TEST-TAKING TIP: The key words are in each option. Eliminate the options that have terms indicative of the qualitative approach. Option 3 contains the phrase "that could best provide data on the phenomenon." Option 4 contains the phrase "participant's meaning." Option 5 contains the phrase "examples provided."

Content Area: *Critiquing Quantitative Research;* ***Cognitive Level:*** *Analysis;* ***Question Type:*** *Multiple Response*

CRITICAL THINKING FACILITATOR:
Review the assumptions and beliefs of the positivist paradigm and identify one or two in the criteria for critiquing quantitative studies.

100. 1. **Beginning studies add evidence that can be used to further knowledge on a topic significant to nursing.**
2. Although a study that strengthens the image of nursing as a scientific discipline is helpful to the profession, it is not important evidence for EBP.
3. **Evidence from research adds to the theoretical knowledge that leads to understanding of phenomena central to the discipline.**
4. **Evidence from research that tests the effectiveness of interventions is critical. It is through tested interventions that excellence in practice evolves.**
5. **As more research is completed, the body of evidence increases. This body of evidence has multiple uses in guiding practice.**

TEST-TAKING TIP: Apply your understanding of research and its role in EBP, and you will be able to answer this question.

Content Area: *Research and EBP;* ***Cognitive Level:*** *Application;* ***Question Type:*** *Multiple Response*

CRITICAL THINKING FACILITATOR:
Using your understanding of research and what you have learned from one or two studies, how can you as a healthcare provider improve patient outcomes?

Glossary of English Words Commonly Encountered on Nursing Examinations

Abnormality — defect, irregularity, anomaly, oddity

Absence — nonappearance, lack, nonattendance

Abundant — plentiful, rich, profuse

Accelerate — go faster, speed up, increase, hasten

Accumulate — build up, collect, gather

Accurate — precise, correct, exact

Achievement — accomplishment, success, reaching, attainment

Acknowledge — admit, recognize, accept, reply

Activate — start, turn on, stimulate

Adequate — sufficient, ample, plenty, enough

Angle — slant, approach, direction, point of view

Application — use, treatment, request, claim

Approximately — about, around, in the region of, more or less, roughly speaking

Arrange — position, place, organize, display

Associated — linked, related

Attention — notice, concentration, awareness, thought

Authority — power, right, influence, clout, expert

Avoid — keep away from, evade, let alone

Balanced — stable, neutral, steady, fair, impartial

Barrier — barricade, blockage, obstruction, obstacle

Best — most excellent, most important, greatest

Capable — able, competent, accomplished

Capacity — ability, capability, aptitude, role, power, size

Central — middle, mid, innermost, vital

Challenge — confront, dare, dispute, test, defy, face up to

Characteristic — trait, feature, attribute, quality, typical

Circular — round, spherical, globular

Collect — gather, assemble, amass, accumulate, bring together

Commitment — promise, vow, dedication, obligation, pledge, assurance

Commonly — usually, normally, frequently, generally, universally

Compare — contrast, evaluate, match up to, weigh or judge against

Compartment — section, part, cubicle, booth, stall

Complex — difficult, multifaceted, compound, multipart, intricate

Complexity — difficulty, intricacy, complication

Component — part, element, factor, section, constituent

Comprehensive — complete, inclusive, broad, thorough

Conceal — hide, cover up, obscure, mask, suppress, secrete

Conceptualize — to form an idea

Concern — worry, anxiety, fear, alarm, distress, unease, trepidation

Concisely — briefly, in a few words, succinctly

Conclude — make a judgment based on reason, finish

Confidence — self-assurance, certainty, poise, self-reliance

Congruent — matching, fitting, going together well

Consequence — result, effect, outcome, end result

Constituents — elements, component, parts that make up a whole

Contain — hold, enclose, surround, include, control, limit

Continual — repeated, constant, persistent, recurrent, frequent

Continuous — constant, incessant, nonstop, unremitting, permanent

Contribute — be a factor, add, give

Convene — assemble, call together, summon, organize, arrange

Convenience — expediency, handiness, ease

Coordinate — organize, direct, manage, bring together

Create — make, invent, establish, generate, produce, fashion, build, construct

Creative — imaginative, original, inspired, inventive, resourceful, productive, innovative

Critical — serious, grave, significant, dangerous, life threatening

Cue — signal, reminder, prompt, sign, indication

Curiosity — inquisitiveness, interest, nosiness, snooping

Damage — injure, harm, hurt, break, wound

Deduct — subtract, take away, remove, withhold

Deficient — lacking, wanting, underprovided, scarce, faulty

Defining — important, crucial, major, essential, significant, central

Defuse — resolve, calm, soothe, neutralize, rescue, mollify

Delay — hold up, wait, hinder, postpone, slow down, hesitate, linger

Demand — insist, claim, require, command, stipulate, ask

Describe — explain, tell, express, illustrate, depict, portray

Design — plan, invent, intend, aim, propose, devise

Desirable — wanted, pleasing, enviable, popular, sought after, attractive, advantageous

Detail — feature, aspect, element, factor, facet

Deteriorate — worsen, decline, weaken

Determine — decide, conclude, resolve, agree on

Dexterity — skillfulness, handiness, agility, deftness

Dignity — self-respect, self-esteem, decorum, formality, poise

Dimension — aspect, measurement

Diminish — reduce, lessen, weaken, detract, moderate

Discharge — release, dismiss, set free

Discontinue — stop, cease, halt, suspend, terminate, withdraw

Disorder — complaint, problem, confusion, chaos

Display — show, exhibit, demonstrate, present, put on view

Dispose — to get rid of, arrange, order, set out

Dissatisfaction — displeasure, discontent, unhappiness, disappointment

Distinguish — to separate and classify, recognize

Distract — divert, sidetrack, entertain

Distress — suffering, trouble, anguish, misery, agony, concern, sorrow

Distribute — deliver, spread out, hand out, issue, dispense

Disturbed — troubled, unstable, concerned, worried, distressed, anxious, uneasy

Diversional — serving to distract

Don — put on, dress oneself in

Dramatic — spectacular

Drape — cover, wrap, dress, swathe

Dysfunction — abnormal, impaired

Edge — perimeter, boundary, periphery, brink, border, rim

Effective — successful, useful, helpful, valuable

Efficient — not wasteful, effective, competent, resourceful, capable

Elasticity — stretch, spring, suppleness, flexibility

Eliminate — get rid of, eradicate, abolish, remove, purge

Embarrass — make uncomfortable, make self-conscious, humiliate, mortify

Emerge — appear, come, materialize, become known

Emphasize — call attention to, accentuate, stress, highlight

Ensure — make certain, guarantee

Environment — setting, surroundings, location, atmosphere, milieu, situation

Episode — event, incident, occurrence, experience

Essential — necessary, fundamental, vital, important, crucial, critical, indispensable

Etiology — assigned cause, origin

Exaggerate — overstate, inflate

Excel — to stand out, shine, surpass, outclass

Excessive — extreme, too much, unwarranted

Exertion — intense or prolonged physical effort

Exhibit — show signs of, reveal, display

Expand — get bigger, enlarge, spread out, increase, swell, inflate

Expect — wait for, anticipate, imagine

Expectation — hope, anticipation, belief, prospect, probability

Experience — knowledge, skill, occurrence, know-how

Expose — lay open, leave unprotected, allow to be seen, reveal, disclose, exhibit

External — outside, exterior, outer

Facilitate — make easy, make possible, help, assist

Factor — part, feature, reason, cause, think, issue

Focus — center, focal point, hub

Fragment — piece, portion, section, part, splinter, chip

Function — purpose, role, job, task

Furnish — supply, provide, give, deliver, equip

Further — additional, more, extra, added, supplementary

Generalize — to take a broad view, simplify, to make inferences from particulars

Generate — make, produce, create

Gentle — mild, calm, tender

Girth — circumference, bulk, weight

Highest — uppermost, maximum, peak, main

Hinder — hold back, delay, hamper, obstruct, impede

Humane — caring, kind, gentle, compassionate, benevolent, civilized

Ignore — pay no attention to, disregard, overlook, discount

Imbalance — unevenness, inequality, disparity

Immediate — insistent, urgent, direct

Impair — damage, harm, weaken

Implantation — to put in

Impotent — powerless, weak, incapable, ineffective, unable

Inadvertent — unintentional, chance, unplanned, accidental

Include — comprise, take in, contain

Indicate — point out, sign of, designate, specify, show

Ineffective — unproductive, unsuccessful, useless, vain, futile

Inevitable — predictable, to be expected, unavoidable, foreseeable

Influence — power, pressure, sway, manipulate, affect, effect

Initiate — start, begin, open, commence, instigate

Insert — put in, add, supplement, introduce

Inspect — look over, check, examine

Inspire — motivate, energize, encourage, enthuse

Institutionalize — to place in a facility for treatment

Integrate — put together, mix, add, combine, assimilate

Integrity — honesty

Interfere — get in the way, hinder, obstruct, impede, hamper

Interpret — explain the meaning of, to make understandable

Intervention — action, activity

Intolerance — bigotry, prejudice, narrow-mindedness

Involuntary — instinctive, reflex, unintentional, automatic, uncontrolled

Irreversible — permanent, irrevocable, irreparable, unalterable

Irritability — sensitivity to stimuli, fretful, quick excitability

Justify — explain in accordance with reason

Likely — probably, possible, expected

Liquefy — to change into or make more fluid

Logical — using reason

Longevity — long life

Lowest — inferior in rank

Maintain — continue, uphold, preserve, sustain, retain

Majority — the greater part of

Mention — talk about, refer to, state, cite, declare, point out

Minimal — least, smallest, nominal, negligible, token

Minimize — reduce, diminish, lessen, curtail, decrease to smallest possible

Mobilize — activate, organize, assemble, gather together, rally

Modify — change, adapt, adjust, revise, alter

Moist — slightly wet, damp

Multiple — many, numerous, several, various

Natural — normal, ordinary, unaffected

Negative — no, harmful, downbeat, pessimistic

Negotiate — bargain, talk, discuss, consult, cooperate, settle

Notice — become aware of, see, observe, discern, detect

Notify — inform, tell, alert, advise, warn, report

Nurture — care for, raise, rear, foster

Obsess — preoccupy, consume

Occupy — live in, inhabit, reside in, engage in

Occurrence — event, incident, happening

Odorous — scented, stinking, aromatic

Offensive — unpleasant, distasteful, nasty, disgusting

Opportunity — chance, prospect, break

Organize — put in order, arrange, sort out, categorize, classify

Origin — source, starting point, cause, beginning, derivation

Pace — speed

Parameter — limit, factor, limitation, issue

Participant — member, contributor, partaker, applicant

Perspective — viewpoint, view, perception

Position — place, location, point, spot, situation

Practice — do, carry out, perform, apply, follow

Precipitate — to cause to happen, to bring on, hasten, abrupt, sudden

Predetermine — fix or set beforehand

Predictable — expected, knowable

Preference — favorite, liking, first choice

Prepare — get ready, plan, make, train, arrange, organize

Prescribe — set down, stipulate, order, recommend, impose

Previous — earlier, prior, before, preceding

Primarily — first, above all, mainly, mostly, largely, principally, predominantly

Primary — first, main, basic, chief, most important, key, prime, major, crucial

Priority — main concern, giving first attention to, order of importance

Production — making, creation, construction, assembly

Profuse — a lot of, plentiful, copious, abundant, generous, prolific, bountiful

Prolong — extend, delay, put off, lengthen, draw out

Promote — encourage, support, endorse, sponsor

Proportion — ratio, amount, quantity, part of, percentage, section of

Provide — give, offer, supply, make available

Rationalize — explain, reason

Realistic — practical, sensible, reasonable

Receive — get, accept, take delivery of, obtain

Recognize — acknowledge, appreciate, identify, aware of

Recovery — healing, mending, improvement, recuperation, renewal

Reduce — decrease, lessen, ease, moderate, diminish

Reestablish — reinstate, restore, return, bring back

Regard — consider, look upon, relate to, respect

Regular — usual, normal, ordinary, standard, expected, conventional

Relative — comparative, family member

Relevance — importance of

Reluctant — unwilling, hesitant, disinclined, indisposed, adverse

Reminisce — to recall and review remembered experiences

Remove — take away, get rid of, eliminate, eradicate

Reposition — move, relocate, change position

Require — need, want, necessitate

Resist — oppose, defend against, keep from, refuse to go along with, defy

Resolution — decree, solution, decision, ruling, promise

Resolve — make up your mind, solve, determine, decide

Response — reply, answer, reaction, retort

Restore — reinstate, reestablish, bring back, return to, refurbish

Restrict — limit, confine, curb, control, contain, hold back, hamper

Retract — take back, draw in, withdraw, apologize

Reveal — make known, disclose, divulge, expose, tell, make public

Review — appraisal, reconsider, evaluation, assessment, examination, analysis

Ritual — custom, ceremony, formal procedure

Rotate — turn, go around, spin, swivel

Routine — usual, habit, custom, practice

Satisfaction — approval, fulfillment, pleasure, happiness

Satisfy — please, convince, fulfill, make happy, gratify

Secure — safe, protected, fixed firmly, sheltered, confident, obtain

Sequential — chronological, in order of occurrence

Significant — important, major, considerable, noteworthy, momentous

Slight — small, slim, minor, unimportant, insignificant, insult, snub

Source — basis, foundation, starting place, cause

Specific — exact, particular, detail, explicit, definite

Stable — steady, even, constant

Statistics — figures, data, information

Subtract — take away, deduct

Success — achievement, victory, accomplishment

Surround — enclose, encircle, contain

Suspect — think, believe, suppose, guess, deduce, infer, distrust, doubtful

Sustain — maintain, carry on, prolong, continue, nourish, suffer

Synonymous — same as, identical, equal, tantamount

Systemic — affecting the entire organism

Thorough — careful, detailed, methodical, systematic, meticulous, comprehensive, exhaustive

Tilt — tip, slant, slope, lean, angle, incline

Translucent — see-through, transparent, clear

Unique — one and only, sole, exclusive, distinctive

Universal — general, widespread, common, worldwide

Unoccupied — vacant, not busy, empty

Unrelated — unconnected, unlinked, distinct, dissimilar, irrelevant

Unresolved — unsettled, uncertain, unsolved, unclear, in doubt

Utilize — make use of, employ

Various — numerous, variety, range of, mixture of, assortment of

Verbalize — express, voice, speak, articulate

Verify — confirm, make sure, prove, attest to, validate, substantiate, corroborate, authenticate

Vigorous — forceful, strong, brisk, energetic

Volume — quantity, amount, size

Withdraw — remove, pull out, take out, extract

References

Amoros, Z. U., Callister, L. C., & Sakrisyan, K. (2010). Giving birth: The voices of Armenian women. *International Nursing Review*, 135-141.

Arieli, D. (2013). Emotional work and diversity in clinical placements of nursing students. *Journal of Nursing Scholarship*, *45*(2), 192-201. doi: 10.1111/jnu.12020.

Bandura, A. (1985). *Social foundations of thought and action: A social cognitive theory.* Englewood Cliffs, NJ: Prentice Hall.

Barroso, J. (2010). Introduction to qualitative research. In G. LoBiondo-Wood & J. Haber (Eds.). *Nursing research: Methods and critical appraisal for evidence-based practice* (7th ed., pp. 85-125). St. Louis, MO: Mosby Elsevier.

Barroso, J. (2010). Qualitative approaches to research. In G. LoBiondo-Wood & J. Haber (Eds.). *Nursing research: Methods and critical appraisal for evidence-based practice* (7th ed., pp. 100-125). St. Louis, MO: Mosby Elsevier.

Bean, M. C., Moskowitz, G. B., Badger, T. A., & Focella, E. (2013). Evidence of nonconscious stereotyping of Hispanic patients by nursing and medical students. *Nursing Research*, *62*(5), 362-367. doi: 1097/NNR.0b01.3e31829e002ec

Beck, C. T., & Watson, S. (2010). Subsequent childbirth after a previous traumatic birth. *Nursing Research*, *59*(4), 241-249.

Beeber, L. S., Schwartz, T. A., Holditch-Davis, D., Canuso, C., & Lewis, V. (2013). Parenting enhancement, interpersonal psychotherapy to reduce depression in low-income mothers of infants and toddlers. *Nursing Research*, *62*(2), 82-90. doi: 10.1097/NNR.0b013e31828324c2

Bobay, K. L., Yakusheva, O., & Weiss, M. E. (2011). Outcomes and cost analysis of the impact of unit-level nurse staffing on post-discharge utilization. *Nursing Economics*, *29*(2), 69-87.

Bolas, N., & Holloway, S. (2012). Negative pressure wound therapy: A study on patient perspectives. *Wound Care*, 530-535.

Boswell, C., & Cannon, S. (2014). *Introduction to nursing research: Incorporating evidence-based practice* (3rd ed.). Burlington, MA: Jones and Bartlett Learning.

Brown, S. J. (2009). *Evidence-based nursing: The research-practice connection.* Boston, MA: Jones and Bartlett.

Burns, N., & Grove, S. K. (2011). *Understanding nursing research: Building an evidence-based practice* (5th ed.). Maryland Heights, MO: Elsevier Saunders.

Cahill, J., LoBiondo-Wood, G., Bergstrom, N., & Armstrong, T. (2012). Brain tumor symptoms as antecedents to uncertainty: An integrative review. *Journal of Nursing Scholarship*, *44*(2), 145-155. doi: 10.1111/j.1547-5069.2012.01445.x

Calzone, K. A., Jenkins, J., Yates, J., Cusack, G., Wallen, G. R., Liewehr, D., & McBride, C. (2012). Survey of nursing integration of genomics into nursing practice. *Journal of Nursing Scholarship*, *44*(4), 428-436.

Cangelosi, P. R., & Moss, M. M. (2010). Voices of faculty of second-degree baccalaureate nursing students. *Journal of Nursing Education*, *49*(3), 137-142. doi: 10.3928/0148384-20090915-02

Carlson, E., Pilhammer, E., & Wann-Hansson, C. (2009). Time to precept: Supportive and limiting conditions for precepting nurses. *Journal of Advanced Nursing*, *66*(2), 432-441. doi: 10.1111/j.1365-2648.2009.05174.x

Carroll, M. D., Kit, B. K., Lacher, D. A., & Yoon, S. S. (2013). Total and high-density lipoprotein cholesterol in adults. National Health Center and Nutrition Examination Survey, 2011-2012. *National Center for Health Statistics Data Brief,* no. 132. Hyattsville, MD: National Center for Health Statistics.

Cashin, A., Newman, C., Eason, M., Thorpe, A., & O'Discoll, C. (2010). An ethnographic study of forensic nursing culture in an Australian prison hospital. *Journal of Psychiatric and Mental Health Nursing, 17,* 39-45. doi: 10.1111/j.1365-2850.2009.01476.x

Chan, M. F., Wong, Z. Y., Onishi, H., & Thayala, N. V. (2011). Effects of music on depression in older people: A randomised clinical controlled trial. *Journal of Clinical Nursing, 21,* 776-783. doi: 10.1111/j.1365-2701.2022.0394.x

Chang, C., Lu, M., Lin. T., & Chen, C. (2013). The effectiveness of visual art on environment in nursing home. *Journal of Nursing Scholarship, 45*(2), 107-115. doi:10.1111.jnu.12011

Cho, S., Lee, J., Mark, B. A., & Yun, S. (2012). Turnover of new graduate nurses in their first job using survival analysis. *Journal of Nursing Scholarship, 44*(1), 63-70. doi: 10.1111/j.1547.5069.2011.01428.x

Choi, S. E., & Reed, P. (2013). Contributors to depressive symptoms among Korean immigrants with type 2 diabetes. *Nursing Research, 62*(2), 115-121. doi: 10.1087/NNR.0b013e31827aec.29

Cohen, R. A., Kirzinger, W. K., & Gindi, R. M. (2013). *Strategies used by adults to reduce their prescription drug costs. National Center for Health Statistics Data Brief,* no. 119. Hyattsville, MD: National Center for Health Statistics.

Davidson, K., & Rourke, L. (2012). Surveying the orientation needs of clinical nursing instructors. *International Journal of Nursing Education Scholarship, 9*(1), 1-11. doi:httpp://dx.doi.org/10.1515/1548-923X2314

Del-Pino-Casado, R., Frias-Osuna, A., Palomino-Moral, P.A., & Ramon Martinez-Riera, J. (2012). Gender differences regarding informal caregivers of older people. *Journal of Nursing Scholarship, 44*(4), 349-357. doi:10.1111/j.154777-5069.2912.01477.x

Demir, D., & Rodwell, J. (2012). Psychosocial antecedents and consequences of workplace aggression for hospital nurses. *Journal of Nursing Scholarship, 44*(4), 376-384. doi: 10.1111/j.15477-5069.2012.01472.x

Edelman, L. S., Yang, R., Guymon, M., & Olson, L. M. (2013). Survey methods and response rates among rural community dwelling older adults. *Nursing Research, 62*(4), 286-291. doi: 10.1097/NNR.ObO13e3182987b.32

Edwards, Q. T., & Siebert, D. (2010). Pre-and posttest evaluation of a breast cancer risk assessment program for nurse practitioners. *Journal of the American Academy of Nurse Practitioners, 22,* 376-381.

Ervin, B. R., & Ogden, C. L. (2013). Consumption of added sugars among U.S. adults, 2005-2010. *National Center for Health Statistics Data Brief,* no. 22. Hyattsville, MD: National Center for Health Statistics.

Fain, J. A. (2009). *Reading, understanding, and applying nursing research* (3rd ed.). Philadelphia, PA: F. A. Davis.

Fakhouri, T. H. I., Ogden, C. L., Carroll, M. D., Kit, B. K., & Fiegal, K. M. (2012). Prevalence of obesity among older adults in the United States, 2007-2010. *National Center for Health Statistics Data Brief,* no. 106. Hyattsville, MD: National Center for Health Statistics.

Fetzer, S. J. (2013). Vital signs. In P. A. Potter, A. G. Perry, P. A. Stockert, & A. M. Hall (Eds.) *Fundamentals of nursing* (8th ed., pp. 441-486). St. Louis, MO: Elsevier Mosby.

Flynn, L., & Liang, Y. (2012). Nurses' practice environments, error interception practices, and inpatient medication errors. *Journal of Nursing Scholarship, 44*(2), 180-186. doi: 10.1111/j.1547-5069.2012.01443.x

Foley, V. C., Myrick, F., & Yonge, O. (2012). A phenomenological perspective on preceptorship in the intergenerational context. *International Journal of Nursing Education Scholarship, 9*(1), 1-23.

Fontenot, H., & Hawkins, J. (2011). The evolution of specialists in women's health care across the lifespan: Women's health nurse practitioners. *Journal of the American Academy of Nurse Practitioners, 23*, 314-319. doi: 10.1111/j.1745-7599.2011.00618.x

Franklin, A. L., & Harrell, T. H. (2013). Impact of fatigue on psychological outcomes in adults living with rheumatoid arthritis. *Nursing Research, 62*(3), 203-209. doi: 10.1097/NNR.0b013e31828.3fch.3

Friese, C. R., & Manojlovich, M. (2012). Nurse-physician relationships in ambulatory oncology settings. *Journal of Nursing Scholarship, 44*(3), 258-265. doi:10.1111/j.1547-5069.2012.01458.x

Garwick, A. W., Seppelt, A., & Riesgraf, M. (2010). Addressing asthma management challenges in a multi-site, urban Head Start Program. *Public Health Nursing, 27*(4), 329-336. doi: 10.1111/j.1525-1446.2010.00862.x

Greene, D., & Dell, R. M. (2010). Outcomes of an osteoporosis disease-management program managed by nurse practitioners. *Journal of the American Academy of Nurse Practitioners, 22*, 326-329.

Haber, J. (2010). Sampling. In G. LoBiondo-Wood & J. Haber (Eds.). *Nursing research: Methods and critical appraisal for evidence-based practice* (7th ed., pp. 220-245). St. Louis, MO: Mosby Elsevier.

Hackney, M. E., Hall, C. D., Echt, K. V., & Wolf, S. L. (2013), Dancing for balance: Feasibility and efficacy in oldest-old adults with visual impairment. *Nursing Research, 62*(2), 138-143. doi: 10.1097/NNR,0b013e318283f68e

Haglund, K., Belknap, R. A., & Garcia, J. T. (2012). Mexican American female adolescents' perceptions of relationships and dating violence. *Journal of Nursing Scholarship, 44*(3), 215-222. doi: 10.1111/j.1547-5069.2012.01452.x

Hall, A. M. (2013). Patient education. In P. A. Potter, A. G. Perry, P. A. Stockert, & A. M. Hall (Eds.). *Fundamentals of nursing* (8th ed., pp. 328-347). St. Louis, MO: Elsevier Mosby.

Hallert, L. R., Friedrichsen, M., Goranson, M., & Hallert, C. (2011). Does a celiac school increase psychological well-being in women suffering from celiac disease, living on a gluten-free diet? *Journal of Clinical Nursing, 21*, 766-775. doi: 10.1111/j.1365-2702.2011.03953.x

Han, L., Li, J. P., Sit, J. W., Chung, L., Jiao, Z. Y., & Ma, W. G. (2010). Effects of music intervention on physiological stress response and anxiety level of mechanically- ventilated patient in China: A randomised controlled trial. *Journal of Clinical Nursing 19*, 978-987. doi: 10.1111/j.1365-2702.2009.02845.x

Happ, M. B., Hoffman, L. A., DiVirgilio, D., Higgins, L. W., & Orenstein, D. (2013). Parent and child perceptions of a self-regulated, home-based exercise program for children with cystic fibrosis. *Nursing Research, 62*(5), 306-314. doi: 10.1097/NNr.0b01.3e.3182a03503

Harris, A. L., Sutherland, M. A., & Hutchinson, K. M. (2013). Parental influences of sexual risk among urban African American adolescent males. *Journal of Nursing Scholarship, 45*(2), 141-150. doi:10.1111/jnu.12016

Hasson, D., & Gustavsson, P. (2010). Declining sleep quality among nurses: A population-based four-year longitudinal study on the transition from nursing education to working life. *PLos ONE, 5*(12), 1-6.

Hawkins, S. Y. (2010). Improving glycemic control in older adults using a videophone motivational diabetes self-management intervention. *Research and Theory for Nursing Practice, 24*(4), 217-232. doi:10.1891/1541-6577.24.217

He, J., Almenoff, P. L., Keighley, J., & Li, Y. (2013). Impact of patient-level risk adjustment on the findings about nurse staffing and 30-day mortality in Veteran Affairs acute care hospitals. *Nursing Research, 62*(4), 226-232. doi: 10.1097/NNR.0b013e318295810c

Hellstrom, A., Fagerstrom, C., & Willman, A. (2011). Promoting sleep by nursing interventions in health care settings: A systematic review. *Worldviews on Evidence-Based Nursing, 8*(3), 128-142. doi:10.1111/j.1741-67687.2010.00203.x

Heron, M. (2010). Deaths: Leading causes for 2009. *National Vital Statistics Reports, 61*(7). Hyattsville, MD: National Center for Vital Statistics.

Jaromi, M., Nemeth, A., Kranicz, J., Laczko, T., & Betlehem, J. (2012). Treatment and ergonomics training of work-related lower back pain and body posture problems for nurses. *Journal of Clinical Nursing, 21*, 1776-1784. doi: 10.1111/j.1365-2702.2012.04089.x

Johnson, J. E. (1999). Self-regulation theory and coping with illness. *Research in Nursing and Health, 22*, 435-448.

Kao, H.-F.S., & An, K. (2012). Effect of acculturation and mutuality on family loyalty among Mexican American caregivers of elders. *Journal of Nursing Scholarship, 44*(2), 111-119. doi:10.1111/j.1547-5069.2012.01442.x

Kaplan, B. G., Abraham, C., & Gary, R. (2012). Effects of participation vs. observation of a simulation experience on testing outcomes: Implications for logistical planning for a school of nursing. *International Journal of Nursing Education Scholarship, 9*(1), 1-15.

Kazemipour, F., Salmiah, M. A., & Poursedi, B. (2012). Relationship between workplace spirituality and organizational citizenship behavior among nurses through mediation of affective organizational commitment. *Journal of Nursing Scholarship, 44*(3), 302-310. doi: 10.1111/j.1547-5069.2012.01456.x

Keall, R. M., Butow, P. N., Steinhauser, K. E., & Clayton, J. M. (2011). Discussing life story, forgiveness, heritage, and legacy with patients with life-limiting illnesses. *International Journal of Palliative Nursing, 17*(9), 454-460.

Keeling, A. W. (2009). "When the city is a great field hospital": The influenza pandemic of 1918 and the New York City nursing response. *Journal of Clinical Nursing, 18*, 2732-2738. doi: 10.1111/j1365-2702.2009.02893.x

Kelly, M., & Dowling, M. (2011). Patients' lived experience of myeloma. *Nursing Standard, 25*(28), 38-44.

Kerr, N. (2013). "Creating a protective picture": A grounded theory of RN decision making when using a charting-by-exception documentation system. *Medsurgical Nursing, 22*(2), 110-118.

Kirton, C. A. (2010). Tools for applying evidence to practice. In G. LoBiondo-Wood & J. Haber (Eds.). *Nursing research: Methods and appraisal for evidence-based practice* (7th ed., pp. 438-463). St. Louis: MO: Mosby Elsevier.

Kwok, C., Fethney, J., & White, K. (2012). Mammographic screening practices among Chinese-Australian women. *Journal of Nursing Scholarship, 44*(1), 11-18. doi:10.1111/j.1547-5069,2011.01429.x

Laguna-Paras, J. M., Jerez-Rojas, M. R., Garcia-Fernandez, F. P., Carrasco-Rodriguez, M. D., & Nogales-Vargas-Machuca, I. (2013). Effectiveness of sleep enhancement nursing intervention in hospitalized mental health patients. *Journal of Advanced Nursing, 69*(6), 1279-1288.

Lam, S. C., Lee, L. Y. K., Wong, S. L., & Wong, A. K. P. (2012). Pedometer-determined physical activity and body composition in Chinese working adults. *Journal of Nursing Scholarship, 44*(3), 205-214. doi:10.1111/j.1547-5069.2012.01460.x

Landrebeau, K., Lee, K., & Landrebeau, M. D. (2010). Quality of life in patients undergoing hemodialysis and renal transplantation: A meta-analytic review. *Nephrology Nursing Journal, 37*(1), 37-45.

Lansiquot, B.A., Tullai-McGuinness, S., & Madigan, E. (2012). Turnover intention among hospital-based registered nurses in the Eastern Caribbean. *Journal of Nursing Scholarship, 44*(2), 187-193. doi:10.1111/j1547-5069.2012.01441.x

Lee, W., Dai, Y., Park, C., & McCreary, L. L. (2013). Predicting quality of work on nurses' intention to leave. *Journal of Nursing Scholarship, 45*(2), 160-168. doi:10.1111/jnu.12017

Levkowicz, R., Whitmore, K. E., & Muller, N. (2011). Overactive bladder and nocturia in middle-age American women: Symptoms and impact are significant. *Urologic Nursing, 31*(2), pp. 106-111.

Lia, H., Li, Y., & Lee, L. (2011). Effects of music intervention with nursing presence and recorded music on psycho-physiological indices of cancer patient caregivers. *Journal of Clinical Nursing, 21*, 745-756. doi: 10.1111/j1365-2702-2011,03916.x

Lin, S. Y. (2013). A pilot study: Fluid intake and bacteriuria in nursing home residents in southern Taiwan. *Nursing Research, 62*(1), 66-72. doi: 10.1097/NNR.0b013e31826901d5

Lindy, C., & Schaefer, F. (2010). Negative workplace behaviors: An ethical dilemma for nurse managers. *Journal of Nursing Management, 18*, 285-292.

Liou, S. R, Cheng, C. Y., Tsai, H. M., & Chang, C. H. (2013). Innovative strategies for teaching nursing research in Taiwan. *Nursing Research, 62*(5). 335-343. doi: 10.1097/NNR.0b013e31829fd827

Liu, F., Williams, R., Liu, H., & Chien, N. (2010). The lived experience of persons with lower extremity amputation. *Journal of Clinical Nursing, 19*, 2152-2161. doi: 10.1111/j.1365-2702.2010.03356.x

LoBiondo-Wood, G. (2010). Introduction to quantitative research. In G. LoBiondo-Wood & Haber, J. (Eds.). *Nursing research: Methods and critical appraisal for evidence-based practice* (7th ed., pp. 157-176). St. Louis, MO: Mosby Elsevier.

LoBiondo-Wood, G., & Haber J. (2010). Non-experimental designs. In G. LoBiondo-Wood & J. Haber (Eds.). *Nursing research: Methods and appraisal for evidence-based practice* (7th ed., pp. 195-219). St. Louis: MO: Mosby Elsevier.

LoBiondo-Wood, G., & Haber J. (2010). *Nursing research: Methods and appraisal for evidence-based practice* (7th ed.). St. Louis, MO: Mosby Elsevier.

LoBiondo-Wood, G., & Haber J. (2010). Reliability and validity. In G. LoBiondo-Wood & J. Haber (Eds.). *Nursing research: Methods and appraisal for evidence-based practice* (7th ed., pp. 285-308). St. Louis, MO: Mosby Elsevier.

Lu, M.-J., Lin, S.-T., Chen, K.-M., Tsang, & Su, S.-F. (2013). Acupressure improves sleep quality of psychogeriatric inpatients. *Nursing Research, 62*(2), 130-137.

Marek, K .D., Stetzer, F., Ryan, P. A., Denison Bub, L., Adams. S. J., Schlidt, A., Lancaster, R., & O'Brien, A. (2013). Nursing care coordination and technology effects on health status of frail older adults via enhanced self-management of medication. *Nursing Research, 62*(4), 269-278. doi: 10.1097/NNR.0b013e318298aa55

McLain, N. E., Biddle, C., & Cotter, J. J. (2012). Anesthesia clinical performance outcomes: Does teaching method make a difference? *AANA Journal, 80*(4), S11-S16.

Melnyck, B. M., & Fineout-Overholt, E. (2010). *Evidence-based practice in nursing and healthcare* (2nd ed.). Philadelphia, PA: Lippincott Williams & Wilkins.

Molanari, D. L., Jaiswal, A., & Hollinger-Forrest, T. (2011). Renal nurse: Lifestyle preferences and education perceptions. *Online Journal of Rural Nursing and Health Care, 11*(2), 16-26.

Monroe, T. B., Kenaga, H., Dietrich, M. S., Carter, M. A., & Cowan, R. I. (2013). The prevalence of employed nurses identified or enrolled in substance abuse monitoring programs. *Nursing Research, 62*(1), 10-15. doi: 10.1097/NNR.0b013e31826ba.3ca

Moreland, S. S., Lemieux, M. L., & Myers, A. (2012). End-of-life care and the use of simulation in a baccalaureate nursing program. *International Journal of Nursing Education Scholarship, 9*(1), 1-15. doi: 10.1515/1548-923X.2405

Naab, F., Brown, R., & Heidrich, S. (2013). Psychosocial health of infertile Ghanaian women and their infertility beliefs. *Journal of Nursing Scholarship, 45*(2), 32-140. doi: 10.1111/jnu.12013

Nadampalli, S. B., & Hutchinson, M. K. (2012). An integrative review of relationships between discrimination and Asian American health. *Journal of Nursing Scholarship, 44*(2), 1217-1135. doi: 10.1111/j.1547-5069.2012.01448.x

Newman. M. (1997). Evolution of the theory of health as expanding consciousness. *Nursing Science Quarterly, 10*, 22-25.

Ni, C., Tsai, W., Lee, L., Kao, C., & Chen, Y. (2011). Minimising preoperative anxiety with music for day surgery patients—a randomised clinical trial. *Journal of Clinical Nursing, 21*, 620-625. doi: 10.1111/j.1365.2702.2010.03466.x

Noble, A., & Jones, C. (2010). Getting it right: Oncology nurses understanding of spirituality. *International Journal of Spirituality, 16*(11), 565-569.

Norris, A. E., Hughes, C., Hecht, M., Perragallo, N., & Nickerson, D. (2013). Randomized clinical trial of a peer resistance skill-building game for Hispanic early adolescent girls. *Nursing Research, 62*(1), 25-35. doi: 10.1097/NNR.0b013e31826138f

Nwankwo, T., Yoon, S. S., Burt, V., & Gu, Q. (2013). Hypertension among adults in the United States: National health and nutrition survey, 2011-2012. *National Center for Health Statistics Data Brief*, no. 133. Hyattsville, MD: National Center for Health Statistics.

Orem, D. E. (2001). *Nursing concepts of practice* (6th ed.). St. Louis, MO: Mosby.

Othman, A. K., Kiviniemi, M. T., Wu, Y. B., & Lally, R. M. (2012). Influence of demographic factors, knowledge, and beliefs on Jordanian women's intention to undergo mammography screening. *Journal of Nursing Scholarship, 44*(1), 19-26. doi: 10.1111/j. 547-5069.2011.01435.x

Park, H., & Wenzel, J. (2013). Experience of social role strain in Korean women with type 2 diabetes. *Journal of Advanced Nursing, 69*(6), 1400-1409. doi: http:/dx.doi.org/ 10.1111/jan.12001

Pender, N. J., Murdaugh, C., & Parsons, M. A. (2011). *Health promotion in nursing practice* (6th ed.). Upper Saddle River, NJ: Prentice Hall.

Phillips, C., Esterman, A., Smith, C., & Kenny, A. (2013). Predictors of successful transition to registered nurse. *Journal of Advanced Nursing, 69*(6), 1314-1322.

Phillips, J. K. (2010). Exploring student nurse anesthetist stressors and coping using grounded theory methodology. *AANA Journal, 78*(6), 474-482.

Plow, M., Finlayson, M., & Cho, C. (2011). Correlates of stages of change for physical activity in adults with multiple sclerosis. *Research in Nursing and Health, 34*, 378-388.

Polit, B., & Beck, C. T. (2014). *Essentials of nursing research: Appraising evidence for nursing practice* (8th ed.). Philadelphia, PA: Wolters Kluwer/Lippincott Williams & Wilkins.

Polit, D. F., & Beck, C. T. (2010). *Essentials of nursing research: Appraising evidence for nursing practice* (7th ed.). Philadelphia, PA: Wolters Kluwer/Lippincott Williams & Wilkins.

Porter, E. J., Matsuda, S., & Lindbloom, E. J. (2010). Intentions of older homebound women to reduce the risk of falling again. *Journal of Nursing Scholarship, 42*(1), 101-109. doi: 10.1111/j.1547-5069.2010.01334x

Powell-Young, Y. M., & Spruill, I. J. (2013). Views of Black nurses toward genetic research and testing. *Journal of Nursing Scholarship, 45*(2), 151-159. doi: 10.1111/jnu.12015

Rao, A. (2012). The contemporary construction of nurse empowerment. *Journal of Nursing Scholarship, 44*(4), 396-402. doi:10.1111/j.1547-5069.2012.01473x

Riegel, B., Dickson, V. V., Cameron, J., Johnson, J. C., Bunker, S., Page, K., & Worrall-Carter, L. (2010). Symptom recognition in elders with heart failure. *Journal of Nursing Scholarship, 42*(1), 92-100. doi: 10.1111/j.1547-5069.2010.01333.x

Rogers, M. E. (1994). The science of unitary human beings: Current perspectives. *Nursing Science Quarterly, 7*, 33-35.

Romeo, E. M. (2013). The predictive ability of critical thinking, nursing GPA, and SAT scores in first-time NCLEX-RN performance. *Nursing Education Perspectives, 34*(4), 248-253.

Ryan, A., Goldberg, L., & Evans, J. (2010).Wise women: Mentoring as relational learning in perinatal nursing practice. *Journal of Advanced Nursing, 19*, 183-191. doi: 10.1111/ j.1365.-2702.2009.02852.x

Rydstrom, L., Ygge, B. M., Tingberg, B., Naver, L., Eriksson, L. E. (2013). The experiences of young adults growing up with innate or early-acquired HIV infection—A qualitative study. *Journal of Advanced Nursing (6)*, pp. 1357-1365. doi: 10.1111/j1365-2648.2012.06127.x

Ryu, M. J., Park, J. S., & Park, H. (2011). Effect of sleep-inducing music in persons with percutaneous transluminal coronary angiography in the cardiac care unit. *Journal of Clinical Nursing, 21*, 728-735. doi: 10.1111/j.1365.2702.2011.03876.x

Sakraida, T. J. (2002). Nola J. Pender: The health promotion model. In A. M. Tomey & M. R. Alligood (Eds.) *Nursing theorists and their work* (5th ed., pp. 624-639). St. Louis, MO: Mosby.

Schmidt, N. A., & Brown, J. A. (2009). *Evidence-based practice: Appraisal and application of research*. Boston, MA: Jones and Bartlett Publishers.

Scholes, C., Mandelco, B., Roper, S., Dearing, K., Dyches, T., & Freehorn, D. (2013). A qualitative study of young people's perceptions of living with type I diabetes: Do perceptions vary by levels of metabolic control? *Journal of Advanced Nursing, 6*(6), 1235-1447. doi: 10/1111/j.1365-2648.2012.06111.x

Schrauf, C. M. (2011). Factors that influence state policies for care givers of patients with kidney disease and how to impact them. *Nephrologic Nursing Journal, 38*(5), 305-402.

Schreiber, R., & MacDonald, M. (2010). Keeping vigil over the patient: A grounded theory study. *Journal of Advanced Nursing, 66*(3), 552-561.

Sheehan, A., Schmied, V., & Barclay, L. (2010). Complex decisions: Theorizing women's infant feeding decisions in the first 6 weeks after birth. *Journal of Advanced Nursing, 66*(2), 371-380. doi: 10.1111/j.1365-2648.2009.05194.x

Simon, M., Klaus, S., Gajewski, B. J., & Dunton, N. (2013). Agreement of fall classifications among staff in U.S. hospitals. *Nursing Research, 62*(2), 74-81.doi: 10.1097NNR/.0b01.3e31827bf8c9

Stanley, M., & Pollard, D. (2013). Relationship between knowledge, attitudes, and self-efficacy of nurses in the management of pediatric pain. *Pediatric Nursing, 39*(4), 165-171.

Streubert, H. J., & Carpenter, D. R. (2011). *Qualitative research in nursing: Advancing the humanistic imperative* (5th ed.). Philadelphia, PA: Wolters Kluwer Lippincott Williams & Wilkins.

Su, C. P., Lai, H. L., Chang, E. T., Yiin, L. M., Perng, S. J., & Chen, P. W. (2013). A randomized clinical trial of the effects of listening to non-commercial music on the quality of nocturnal sleep and relaxation indices in patients in medical intensive care unit. *Journal of Advanced Nursing, 69*(6), 1377-1389. doi: http://dx.doi.org/10.1111/j.1365-2648.2012.06130.x

Sullivan-Bolyai, S., & Bova C. (2010). Data-collection methods. In G. LoBiondo-Wood & J. Haber (Eds.). *Nursing research: Methods and critical appraisal for evidence-based practice* (7th ed., pp. 268-284). St. Louis, MO: Mosby Elsevier.

Taylor, H., & Reyes, H. (2012). Self-efficacy and resilience in baccalaureate nursing students. *International Journal of Nursing Education Scholarship, 9*(1), 1-13. doi: 10.1515/1548-923X.2218

Thornton, K., Parrish, F., & Swords, C. (2011). Topical vs systemic treatments for acute otitis media. *Pediatric Nursing, 37*(5), 263-242.

Toma, L. M., Houck, G. M., Wagnicki, G. M., Messecar, D., & Jones, K. D. (2013). Growing old with fibromyalgia: Factors that predict physical function. *Nursing Research, 62*(1), 16-24. doi: 10.1097/NNR.ObO13e318273b853

Tunnah, K., Jones, A., & Johnstone, R. (2012). Stress in hospice at home nurses: A qualitative study of their experiences of their work and well-being. *International Journal of Palliative Nursing, 18*(6), 283-289.

Turner, A., Hochschild, A., Burnett, J., Zulfiqar, A., & Dyer, C. B. (2012). High prevalence of medication non-adherence in a sample of community-dwelling older adults with protective services-validated self-neglect. *Drugs Aging, 29*, 741-749.

Urrutia, M., & Hall, R. (2013). Beliefs about cervical cancer and Pap test: A new Chilean questionnaire. *Journal of Nursing Scholarship, 45*(2), 126-131. doi: 10.1111/jnu.12009

Vieira, F., Bachion, M. M., Mota, D. D., & Munari, D. B. (2013). A systematic review of interventions for nipple trauma in breastfeeding mothers. *Journal of Nursing Scholarship, 45*(2), 116-125. doi: 10.1111/jnu.12010

Walker, L. O., Sterling, B., Guy, S., & Mahometa, M. J. (2013). Cumulative psychosocial and behavioral health among low-income women at six weeks postpartum. *Nursing Research, 62*(4), 233-242. doi: 10.1097/NNR.0b013e31829499ac

Wang, P. (2013). The effectiveness of cranberry products to reduce urinary tract infections in females: A literature review. *Urologic Nursing, 33*(1), 38-45.

Ward, E. C., Wiltshire, J. C., Detry, M. A., & Brown, R. L. (2013). African American men and women's attitudes toward mental illness, perceptions of stigma, and preferred coping behaviors. *Nursing Research, 62*(3), 185-194. doi:10.1097/NNR.ObO13e31827bf533

Whisenant, D. P., & Woodring, B. (2012). Improving attitudes toward organ donation among nursing students. *International Journal of Nursing Education Scholarship, 9*(1), 1-15. doi: http:/dx.doi.org/10.1515/1548-923X.2404

Wilson, B., Harwood, L., Oudshoorn, A., & Thompson, B. (2010). The culture of vascular access cannulation among nurses in a chronic hemodialysis unit. *The CANNT Journal, 20*(3), 35-42.

Yancey, V. (2013). The experience of loss, death, and grief. In P. A. Potter, A. G. Perry, P. A. Stockert, & A. M. Hall (Eds.) *Fundamentals of nursing* (8th ed., pp. 708-730). St. Louis, MO: Elsevier Mosby.

Yang, H. L., Lee, H. F., Chu, T. L., Su, Y. Y., Ho, L. H., & Fan, J. Y. (2012) The comparison of two recovery room warming methods for hypothermia patients who have undergone spinal surgery. *Journal of Nursing Scholarship, 44*(1), 2-10. doi: 10.1111/j.1547-5069.2011.01426.x

Yoon, S. L., & Kim, H-H. (2013). Job-related stress, emotional labor, and depressive symptoms among Korean nurses. *Journal of Nursing Scholarship, 45*(2), 169-176.

Zellani, R., & Seymour, J. E. (2012). Muslim women's narratives about bodily change and care during critical illness: A qualitative study. *Journal of Nursing Scholarship, 44*(1), 99-107. doi: 10.1111/j.1547-5069.2011.01427.x

Zhuang, S., An, S., & Zhao, Y. (2013). Yoga effects on mood and quality of life in Chinese women undergoing heroin detoxification. *Nursing Research, 62*(4), 260-268. doi: 10.1097/NNR.0b013e38292379b

RECOMMENDED RESOURCES ON CRITICAL THINKING AND TEST TAKING

Alfaro-LeFevre, R. (2009). *Critical thinking and clinical judgment* (4th ed.). St. Louis, MO: Saunders Elsevier.

Nugent, P. M., & Vitale, B. A. (2011). *Test success: Test-taking techniques for beginning nursing students* (6th ed.). Philadelphia, PA: F. A. Davis.

Index

F

G

H

I

J

K

L

M

N

O

P

V